Indigenous Knowledge and Mental Health

David Danto • Masood Zangeneh
Editors

Indigenous Knowledge and Mental Health

A Global Perspective

Springer

Editors
David Danto
Psychology
University of Guelph-Humber
Toronto, ON, Canada

Masood Zangeneh
Faculty of Liberal Arts & Sciences and Innovative Learning
Humber College
Toronto, ON, Canada

ISBN 978-3-030-71344-7 ISBN 978-3-030-71346-1 (eBook)
https://doi.org/10.1007/978-3-030-71346-1

This Springer imprint is published by the registered company Springer Nature Switzerland AG
The registered company address is: Gewerbestrasse 11, 6330 Cham, Switzerland

Endorsement

This text represents a wholly refreshing, important, challenging, and creative contribution to the literature addressing the impacts of colonization on the well-being of Indigenous Peoples and the role of Indigenous knowledge(s) in healing and well-being. If this collection's breadth of representation loads the bases, the scholarly depth of these contributions hits the ball out of the park. The global voices we hear are of Indigenous Peoples themselves, and of health workers, activists, and allies embedded within those communities by the suffering of a passion, and a commitment of understanding unafraid to be taught. As such, the book claims the all-important promise of its title, of Indigenous knowledge(s) by which our predominantly Western and positivistic understanding of mental health, inclusive of its praxis implications, can and must be challenged, refigured, adapted, and sometimes even abandoned. A radical teaching, this. This text moves us away from abstractions and platitudes to show us just how, just what, it might mean in practice to be "sensitive" to the other, to be "responsive," and to be open to creative invention and respectful collaboration. We learn about innovative therapies, interventions, and research methodologies: land-based interventions, anti-oppressive therapy, body work, using dance and rituals in therapy, conducting clinical ethnographic, auto-ethnographic, or performance ethnographic research, analyzing songs and folk tales, and what it means to be allies and companions in research and therapy. We learn of a therapy and research of the heart, of a therapy and research for, from, and of the other. In the end, this book does everything it sets itself to, and exceptionally so. Now it is our turn. Having spoken so eloquently and powerfully, the test of our listening is in our response, which is also to say our responsibility.

Leswin Laubscher
Duquesne University
Pittsburgh, PA, USA

Foreword

In these very challenging times, as the global population weathers a pandemic that has triggered significant death tolls and intense mental health consequences, we are also observing deepening social conflict. Long-term social isolation, whether sought or imposed, can generate fear and distrust. In response, Canadian society has had to revive uncomfortable conversations on equity, diversity, and inclusion, readdress concepts like "cultural safety" in health care, and confront why black lives and Indigenous lives matter. This may be true in every society referenced in the stories of this book. I am gazing through the lens of an Indigenous woman in Canada, and it is Canada I am watching respond to this crisis in health, mental well-being, and social/economic paralysis. Unfortunately, these crises are also manifest around the globe.

It is comforting however, albeit deeply ironic, to know there are solutions to the conflicts we are being confronted with, many embedded in the very cultures this country and others have frequently driven to the edge of survival. There are lessons in these cultural stories, lessons about how historically inherent strengths, resilience, knowledge, and coping mechanisms, used since time immemorial, can provide viability and hope for our mutual future.

The pages of this book contain powerful examples of possibility, of rising from genocide and hatred, of protecting and sharing, and of reconstituting hope and a new way forward. Many of the cultures addressed in these stories have experienced the pain of exile, the trauma of genocide, and for some, unrelenting death into contemporary times. But, there is inspiration here, and a poignant reminder that if you don't know who you are and what you stand for, you are going to find it very difficult to not only survive but also recover from what we are presently experiencing. Severe weather events, intensifying temperatures, highly contagious diseases, growing economic disparity, food shortages, and increasingly unstable governments are now becoming normative.

Here you will find candid expression and recognition of a need to return to a reliance on land as a source of life and the value of maintaining a symbiotic relationship with forest ecosystems. We cannot live without food, water, and each other. Each chapter calls forth the value of land-based healing and the roles of Elders, knowledge transfer, language, identity, and culture as healing. Each author makes a strong case for not only reviewing historical challenges and highlighting cases of resilience but also promoting healing and growth through the revival of communal life. The kind of living that supports and draws forth the gifts of every culture, puts down the need to divide and conquer, or worse kill, and embraces the notion of all being in this together. It doesn't mean giving up everything you may know and understand, it means acknowledging Indigenous culturally grounded approaches can be integrated with Western approaches to create a powerful force for healing and change.

A strong message of resilience and hope runs through this entire book, a message that asks us to embrace the reconstitution and use of traditional practices and knowledge as a way to change the present trajectory of planetary (and human) destruction. We are living in challenging times, witnessing social disintegration, and far too much fear, we have a chance to do better, to live better, and ensure a brighter future for many generations to come.

CynthiaWesley-Esquimaux
Lakehead University
Orillia, ON, Canada

Introduction

Indigenous people span the world and number in the hundreds of millions. Rich in diversity and distinctiveness, Indigenous cultural groups are spread across nearly every continent and country. Indigenous Peoples exhibit diversity in lifestyle, culture, socio-political organization, and history; however, many of these groups have shared rapid culture change, marginalization, and absorption into a colonial economy with little regard for their autonomy. This cultural discontinuity has been linked to high rates of depression, substance abuse, suicide, and violence in many communities, with the most dramatic impact on youth. Nevertheless, many Indigenous communities provide remarkable examples of resilience, community cohesion, and happiness.

Recently in Canada, ground penetrating radar was used to explore the sites of several "Indian Residential Schools," institutions funded by the federal government of Canada and administered by churches between the 1880s and mid-1990s. For over 100 years, these schools undertook the project of forced "education" of Indigenous children in Euro-Western values and religion. Many stories of horrific abuse and mistreatment emerged from this system of approximately 150 such "schools" across the country. More recently the term "cultural genocide" has been used in Canada to define the motives and sequelae of this oppressive system. Indeed the use of the term "genocide" is being debated as well.

Beginning in May of 2021, the ground penetrating radar investigations revealed the remains of children buried on the sites of several residential schools. At the time of the publication of this book, approximately 1000 bodies have been found; however, estimates vary regarding how many bodies will eventually be found. Certainly, the number of Indigenous lives lost as a result of contact with Euro-Western settlers in the territories now known as Canada will dwarf the numbers of remains found and identified. When we take a global perspective, however, humanity's crimes against its own Indigenous people become truly unfathomable. Yet this global perspective is necessary to respect and acknowledge those lives that were taken and because an investigation of the crime informs us of the motives of the perpetrator, which is a painful but necessary step in looking toward a brighter future.

In the spring of 2018 the University of Guelph-Humber held its first annual International Symposium on Indigenous Mental Health at the Native Canadian Centre of Toronto, in Canada, on the traditional territory of the Mississaugas of the New Credit. Many attended to explore indigeneity in a global context, learn about the role of culture and tradition in healing the wounds of colonization and trauma, and better understand the incredible strength and resilience of Indigenous communities around the world. This book developed out of that meeting and hopefully extends that spirit of dialogue, support, and collaboration.

We bring together the perspectives of Indigenous researchers and allies around the world whose interests focus on the well-being of Indigenous Peoples. Through a strength and resilience-oriented approach, chapters will explore the challenges, cultural values, and traditions that inform how these communities facilitate mental health among their members.

The reader may notice that some chapters do not flow neatly into subsequent chapters in the way that some are accustomed. In soliciting chapters from the authors, we chose to remain minimally directive, preferring that authors feel free to express themselves in the way most appropriate to their context. There are, of course, vast differences in the contexts of Indigeneity and mental health around the world. In reading the following chapters, we encourage the reader to contemplate these contexts and consider the historical, political, economic, and social situations which not only gave rise to the current challenges and strengths of a particular Indigenous group, but which also provide the ground for the authors and the chapters themselves.

This book takes the reader on two simultaneous journeys. The first is a trip around the world meeting with Indigenous scholars and allies to learn about the work that is being done in the field. The second is a path toward reconciliation, from acknowledgement of truth, to giving voice to the suffering, to the importance of culture, to the process of healing, and lastly to reconciliation. Both these journeys merely scratch the surface regarding the wealth of reports and stories around the world and the work to be done, as we as a species reflect upon our historical and ongoing interactions with one another.

We begin with a difficult look at the harsh reality of genocide, exile, and trauma experienced by several Indigenous Peoples around the world. In his chapter titled Yazidi Mental Health and Collective Trauma and Terror, Jan Ilhan Kizilhan examines the brutal genocide of the Yazidi people, one of the Indigenous nations in Iraq, by the mercenary group known as ISIS, which took place in 2004. Kizilhan discusses the importance of cultural and socio-political considerations when helping the survivors.

In the next chapter titled The Health and Well-Being of Indigenous Khmer Displaced and in Exile, Gwynyth Øverland recalls her experiences with a number of Cambodian Khmer members in Norway and discusses how Indigenous groups scattered in diaspora manage to guard, maintain, and sustain the mental health of their peoples. In this chapter, Øverland seeks to understand how survival and recovery are related to strength and resilience among these members.

In the chapter titled the Psychology of Mussar: Cultural Safety as a Verb, Silvia Tenenbaum examines the memory of historical and geographical cycles of exile among Uruguayan individuals claiming Indigenous roots. Using a decolonizing, anti-hegemonic frame informed by psychological research on the ethical teachings of the Mussar movement, Tenenbaum discusses the notion of "cultural safety" and the potential benefits of a post-traumatic growth approach to Indigenous communities in general and Uruguayan individuals in particular.

Our focus then shifts toward approaches to healing and the relevance of the land to a number of distinct Indigenous groups.

In the chapter titled Healing Practices and Rituals of the Forest-Dwelling Rabha Community in Modern Times, Chinmayi Sarma discusses health and well-being practices among the Rabhas of Assam, an Indigenous community of forest dwellers from India's North East who share a symbiotic relationship with their forest ecosystem. Sarma examines the nature of healing rituals and process and explores the implications of a Western medical approach for the Traditional Knowledge systems and healing practices of the forest-dwelling Rabhas.

In the following chapter in this section, Danto, Walsh, and Sommerfeld interview individuals directly involved with land-based healing programs in one First Nation community in Canada, within Mushkegowuk Territory in northern Ontario. They identify shared and distinct features across land-based approaches to healing in the region. Themes that arise include the roles of Elders, knowledge transfer, language, identity, and culture as healing.

We then investigate the impact of cultural knowledge and identity on resilience. In their chapter titled Mental Health and the San of Southern Africa, Chris Low and Joram Useb examine the colonial and postcolonial changes that have impacted San mental health and well-being by examining various social and geographical spaces that allow traditional rituals to interface with new practices.

In the chapter titled Indonesia's Political Reform: Challenges and Opportunities for the Adat Community's Mental Well-Being, Tody Sasmitha, Jiwa Utama, Isnenningtyas Yulianti, and Nurul Saadah discuss the legal and political discourse on the resurgence of adat revivalism and Indigenous development projects, and their impact on the psychological well-being of community members. The authors examine opportunities to enhance adat community members' well-being through common cultural practices and local knowledge.

In their chapter titled Happiness, Underdevelopment, and Mental Health in an Andean Indigenous Community, Jorge Yamamoto, María Victoria Arevalo, and Sebastian Wendorff explore subjective well-being, mental health, and the natural landscape in a small traditional Andean Peruvian village. To that end, the authors examine the complex interactions among subjective life satisfaction, the natural landscape surrounding the village, and supportive social interactions with friends and family members to address well-being among the community members and contrast this with popular fallacies about happiness in consumer-driven societies.

In the next chapter titled The Jewish People and Indigenous Resilience, Havatzelet Yahel examines the Jewish people's survival strategies and achievements within the framework of Indigenous resilience. Yahel examines her thesis by reviewing historical challenges, cases of resilience, healing and growth through the revival of communal life.

We then turn our attention to the relationship between culture and treatment in several Indigenous contexts. In the chapter titled Alcohol Use and Resilience Among the Indigenous People of Siberia, Anastasia Peshkovskaya, Nikolay Bokhan, Anna Mandel, and Irina Badyrgy discuss the loss of cultural, religious, and ecological values by Tuvinians, Indigenous People in Siberia, and implications for alcohol-related problems among the community members. The authors also discuss the role of clan communities in promoting a healthy lifestyle and building resilience. Moreover, the authors highlight the importance of traditional occupations and belief systems that have become a source of strength for Tuvinians and the importance of cultural sensitivity in relation to therapy and treatment.

In his chapter titled Reclaiming Our Identity Through Indigenous Cultural Generative Acts to Improve Mental Health of All Generations, Jordan P. Lewis discusses Erikson's concept of "Generativity" which includes sharing knowledge with younger people, and its implication for mental health. Lewis examines four Indigenous cultural generative acts used by Alaska Native Elders both to achieve sobriety and to fill the role of an Elder in their family and community. Furthermore, Lewis discusses how these cultural factors can be used to guide development of culture-specific treatment and mental health strategies, and argues for the role of intergenerational healing in improved mental health for Indigenous Peoples of all ages.

In their chapter titled Ka Huri Te Ao, a Time of Change: Māori Mental Health and Addiction in Aotearoa, New Zealand, Kahu McClintock, Terry Huriwai, and Rachel McClintock discuss the impacts of substance misuse and problem gambling among Māori, the Indigenous population of Aotearoa. The authors examine policy initiatives that have been dedicated to address socio-economic service development and delivery for improving health outcomes for the Māori population.

In their chapter titled I Remember Who I Am: Deg Xit'an Athabascan Perspectives on Wellness, LaVerne Xilegg Demientieff and Patrick Frank discuss the importance of culture and traditional practices for the well-being and quality of life of Indigenous People. The authors emphasize the historically inherent strengths, resilience, knowledge, coping mechanisms, and practices of Indigenous People where they serve as grounds for wellness and healing practices. The authors further highlight ancestral wisdom for health and wellness prevention and intervention, and ways to align Western health and mental health systems with grassroots, community-led and community-based approaches to meet the needs of Indigenous People.

Increasingly Indigenous culturally grounded approaches are being integrated with Western approaches to treatment in ways that are respectful of Indigenous knowledge and facilitate mental health and healing. In their chapter titled Traditional Aboriginal Healing in Mental Health Care, Western Australia, Jocelyn Jones, Hannah McGlade, and Sophie Davison discuss mental health services for Aboriginal and Torres Strait Islander Peoples and the requirements for these services under Western Australian (WA) law. The authors describe the experiences and the role of Traditional Healers working with Aboriginal mental health patients. The authors highlight cultural factors in Indigenous healing practices that could inform Western mental health caregivers when caring for Indigenous people. The authors argue for research-informed collaboration between Indigenous healers and Western mental health practitioners.

In the chapter titled Integrating Indigenous Healing and Western Counselling: Clinical Cases in Culturally Safe Practice, Teresa Beaulieu and Allison Reeves discuss culturally safe mental health services for Indigenous clients. By using case studies from Toronto, Canada, the authors examine the context for this integrative healing movement and describe environments that can support the work of Indigenous Healers, Elders, and counselors, alongside Western practitioners.

Lastly, we explore the importance of addressing reconciliation in mental health. In their chapter titled Reconciliation Social Work: Sustainable Community Development, Cynthia Wesley-Esquimaux and Steven Koptie discuss the incorporation of 16 principles that were developed by Phil Lane, Jr., Michael Bopp, and Judith Bopp in the context of the 94 Calls for Action tabled by the Canadian Truth and Reconciliation Commission (TRC). The authors argue the importance of their consideration for Indigenous Peoples to embrace internal personal and community change to prompt external change and reconciliation in social work practice.

In their chapter titled A Canadian Psychology Task Force Response to the Truth and Reconciliation Commission Report: Summary and Reflections, Christine Maybee, Fern Stockdale Winder, and David Danto recall their experiences leading up to the formation of their task force and then summarize the process and outcomes of their meetings which resulted in a report. In addition to a formal apology, the report makes a number of recommendations regarding the intersection between the profession of psychology in Canada and the Indigenous Peoples who inhabit this land.

It is our hope that whether the reader is Indigenous or an ally, a new student or experienced academic, a clinician or simply a concerned global citizen, that the experiences and accounts presented in this text will resonate and serve to contribute to the long overdue literature on the impacts of colonization on the well-being of Indigenous Peoples and the role of Indigenous knowledge in healing and well-being. Finally, we hope that the reader will find inspiration in these pages, to contribute to the collective effort toward truth and reconciliation that is already underway.

David Danto
University of Guelph-Humber
Toronto, ON, Canada

Masood Zangeneh
Faculty of Liberal Arts and Sciences
and Innovative Learning
Humber College
Toronto, ON, Canada

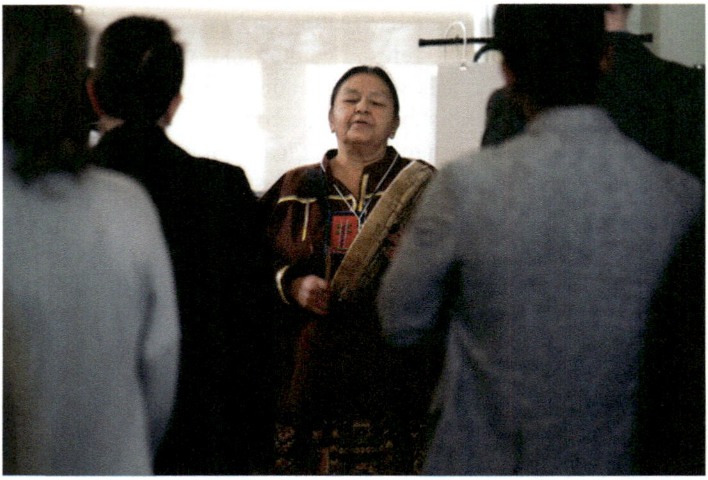

Photos taken at the 2018 University of Guelph-Humber International Symposium on Indigenous Mental Health, Native Canadian Centre of Toronto.
Photographer: George Nikitaras, University of Guelph-Humber

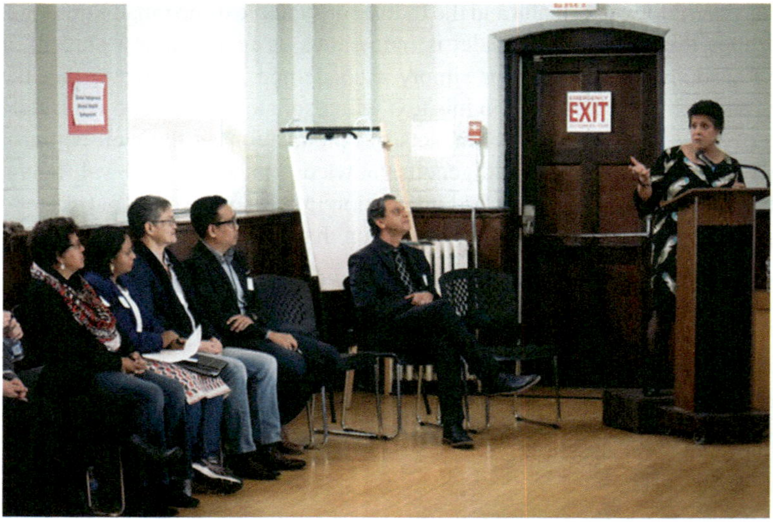

Photographer: George Nikitaras, University of Guelph-Humber

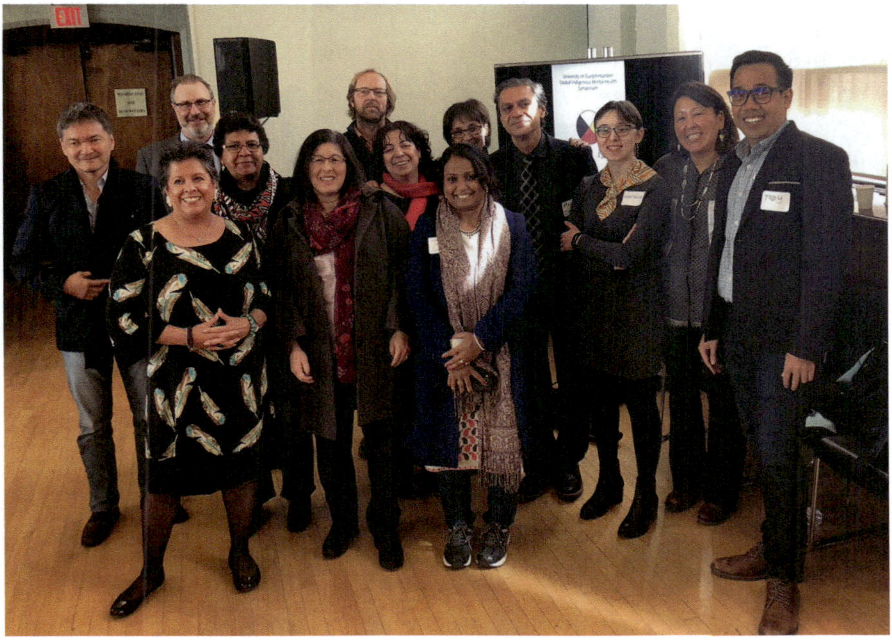

Photographer: George Nikitaras, University of Guelph-Humber

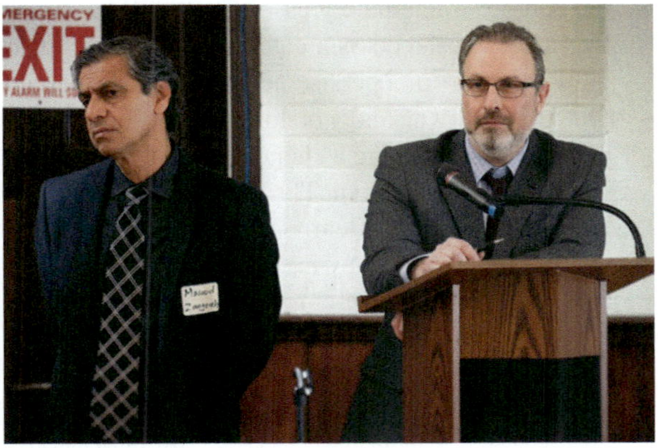

Photographer: George Nikitaras, University of Guelph-Humber

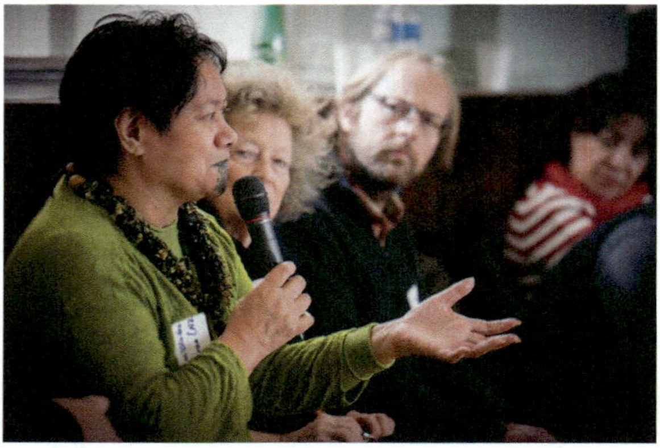

Photographer: George Nikitaras, University of Guelph-Humber

Contents

Contributors

Nurul Saadah Andriani SAPDA Foundation (Yayasan SAPDA), D.I. Yogyakarta, Indonesia

María Victoria Arevalo Department of Psychology, Pontificia Universidad Católica del Peru (PUCP)/Peruvian Institute of Cognitive Behavioral Therapy, San Miguel, Peru

Irina Badyrgy Social Policy Committee, Kyzyl, Republic of Tyva, Russia

Teresa Beaulieu Weaving Wellness Centre, Toronto, ON, Canada

Nikolay Bokhan Mental Health Research Institute, Tomsk National Research Medical Center of the Russian Academy of Sciences, Tomsk, Russia

Siberian State Medical University, Tomsk, Russia

David Danto Psychology Department, University of Guelph-Humber, Toronto, ON, Canada

Sophie Davison Department of Psychiatry and Clinical Neurosciences, University of Western Australia, Perth, Australia

LaVerne Xilegg Demientieff Social Work Department, University of Alaska Fairbanks, Fairbanks, AK, USA

Patrick Frank Anchorage, AK, USA

Terry Huriwai Te Rau Ora, Hamilton, New Zealand

Jocelyn Jones National Drug Research Institute (NDRI), Faculty of Health Sciences, Perth, Western Australia

Jan Ilhan Kizilhan Institute for Transcultural Health Science, State University Baden-Württemberg, Stuttgart, Germany

Steven Koptie Mamaway Wiidokdaadwin, Orilla, ON, Canada

Jordan P. Lewis University of Minnesota Medical School, Duluth Campus, Memory Keepers Medical Discovery Team, Duluth, MN, USA

Christopher Low !Khwa ttu San Heritage Centre, Research Affiliate, Pitt Rivers Museum, University of Oxford, London, UK

Anna Mandel Mental Health Research Institute, Tomsk National Research Medical Center of the Russian Academy of Sciences, Tomsk, Russia

Christine Maybee Payukotayno James and Hudson Bay Family Services, Moosonee, ON, Canada

Kahu McClintock Te Rau Ora, Hamilton, New Zealand

Rachel McClintock Te Rau Ora, Hamilton, New Zealand

Hannah McGlade Curtin Law School, Faculty of Business and Law, Perth, Western Australia

Gwynyth Overland Interim Secretary General of the International Society for Health and Human Rights, Kristiansand, Norway

Anastasia Peshkovskaya Mental Health Research Institute, Tomsk National Research Medical Center of the Russian Academy of Sciences, Tomsk, Russia

Tomsk State University, Tomsk, Russia

Allison Reeves Department of Psychology, University of Guelph, Toronto, ON, Canada

Chinmayi Sarma Centre for North East Studies and Policy Research, Jamia Millia Islamia, New Delhi, India

Jocelyn Sommerfeld Department of Psychology, Trent University, Peterborough, ON, Canada

Silvia Tenenbaum Dalla Lana School of Public Health, University of Toronto, Toronto, ON, Canada

Joram |Useb !Khwa ttu San Heritage Centre, Grootwater Farm, Yzerfontein, South Africa

Tody Sasmitha Jiwa Utama Faculty of Law, Universitas Gadjah Mada, D.I. Yogyakarta, Indonesia

Russ Walsh Psychology Department, Duquesne University, Pittsburgh, PA, USA

Sebastian Wendorff Wellbeing, Culture and Development Research Group, Pontificia Universidad Católica del Peru (PUCP), San Miguel, Peru

Cynthia Wesley-Esquimaux Office of the President, Lakehead University, Orillia, ON, Canada

Fern Stockdale Winder Operational Stress Injury Clinic, Saskatchewan Health Authority, Saskatoon, SK, Canada

Havatzelet Yahel Ben-Gurion Institute for the Study of Israel & Zionism, Ben-Gurion University of the Negev, Midreshet Ben-Gurion, Israel

Jorge Yamamoto Department of Psychology, Pontificia Universidad Católica del Peru (PUCP), San Miguel, Peru

Isnenningtyas Yulianti Researcher on Center for Research and Development of Social Welfare Services (B2P3KS), D.I. Yogyakarta, Indonesia

About the Artist

Betty Albert Wabimeguil (White Feather) is the Cree name of the Canadian Indigenous artist Betty Albert. Betty has been a painter since 1992. Her preferred medium is acrylic on canvas although she does, on occasion, experiment with mixed mediums. Betty's distinctive style is rooted in the life experiences she had prior to her decision to become a full-time artist. Adopted and raised by French-Canadian parents in Northern Ontario, she eventually spent time on Vancouver Island where her interests in art and spirituality emerged. During the next ten years she explored her artistic talent through images of wildlife using pencil and ink. Circumstances led to a happy reunion with her father and she became aware of her Indigenous, Cree roots. He encouraged her to continue to pursue her development as an artist on the basis of her newfound identity. A fortuitous encounter with Norman Knott, a fellow Canadian Indigenous artist, led to a crucial realization: that in order to evolve as an artist, she would have to confront her fear of color, let go of the pencil, and develop an "abstract" style using paint. A period of agonizing growth ensued, as she ventured with uncertainty into the unknown. With the support and encouragement of her family, she successfully navigated this artistic-spiritual transformation. Betty emerged with the determination to continue her life as an artist and began to produce artwork in a style that was her own. In 1992, with her father as business partner, she quit her day job. Betty has been a full-time artist, mother, and inspiration to other artists ever since.

Betty's artwork is distinguished by its bold colors and broad strokes combined with minute detail and vivid backgrounds. The colors of dusk and dawn in the northern sky inspire her backgrounds—and they serve as a backdrop for starkly contrasted images that manifest her experience of art as a deeply spiritual experience. Betty's dreams have exerted a fateful influence throughout the different phases of her career as an artist. The distinctive style of her first paintings was inspired by a dream in which the people appeared faceless. Later, the beauty of the spiritual teachings of the Thirteen Clan Mothers had a critical impact on her development. They led to a series of paintings that have been recreated in several cycles over the years. This series also served as the basis for her Moon Journal. She is most productive in the solitude of nature, alone with her tools. Her artwork gives expression to the peace that she experiences when she enters this sacred space of creation. Through her art, Betty attempts to represent the strength and the beauty of the feminine when it is grounded in the Great Spirit—women as sacred, dignified, and self-defining spiritual beings. Very recently, Betty has shifted her focus to the wildlife and wilderness of the James Bay Coast. In this phase, Betty honors her roots by revisiting the subject matter that marked the beginning of her spiritual journey as an artist.

Alongside her work as an artist, Betty has spent the last twenty years studying the art of healing and self-empowerment. Her journey as a healer began in 1984, with an evening course that she created and taught under the auspices of a college in Northern Ontario. "Assertiveness Training for Women" was a tremendous success and the college kept the course going for three years. This course was taught during a time in Canada's history when women were beginning to assert their rights to be equal participants in the workforce and it was as much of a learning experience for Betty as it was for her students. Betty learned that by being assertive and focusing your thought on what you want to become can lead to self-empowerment, healing, and the capacity for women to live a good life. Teaching the course changed Betty's life. She soon became director of a women's shelter and shortly after that decided to honor her talents and become a full-time artist. This was all made possible on the basis of the lessons of self-empowerment and healing that she learned while teaching the course.

In 1995 Betty began to learn about the teachings of the Sweat Lodge and also went on her first fast. Since then, Cree ceremonies have become a fixed part of her life. Betty now runs her own Sweat Lodge, is a Sun Dancer (she completed her fourth year in 2005 at the Sprucewoods Sun Dance in Manitoba), and was recently given the right to conduct the Shake Tent ceremony. Betty's life as an artist and as a healer coalesced in the discovery of the Haudenosaunee teachings of the Thirteen Clan Mothers. In addition to using these teachings as inspiration for numerous paintings, Betty has recently developed a life-coaching workshop that helps individuals to use the Teachings as a path to self-empowerment and self-realization. In 2012, upon moving to the Winnipeg area, Betty enrolled in a life-coaching program, from which she graduated in September 2014. She is currently in the process of building a coaching practice and offers online courses, tele-seminars, and workshops that are inspired by the Thirteen Clan Mother Teaching, the teachings of ceremony and the lessons of self-assertiveness that she learned while teaching her college course. Betty is also a certified Usui Reiki Master Teacher and continues to learn about ceremonies, run Sweat Lodges, and to help out every year at the annual Sprucewoods Sun Dance.

Part I
Genocide, Exile and Trauma

Yazidi Mental Health and Collective Trauma and Terror

Jan Ilhan Kizilhan

Among the ethnic group of the Kurds, the Yazidi people constitute a minority, with differences that are mainly expressed in aspects of religion. While most Kurds have been converted to Islam (see below), the Yazidi people have adhered to the principles of what they consider the oldest religion in the world. Most Yazidi people live in the Northern region of Iraq. Estimates figure their global population at 800,000–1,000,000 people [1].

Who Are the Yazidis?

The Yazidi people have existed as a religious group for centuries and are descended from the followers of the ancient religion of Mithraism, which dates back to the Sumerian period [2]. Their faith has been passed mostly by way of oral tradition for centuries. Their customs combine elements from several different religious points of view, incorporating Islamic elements, the principles of Zoroastrianism, elements of which were crucial to ancient Persians, and the religious practices and beliefs of Mithraism [3].

The Yazidis are Kurds and, as regards their political and social situation in their country of origin, they share the same fate. The Yazidis belong, however, to a small group of Kurds, distinguished not ethnically or linguistically, but by religion. They live as farmers and cattle breeders, scattered throughout Turkey, Syria, Iraq, and the former Soviet Union. With the spread of Islam in the Kurdish areas led by Caliph Umar in the year 637, they shared the same fate as the Kurds. The majority of Kurds were forced to convert to Islam [1, 3]. The Yazidis, who opted to stay outside this movement, regard themselves as followers of the oldest religion in the world, one which existed before Adam and Eve. Owing to the migration of labour in the 1970s, the Yazidis made their way from the Middle East to Europe, mostly to Germany, where some 120,000 live today [1].

The period when the settlement areas of the Kurds in Turkey, Syria, Iraq, and Iran were Islamized was a time of systematic and extensive persecution. The Kurds,

J. I. Kizilhan (✉)
Institute for Transcultural Health Science, State University Baden-Württemberg, Stuttgart, Germany
e-mail: kizilhan@dhbw-vs.de

D. Danto, M. Zangeneh (eds.), *Indigenous Knowledge and Mental Health*,
https://doi.org/10.1007/978-3-030-71346-1_1

including the Yazidis, were forced to convert to Islam. This happened not with the onset of ISIS terror but with the overall Islamization of the Middle East. Islamized groups and states have carried out an estimated 74 genocides against the Yazidis in the past 800 years. To date, according to conservative estimates, some 1.8 million Yazidis have been forced to convert to Islam and some 1.2 million Yazidis have been killed [4]. Numerous fatwas have "legitimized" their killing, looting, abduction and, since their religion was not recognized, their forcible conversion to Islam. ISIS also use such spurious arguments to carry out genocide against the Yazidis [5].

Systematic Destruction of the Yazidi Community

From August 3, 2014, onward, ISIS began terrorizing Yazidi villages and soon gained control of the area. The Iraqi army and the Kurdish Peshmerga retreated and the people were left helpless at the mercy of Islamic State terror. ISIS herded people into buildings such as schools and town halls and confiscated their jewellery and valuables, then separated the men from the women. Many men were executed immediately. More than 150 women I interviewed reported that in the village of Kocho, for example, more than 413 men were executed on August 15, 2015. After that, the older women, women with children, married women without children, young boys and girls between 8 and 14 years had to form groups and were taken to various locations. Older women and women with children were interned in mass accommodation or in villages, near Tel Afar or Mosul for instance, where the Shiites had previously lived. They were guarded by ISIS fighters, humiliated, beaten, and raped. Every evening not only ISIS fighters but also male civilians from Syria, Saudi Arabia, Egypt, Qatar, Tunisia, and other countries turned up because they wanted to buy the women and take them with them [4].

Case Study: Delal

Delal, 28, reports that "Islamic State" took her family prisoner and killed them. She herself was repeatedly raped and sold before she was able to escape from the hands of her tormentors. ISIS trained her 8-year-old son as a child-soldier.

She reports how the ISIS fighters took her prisoner; she talks of violence, rape, escape, and unimaginable suffering. She says she was sold 12 times to ISIS fighters in Iraq and Syria, and beaten and raped again and again. ISIS women in Mosul punished her with beatings, tied her up, and deprived her of food.

She goes on: "An Islamic woman watched me being raped. She said I had now become a Muslim." Finally, after 6 months being held hostage, she managed to flee from Syria.

Her 6-year-old daughter and her son are still in the hands of ISIS. She doesn't know where they are at the moment. She only talks in passing about her husband, who was executed along with several other men near Sincar.

ISIS perpetrators tried to convert women to their understanding of Islamic religion, forcing them to say their prayers in the Arabic language, which the women had not mastered. Their treatment of children was characterized by inhumanity. Imitating the procedures applied to child soldiers in Africa, ISIS used camps to train children to become soldiers whose behaviour is characterized by extreme brutality, including violence toward their own loved ones. Children were drilled to beat other children and forced to crucify or bury alive those who do not comply with ISIS. Those trained fighters who are not deployed during military campaigns are used to serve and protect the emirs or to work as guards or spies in camps and villages where they hold Yazidi people and members of other minority groups captive.

Ever since ISIS launched their military offensive in August 2014, they have killed more than 7000 Yazidi people and have held numerous families hostage in their home villages. Agents of ISIS kill anyone who is reluctant to convert to Islam. Moreover, they have kidnapped and enslaved more than 5800 young girls whom they frequently abuse sexually as well as violently and sell

Mental Health of the Yazidi Population

There have been few epidemiological studies published on the psychological disorders of the Yazidi genocide. Ceri et al. [5] interviewed children and adolescents in a refugee camp in Turkey approximately 2 years after the genocide and concluded that 43% of the survivors showed moderate to severe posttraumatic stress disorder (PTSD) reactions [5]. PTSD reactions of children and young adolescents were associated with parental loss, exposure to violence, and, most important, the feeling that their life was perpetually in danger. More women than men suffered from PTSD, and more women than men with PTSD or depression reported having experienced rape or witnessed the death of a spouse or child [7, 8].

The medical and psychological treatment of traumatized refugees presents therapists with enormous difficulties [9]. In addition to the problem of language, these include culture-specific perceptions of illness and how the patients describe it, their relationship to the therapist, how they structure their reporting of events, political constellations (residence permits, refugee status, access to health services, and so on), and sex-specific aspects, all of which go to make the examination, diagnostics, and treatment more difficult [4].

In addition to their traumatic experiences, it can be assumed that the Yazidi refugees carry an increased mental burden as a result of additional stress factors during their flight and their adaption to migration [10, 11]. For several generations, the Yazidis have suffered repressive measures in their homeland on account of their ethnicity or religion [4, 12].

The Yazidis have different conceptions of health and illness [13]. Their ideas of dealing with traumatic experiences are influenced by their respective cultures and their traditional medicine [14, 15]. The therapist must therefore be very conscious of his or her own Western constructs, and adapt them, and integrate alternative concepts when encountering traumatized individuals from other cultures [13, 14].

Transgenerational Traumata and the Consequences for the Current Generation

For the Yazidi people, their current traumatization by genocide at the hands of ISIS brings back to mind the genocide and massacre of their ancestors [15]. Thus, they experience a double or multiple traumatizations and may come to the conclusion that they cannot defend themselves and that they will, again and again, be victims of Islamic terror (Gerdau et al. 2015). The distance between the Yazidi and Muslims has become significantly greater because the violence they have experienced at the hands of different groups and states is always being done in the name of Islam. Out of fear of their Muslim fellow countrymen, they keep quiet and say nothing, yet they have lost their trust, because once more, in the name of Islam, they are being subjected to a collective massacre just as they were in the eighteenth and nineteenth centuries [13, 16, 17].

We can see similar types of behaviour as with those who experienced the Holocaust (Lazar et al. 2006). They are unsure and tense; they worry that their children cannot survive and have feelings of being powerless and helpless [18]. They experience their individual traumata and were collectively traumatized on August 3, 2014, and remember the transgenerational traumata of their ancestors.

We can observe three types of trauma with the Yazidi. Through narrative, the genocides, connected with fear and insecurity, have been passed on from one generation to another via stories, songs, and prayers. The term *Ferman* is synonymous with eradication and genocidal as well as traumatic events. For Yazidi people, this term reminds them of all of the cruel mass killings perpetrated against them. As the word is passed down from one generation to another through oral tradition, it has become well-known to every member of the Yazidi people. In the course of the brutal and cruel military campaigns by ISIS, the word *Ferman* has become increasingly significant again, as can be seen in Yazidi expressions of feelings of mourning and fear caused by the term [19]. It is against this background that the Yazidis experienced the genocide at the hands of the ISIS, beginning on August 3, 2014, as a continuation of the collective traumatization of their community [20].

These collective experiences are part of the collective memory of the Yazidi; however, as bad as they may be, during therapy they can probably “help” a person come to terms better with his or her individual traumata by providing resilience strengthening. In treating the survivors of terror, resilience strengthening is of great significance [20, 21].

Preconditions for Mental Health Treatment

The diagnostics of mental disorders and the diagnostics of posttraumatic stress disorders orient toward the criteria of ICD-10 and DSM-V. This assumes comparable burdens and reactions in all people who have lived through a traumatic event.

However, this assumption is not confirmed by clinical experience or by the findings of transcultural psychiatry [9].

In principle, the concepts of PTSD and cognitive behavioural therapy are generally applicable to all ethnic groupings. However, the differing conceptions of health, illness, and cultural-traditional medical treatment in dealing with traumatic experiences demand alternative approaches or additions [22].

A basic prerequisite is a secure environment in which the person does not feel threatened by persecution or any other danger or, in the case of refugees, does not have to fear that he will be deported to his homeland. Only when this safe environment has been established can the person speak about the critical events in his or her life and accept the therapy and therapists [23].

Even the working out of thoughts, emotions, the definition of the self, individual, and collective identity, and the way the problems are presented (e.g., when taking the case history, some groups of patients only report pain in their body) can make treatment difficult because there is often no match with the known diagnostic criteria [24]. Therapists often report that, when taking the initial case history, patients from a community that places a lot of importance on family loyalty, first of all talk in great detail about their ancestors' problems and only later may connect this to their traumatization. This can lead to a lack of understanding and impatience on the part of the therapist [25, 26].

Behavioural Case History

The psychotherapeutic interview is of central importance to the treatment of mental illnesses. Indigenous Patients or those from other cultures come to the first meeting perhaps with different expectations than those of patients within the dominant culture [27]. It is essential to recognize these and, within the realms of what is possible, to focus on them in order to create a good starting point for the treatment [28]. There can be misunderstandings, for instance, when the relatives accompanying the patient want to be present at the initial interview. In this case, Lersner und Kizilhan [23] recommend having everybody in the treatment room and doing the first session with the whole family, even if this setting is unusual [23]. At this point, we must remember that socio-centric-oriented people experience life as part of a social system. They think, feel, and act within this system. Everyday reality is in the family and is always linked to the "others"; the "collective thought" outweighs and influences their thoughts and actions. Concepts relating to the "ego" are not individualist as in Western thinking [25, 29].

When recording their case history, people from family-oriented communities, such as many Indigenous communities, do not relate events in a chronological or individual way regarding a particular focal incident. Instead, they may link these to the collective, that is, they refer to their ancestors, to their family, to clan structures, and so on [30]. This can lead to a stress situation for the Western-trained therapist, since he or she is used to a linear storyline, with a beginning and an end, and the patient has not finished within the time allocated for the therapy. Pushing the patient to "get to the point" can be understood by him or her as an insult or rejection. This can put a strain on the patient–therapist relationship right from the start. In such cases, it is advisable to allocate a double session for the biographical history [29, 30].

Forming Relationships

As a result of their traditional upbringing and socialization, the members of a family-oriented communities may regard the relationship to other people is very significant [28]. This also applies to their relationship to the doctor or therapist administering treatment since many patients have already [31] sought help from Traditional Healers in their homeland who are able to communicate effectively [32, 33]). With traumatized people in particular, the therapist's qualities such as understanding, patience, respect, politeness, attentiveness, friendliness, and openness are often more highly regarded than specialist knowledge [23, 25].

A relationship based on trust, which above all means accepting the patient's problems, is especially important. In the case of patients from family-oriented communities, the doctor (the clinical psychologist is also regarded as a "doctor") is traditionally seen as a fatherly friend of the family [34]. He is a figure of authority who deals with the patient and his family in an active, knowledgeable, and advisory capacity. He has to accept this cultural transmission so as not to cause considerable insecurity in the patient. Female therapists also enjoy great authority and male patients allow these women to treat them. Both male and female therapists are highly regarded in traditional communities, and in everyday conversations you often hear the phrase "First God, then the doctor" [34]. Men and women have no problem with undergoing a physical examination by either male or female doctors. In the case of patients severely traumatized due to sexual violence, for instance, it is advisable to ask, prior to treatment, if they will accept treatment from a male therapist [15]. In such cases, feelings of shame and transference phenomena play an important role, and this should be taken into consideration [35]. Unlike when dealing with patients from Western countries, where it is very important for patients to mobilize their own potential, to learn how to help themselves, the patients mentioned above have to be offered more help by the psychotherapists and, in fact, they expect this [36]. This means, however, that the therapist has to develop an awareness of his or her own cultural dependence. From this position he or she should be in a position to be aware of his (counter)-transferences toward the patients. He must acknowledge all his individual and social prejudices and stereotypes, which are present in the shape of collective transferences, before they begin to have a destructive effect on the treatment [27, 37]. Only then is it possible for the patient to be willing to change his physical and mental behaviour.

Disorders and burdens are not individualized and pathologized a priori, but are linked to the social environment. The individual's history is seen in the context of his family and his community within a cultural socio-political context. This applies in particular to politically motivated experiences of violence since these people become the victims of violence on account of their belonging to a social or political group [37]. Together with an appreciation of the migration and flight experience as a necessary developmental process, this is the basis for a productive trauma therapy for patients from family-oriented communities.

If the family and the role of each member of the extended family are included as a factor, this can lead to a better appreciation of any possible family conflicts and dependence on relationships. In cases of sexual violence, outside or within the family, the strong solidarity of the family with a traumatized patient can, in certain circumstances, prevent an improvement and even make the symptoms worse [25, 26].

Whereas contact with a different culture as a result of migration does have an influence on the explanation models of illness and health, it does not essentially influence attribution patterns. As we know from studies on migration, flight and war, groups abroad or in refugee camps tend to intensify their values and attitude systems [11]. On the other hand, attribution patterns which have been experienced positively are adopted and are integrated into their own concept of illness.

Mental Health Treatment

An interculturally proven helpful method is the combination of narration and exposure therapy, such as in Narrative Exposure Therapy and Culture-Sensitive Narrative Trauma Therapy [26, 29]. A different understanding of health and illness, traditional medical care in the homeland, and the role of the individual and the collective can all play a major role in the diagnostics and treatment of people from other cultures with mental reactions to extreme stress [37]. Therefore, people from traditional-rural regions as a rule are steeped in a collective way of thinking, in which personal desires, interests, and the complaints of a single member are valued as secondary. Harmony and security in the family and peer group are considerably more important than individual autonomy. The individual sees himself as part of a mutually supportive group from which arise the appropriate tasks and obligations. Therefore, he has to make sure that this solidarity group, especially the core and extended family, does not come to any harm. As a result, personal feelings and complaints are not expressed, so as not to burden or cause any possible harm to the family [11].

Case Study: Sari

Sari is 16 years old and a Yazidi. She was taken prisoner by the ISIS along with her family. Her father and two brothers, together with other men, were executed before her very eyes. She herself was guarded, humiliated, beaten by IS fighters, and repeatedly raped in Mosul. Every evening IS fighters and also civilian men from Syria, Saudi Arabia, and other Arab countries turned up, looked at the girls, and bought them for themselves. She was bought by a Tunisian and taken to Syria. In Syria she was raped again and again, and then sold on. In total, she was sold 12 times to IS fighters in Iraq and Syria. Finally, after 10 months as a hostage, she managed to flee from Syria. Two of her sisters are still in the hands of the ISIS. She does not know where her mother is at the moment. She says, "When the ISIS came to our village, my mother told me that we Yazidi were facing another disaster just as we had done 73 times before in our history." Sari reports stories of previous massacres and that she has learned never to trust Muslims, to be polite to them but always distanced, since her ancestors suffered greatly at their hands. She is suffering from posttraumatic stress disorders and has dissociative cramp spasms nearly every day.

The experience of being a target of sexually violent behaviour is particularly significant, as it causes those affected to be extensively ashamed and to be afraid of being excluded from their community because of what happened to them.

In this context, many patients report that they are ashamed of the sexualized violence they have experienced, but society also indirectly shows them that they are "different" and they are often excluded. High moral ideas and restrictions, especially with women, lead to great worry and anxiety, since the victims of sexual assault are in danger of being ostracized by the collective. Feelings of shame play a special role in this, because in a "shame culture," it is not so much the incident and the committing of a possible violation of the norm which plays a part but the need to save one's face in front of the others. The rape of a young woman can be evaluated by the collective as disgraceful and the victim can be ostracized. The role of the perpetrator is also regarded as a violation of the norm, but in the collective it is only of secondary importance. It is not uncommon that unmarried young women who have been raped want to have their hymen recreated so that, in the event of marriage, they can appear as "virgins" and not be ostracized by their society [8].

As regards the Yazidi people, the following must be emphasized. Apart from feeling ashamed, the Yazidi people see an experience of sexual assault as a person's disregard for the religious principles of their Yazidi community [3]. These principles are supposed to prohibit Yazidi people from having a sexual relationship with non-Yazidis, which is synonymous with being excluded from a Yazidi community. This exclusion also comes into effect even if non-Yazidis rape Yazidi individuals. The high council of the Yazidi people did not abolish this principle, until after ISIS abducted and sexually abused several thousands of Yazidi women [10].

Family-oriented societies often broach the subject of traumatic experiences via expressions of pain [33]. From a psychodynamic perspective, somatization offers people with severe traumatic experiences a chance to shift ostracism, social hurt, feelings of guilt and inferiority from the conscious experience to a physical level. In this way, they retain their self-respect and at the same time hope that the doctor and some medicine can help them [38].

In individual psychotherapy, the following culture-specific components can be helpful when encountering people from other cultures with PTSD. The various steps do not always have to be in this sequence but can be adapted individually [20, 38].

Summary and Conclusion

An individual and culture-sensitive treatment which takes the relationship structure between the survivors and therapist into consideration is especially important, whereby traumatologists and doctors co-operate with other professional groups (sport therapists, physiotherapists, creative therapists, and so on) and look at the patient's cultural imprint.

If aspects specific to language, cultural, flight, and migration are included in the consultation, treatment, and social support of survivors with PTSD, it is possible to fundamentally improve their care and integration. Specific transcultural knowledge and the consideration of the social and political structures of the health institutes are therefore necessary, on the part of both the therapist and the health institutes, in order to be able to treat these patients early enough and adequately—and, in this way, for instance, to prevent a chronification of the illness. In addition to ensuring multicultural teams of therapists, it is above all necessary to make all staff aware of the need to take a transcultural, culture-sensitive perspective.

Treating survivors with PTSD is not about learning a new form of psychotherapy. It is about understanding and learning the skills of culture-sensitive use of psychotherapeutic treatment in general and especially in behavioural trauma therapy methods. Individual therapy is also about recognizing people from different cultures, with a different concept of illness and how to deal with it. This requires being willing to reflect and possessing a critical attitude to one's own work while at the same time remaining impartial and open to the patients' concerns. Transcultural competence is needed and means that it is necessary to reflect on one's own culture in order to understand other cultures. In addition, the therapist must have the ability to change perspective, must deal in an unbiased way with people from different cultures, must employ curiosity and enquiry, flexibility, and a variety of methods, and must deal with mistrust and distance caused by the traumatic incidents which the refugees have experienced.

When dealing with Yazidi survivors with PTSD, it is necessary to consider cultural, historical (trauma), and socio-political aspects, the perception of illness and dealing with it, and the way in which a relationship can be formed with the patient. In addition, alternative therapy approaches are important, involving an interdisciplinary and culture-sensitive focus among the psychiatrists and psychotherapists, as well as close co-operation with other professional groups. All these groups and professionals must take seriously the patient's concept of illnesses and the ways in which the patient approaches and deals with illness.

References

1. Kreyenbroek PG. Yezidism in Europe: different generations speak about their religion. In: Collaboration with Z. Kartal, Kh. Omarkhali, and Kh. Jindy Rashow. Wiesbaden: Otto Harrassowitz; 2009.

2. Hanish SC. Yazidis, and Mandaeans in Iraq: a survival issue. Dig Middle East Stud. 2009;18(1):1–16.
3. Omarkhali K. The Yezidi religious textual tradition: from Oral to Written. Categories, transmission, scripturalisation and canonisation of the Yezidi Oral religious texts. Wiesbaden: Harrassowitz; 2017.
4. UN Human Rights Council. "They came to destroy": ISIS crimes against the Yazidis. A/HRC/32/CRP.2; 2016. https://www.refworld.org/docid/57679c324.html
5. Ceri V, Özlü-Erkilic Z, Özer Ü, Yalcin M, Popow C, Akkaya-Kalayci T. Psychiatric symptoms and disorders among Yazidi children and adolescents immediately after forced migration following ISIS attacks. Neuropsychiatrie. 2016;30(3):145–50.
6. Guest JS. The Yezidis. A study in survival. New York: Routledge and Kegan Paul; 1998.
7. Tekin A, Karadag H, Suleymanoglu, et al. Prevalence and gender differences in symptomatology of posttraumatic stress disorder and depression among Iraqi Yazidis displaced into Turkey. Eur J Psychotraumatol. 2016;7:28556.
8. UN Human Rights Office of the High Commissioner. UN Commission of Inquiry on Syria: ISIS is committing genocide against the Yazidis. 2016. http://www.ohchr.org/en/NewsEvents/Pages/DisplayNews.aspx?NewsID=20113&LangID=E. Accessed 10 Oct 2017.
9. Schouler-Ocak M. Trauma and migration. Cultural factors in the diagnosis and treatment of traumatised immigrants. Berlin: Springer; 2015.
10. Mohammadi D. Help for Yazidi survivors of sexual violence. Lancet Psychiatry. 2016;3(5):409–10.
11. Pagotto LF, Mendlowicz MV, Coutinho ES, Figueira I, et al. The impact of posttraumatic symptoms and comorbid mental disorders on the health-related quality of life in treatment-seeking PTSD patients. Compr Psychiatry. 2015;58:68–73.
12. Maercker A. Psychologische Modelle. In A. Maercker (Hg.), Posttraumatische Belastungsstörungen (Psychological models). In: Maercker A, editor. Posttraumatic stress disorders. Heidelberg: Springer Medizin; 2009. p. 33–50.
13. Hinton D, Kirmayer LJ. The flexibility hypothesis of healing. Cult Med Psychiatry. 2016;2016 https://doi.org/10.1007/s11013-016-9493-8.
14. Kirmayer LJ, Ryder A. Culture and psychopathology. Curr Opin Psychol. 2016;2016(8):143–8.
15. Kizilhan JI, Null-Hussong M. Individual, collective, and transgenerational traumatization in the Yazidi. BMC Psychiatry. 2017;15:198. https://doi.org/10.1186/s12916-017-0965-7.
16. Kizilhan JI. Patient form middle east and the impact of culture on psychological pain-treatment. Fibrom Open Access. 2017a;2:1.
17. Kizilhan JI. The Yazidi—religion, culture and trauma. Adv Anthropol. 2017b;7:333–9. https://doi.org/10.4236/aa.2017.74019.
18. Hassan G, Ventvoegel P, Jeffee-Bahloul H, et al. Mental health and psychosocial wellbeing of Syrians affected by armed conflict. Epidemiol Psychiatr Sci. 2016;25(2):129–41.
19. Kizilhan JI. Wer sind Eziden? Berlin: VWB; 2013.
20. Gerdau I, Kizilhan JI, Noll-Hussong M. PTSD and related disorders among female Yazidi refugees following ISIS attacks—a case series and mini-review. Front Psych. 2017; https://doi.org/10.3389/fpsyt.2017.00282.
21. Clay A. Treating Yazidi rape survivors. APA. 2016;47(8)
22. Kira IA. Etiology and treatment of post-cumulative traumatic stress disorders in different cultures. Traumatology. 2010;16(4):128–41.
23. Lersner U, Kizilhan JI. Kultursensitive Psychotherapie (Cultursensitive Psychotherapy). Göttingen: Hogrefe; 2017.
24. Summerfield D. The invention of post-traumatic stress disorder and the social usefulness of a psychiatric category. Br Med J. 2001;322:95–8.
25. Droidek B. How do we salve our wounds? Intercultural perspectives an individual and collective strategies of making peace with own past. Traumatology. 2010;16(4):5–16.
26. Schauer M, Neuner F, Elbert T. Narrative exposure therapy. A short-term treatment for traumatic stress disorders (2nd, rev. and exp. edition). Cambridge: Hogrefe; 2011.

27. Ford JD, Courtois C, van der Hart O, Nijenhuis E, Steele K. Treatment of complex posttraumatic self-dysregulation. J Trauma Stress. 2005;18:467–77.
28. Neuner F, Schauer M, Klaschik C, Karunakara U, Elbert T. A comparison of narrative exposure therapy, supportive counseling, and psychoeducation for treating posttraumatic stress disorder in an African refugee settlement. J Consult Clin Psychol. 2004;72(4):579–87.
29. Kirmayer LJ. Landscapes of memory: trauma, narrative and dissociation. In: Antze P, Lambek M, editors. Tense past: cultural essays on memory and trauma. London: Routledge; 1996. p. 173–98.
30. Pennebaker JW. Writing about emotional experiences as a therapeutic process. Psychol Sci. 1997;8(3):162–6.
31. Slobodin O, De Jong TJ. Mental health interventions for traumatized asylum seekers and refugees: what do we know about their efficacy? Int J Soc Psychiatry. 2015;2015(61):17–26.
32. Buhmann CB. Traumatized refugees: morbidity, treatment and predictors of outcome. Dan Med J. 2014;61:48–71.
33. Kirmayer LJ, Sartorius N. Cultural models and somatic syndromes. Psychosom Med. 2007;69(9):832–40.
34. Machleidt W, Gül K. Kulturelle und transkulturelle Psychotherapie—Tiefen-psychologische Behandlung (Cultural and transcultural Psychotherapy—psychoanalytic treatment). In: Machleidt W, Heinz A, editors. Praxis der interkulturellen Psychiatrie und Psychotherapie, pp 401–413 (Practice of the intercultural Psychiatry and Psychotherapy). München: Elsevier; 2010.
35. Wilson JP, Drozdek B, Turkovic S. Posttraumatic shame and guilt. Trauma Violence Abuse. 2006;7:122–41.
36. Kinzie DJ. Immigrants and refugees: the psychiatric perspective. Transcult Psychiatry. 2006;43:577–91.
37. Wenk-Ansohn A, Gurris N. Intercultural encounters in counselling and psychotherapy—communication with the help of interpreters. Torture. 2011;2011(21):182–5.
38. Cetorelli V, Burnham G, Shabila N. Prevalence of non-communicable diseases and access to health care and medications among Yazidis and other minority groups displaced by ISIS into the Kurdistan Region of Iraq. Confl Heal. 2017;11:4.
39. Butler EA, Lee TL, Gross JJ. Emotion regulation and culture: are the social consequences of emotion suppression culture-specific. Emotion. 2007;2007(7):30–48.
40. Hofstede G. Culture's Consequences, 2004. Thousand Oaks: Sage Publications; 2004.
41. Kirmayer LJ, Looper KJ. Somatoform disorders. In: Hersen M, Turner S, Beidel D, editors. Adult psychopathology. New York: Wiley; 2007. p. 420–75.
42. Lazar A, Litvak-Hirsch T, Chaitin J. Between culture and family: Jewish-Israeli young adults' relation to the holocaust as a cultural trauma. Traumatology. 2008;14:93.

Jan Ilhan Kizilhan is Prof. Dr. Rer Nat. Dr. Phil, Dipl.-Psych., at the Institute for Psychotherapy and Psychotraumatology, University of Duhok/Northern Iraq. He is also affiliated with the Institute for Transcultural Healths Science at the State University Baden-Württemberg, Germany, and MediClin Clinic Donaueschingen, Department of Transcultural Psychosomatic, Germany.

Dr. Kizilhan is a psychologist, psychotherapist, and orientalist. His expertise is in psychotraumatology, social medicine, culture-sensitive psychiatry and psychotherapy, forensic and ethnological studies. He was chief psychologist of the Special-Quota Project, a programme funded by the State Government of Baden-Württemberg. The project's aim is to bring 1100 women and children who have been held hostage by Islamic State to Germany for medical treatment. He has published more than 27 books and 120 research articles in international journals. He has been awarded many times nationally and internationally for his work.

The Health and Well-Being of Indigenous Khmer Displaced and in Exile

Gwynyth Overland

Setting the Stage

As a refugee worker and clinical sociologist in Southern Norway in the 1980s and 1990s, I found it easy to get to know the first Khmer refugees in Norway rather well, both professionally and socially, because all received refuge in our district. Yet few ever showed up at our outpatient clinic for traumatized refugees.[1] Had they really managed so well that they needed no psychosocial support? If this was the case, where did they find their strength? Forms of behaviour, attitudes, and motivations always exist in some context or setting, and a war cohort will inevitably pass through several contextual shifts on the way into and out of a war zone. The influence of past and present settings on displaced Indigenous groups such as the Khmer therefore needs to be understood from setting to setting. The study of such peoples benefits from a perspective that views "war, flight, camp life and resettlement as a series of distinctive cultural experiences that have a far-reaching impact" ([1], p. 19).

To describe and understand the experience and behaviour of Khmer survivors in contextual rather than essentialist and static terms, we must be familiar with the changing contexts, or environments. Understanding the cultural, religious, social, geographical, and economic contexts involves first describing them, preferably with "thick description" ([2], p. 10). I begin this chapter with descriptions of experiential contexts, a series of sets of relationships between individuals, events, practices, and language. Who were the Khmer war cohort, what were their experiences, and how did they manage to deal with them?

[1] Psychosocial Team for Refugees in Southern Norway, 1998–2008.

G. Overland (✉)
Interim Secretary General of the International Society for Health and Human Rights, Kristiansand, Norway

D. Danto, M. Zangeneh (eds.), *Indigenous Knowledge and Mental Health*,
https://doi.org/10.1007/978-3-030-71346-1_2

Shared Life Experience of the Khmer War Cohort

Whether or not the Khmer are an Indigenous People may be at issue, but written history places them in India from the late Iron Age and in Western Cambodia from mid-sixth century CE.[2] Since then, they have become the majority population in the area known today as Cambodia.

The Khmer war cohort of the interviewees selected for this project lived through the Khmer Rouge period with full consciousness of its character. They were born in Cambodia before 1965 and passed their childhood before the great changes that engulfed the country from 1975. The youngest informants were teenagers by the end of the Pol Pot experiment, in 1979.

The interviewees were selected from this cohort, in three samples of 10 persons each. The first sample came as refugees in the 1980s and 1990s and had been living in small towns in Norway for 20 years; the second fled from Cambodia after recent political oppression, arriving in Norway after 2000; and the third consisted of Internally Displaced Persons (IDPs) who returned to their villages in Cambodia after the Pol Pot regime and remained there.

All interviewees experienced at least three radically different cultural settings: first, a Cambodian village; next, the Khmer Rouge regime with its forced labour and summary executions in re-education camps; and then, the refugee camps along the Thai border. The first two sample groups also experienced a fourth setting, resettlement in Norway.

Context 1: The Village in the Lowlands

> Former environments are always with us and since we live in a continual process of making the present "former" we never … meet any environment as a person who never had an environment. ([3], p. 24)

The memory of a village appears to be ever-present for most Khmer, whether they left it long ago or live there still. Even today, city dwellers in Cambodia return to the villages they may have left decades ago to celebrate Cambodian New Year. For that reason, I have called the Cambodian site for this study "Phum Puon," and described it in some detail as an example of a village archetype. I updated my first description of the village, written while I was active in fieldwork in 1997–1998, during field trips in 2005, 2007, and 2009 [4, 5].

Phum Puon village is by Cambodian standards a rather poor village lying about 8 km from the market town along a clay track. In the village, there are approximately180 families, 716 people living in houses of palm-leaf-covered frames or

[2] Sanskrit and Pali inscriptions and the monoliths of Ashoka, the third-century BCE king who converted to Buddhism. *Brittanica*, accessed March 19, 2018.

wood on pylons, at intervals of 10–50 m (interview with village leaders, 2009).[3] The villagers are ethnic Khmer rice farmers. Under the houses, between the pillars that support them, are wide wooden beds on which several people can eat, work, talk, and sleep. Families of pigs, chickens, dogs, and, sometimes, one or two oxen that pull carts and ploughs typically share the under-house space.

As the main track from the village rolls out into paddy land and grazing fields, it arrives at the pagoda, with its cloister school for the religious training of teenage boys. The scene seemed rather idyllic in 1998, even more so in 2009. In the Pol Pot era, however, during the years 1975–1978, the school and its grounds were out of bounds under pain of death. Destroying school and temple, the Khmer Rouge used the site as a torture and extermination centre. "This area was one of the killing fields. When we excavated to build this school, we found two mass graves; the pagoda was the first thing we rebuilt" (Headmaster, cited in a field note, May 9, 2009).

Returning in 1989 to the village where she had done fieldwork in the 1950s for the first full-length monograph on Cambodian society, Ebihara noted that people who had formerly lived in "comfortable wooden houses" now lived in small thatched dwellings built directly on the ground ([6], p. 69). By 1998, the people of Phum Puon had gradually replaced the thatched houses with wooden houses on pylons, and by 2007 the process was complete (field notes, February 1998 and May 2007).

An important aspect of village life I noted during my field trips from 1998 to 2009 was the activity that emanated from the pagoda. The pagoda provided schooling, spaces for ceremonies, rituals, rites of passage and commemorations, community meetings, a place of retreat, and, for the elderly, an opportunity to give service.

Context 2: War Experience

The early 1970s were chaotic. As US planes bombed southeastern Cambodia in an attempt to obliterate the Ho Chi Minh Trail, city populations swelled to several times their size. All members of the war cohort interviewed experienced a violent cultural transition on April 17, 1975, when Pol Pot assumed power. When the Khmer Rouge evacuated the urban population to the countryside, people were forced to go back to their ancestral villages (see, for example, [7–12]). Youk Chhang, a city boy who lost contact with his family during the mass evacuation, recounts: "I remembered the name of my mother's village in Takeo and just began walking that way, asking where it was. It took three to four weeks to get there. People recognized me—'Oh, your parents are so-and-so'—and put me to work" (Youk Chhang cited in a field note, September 26, 2008).

All—including, in the end, Khmer Rouge soldiers—then experienced Pol Pot's work-communes, hard labour and hunger, flight through mine-studded jungles, and

[3] In 1998, there were 197 families, roughly 1000 people (interview with village leaders, 1998).

the loss of family members, including husbands, wives, and children. Every fourth person in Cambodia died. After 3 years, 8 months, and 20 days, the Vietnamese invaded, driving out the Khmer Rouge. Some survivors struggled and fought their way to the refugee camps along the Thai border. Some escaped from the Khmer Rouge labour camps, known as "production units" before the fall of Pol Pot and joined various military factions in the forest. Some displaced persons, who often took many months to arrive, straggled back to the places where their homes had been, starved and exhausted. They reconstructed their homes and livelihoods and continue to live in a village like Phum Puon.

Many tried instead to get to the refugee camps, hoping for resettlement in a peaceful place.

Context 3: The Refugee Camps

Scholars have described living conditions in the refugee camps along the Thai-Cambodian border, where many Khmer stayed for years, including Site 2, Site 8, and Khao I Dang (KiD) ([13–18]. Danger, hunger, sickness, and death continued to be a part of everyday life. The psychiatrist Richard Mollica, who visited the camps with a relief and research team in 1989, relates how he looked out over the refugee camp at Site 2. Faced with the monumental task of bringing relief in a desperate situation, he wrote, "I felt myself slip and saw myself fall out of the tree and down to my death, engulfed by despair" ([15], p. 93).[4]

The refugee experience, as shared by Khmer refugees in Norway, has been described as extended liminality, a limbo of betwixt-and-betweenness ([19], p. viii; [1]). Stripped of the symbols of their identity, they were subject to traumatic dispersal, moved by events wholly outside of their control, "events in which the suddenness, scale, and intensity of exogenous factors unambiguously impel migration or flight" ([20], p.180).

In the early 1980s, those refugees Norway had selected for resettlement began to arrive.

The sky was different: the stars were different, even the shapes of clouds were different. Trees, plants, and fruits were different. Food was different. The length of the day, of the night, and of the seasons were different. Clothes were very different. A refugee officer was amazed to see a Khmer trying the unfamiliar garment, the underpants, on her head. If one wished to brainwash, depersonalize, and estrange people, so that their actions and relations become confused and unclear, one could hardly do better than to give them the standard refugee experience. Tear them out of

[4] Mollica and his team developed the Harvard Trauma Questionnaire, which is still widely used for refugee patients.

the accustomed gestalt, transport them halfway around the world in a mystical machine, and dump them down in "inside-out-land."[5]

Context 4: The Suburbs on the Hills

Several hundred thousand Cambodians became refugees and have lived in diaspora since the 1980s. This section describes the context of those selected for resettlement in Norway. In contrast to the United States, for example, Norway elected to take on its UN quota of "20 or More" refugees with physical and psychological challenges. The few professionals who survived Pol Pot's systematic eradication were little inclined to stick their necks out, but were glad to have arrived at all. Thus, the group as a whole appeared very much reduced in the first year or two.

In contrast to the village life described at the beginning of the chapter, which is still the context, or environment, for much of the Cambodian population, Khmer refugees in Norway now live in small detached homes, flats, or semi-detached houses on the outskirts of small- and medium-sized towns. In contrast to present examples of global poverty, they are far from indigent. Concerted attempts on the part of the local housing authority have made these neighbourhoods relatively homogeneous, even classless. The Norwegian immigration authorities made the untypical decision to resettle the first Khmer refugees in the same part of the country, to foster mutual support within the group. Yet, abruptly thrust into the intimacy of the nuclear family after the enforced "solidarity" of the Khmer Rouge and 5–10 years in the enormous, overcrowded, and dangerous tropical camps, the first Khmer refugees in Norway were relatively isolated from each other, compared to their traditional lifestyle in rural Cambodia. They found themselves restricted by unfamiliar weather, architecture, residential patterns, and de facto segregation to the four walls of their homes (field note, October 7, 1997). And yet there were opportunities for social contact with each other because they had found refuge in the same local communities.

Contexts for Indigenous Cultural and Religious Practices

Religion and culture played a role in each of the different contexts the Khmer described. For this reason, I also consider the contextual perspective of local religious beliefs and practices. Ninety-four percent of Cambodians are Khmer Buddhist. They belong to the Theravada tradition of Southeast Asia, but their faith is also syncretic, containing elements of Hinduism, ancestor-spirit worship, and the use of shamans, the *gru parami,* who perform many kinds of healing rituals. According to

[5] A common self-deprecating saying among Norwegians about their country.

some, the *gru* have been chosen "To pacify and educate all the souls of the dead killed under Pol Pot, who continue to roam and distress people. For the mediums, the *parami*[6] have come to make order among the living and the dead and to repair a collective trauma" ([21], p. 166).

These shamanic practices appear to have become an integral part of the Khmer Buddhist universe (see, for example, [22]).

Described as "endemic" [23] in Traditional Khmer society, Khmer Buddhism with its worldview and codes of conduct was a community practice with its own framework and discourse, forming part of the unconscious environment for socialization. The interviewees represented the last Khmer population to receive this religious ontology in its traditional form. They spent their childhoods in a "post-figurative culture," in Margaret Mead's terms, one that answers for its members the existential questions: "In which gods shall I believe, how should I speak and move, eat and sleep, make love, earn a living, become a parent, meet death" ([24], p. 39).

How Did They Manage?

Like the rest of the Khmer diaspora, Norwegian Cambodians experienced rapid cultural change, marginalization, and official attempts to integrate them into alien cultures and lifestyles. Among the Khmer now resident in Norway, however, there have been few instances of substance abuse, family violence, criminality, suicide, and depression. The vast majority have, quite simply, managed remarkably well given the radical changes they have endured. They demonstrate an exceptional resilience, an ability to recover after life-threatening events. How exactly this community—now 450 strong in a collection of neighbouring Norwegian towns—facilitates mental health among its members is a question closely related to the topic of my original research, "What have resilient Cambodian survivors found useful for their recovery and normalisation after the traumatic events of the Khmer Rouge regime?" [5].

How to explain their collective resilience? This was a compelling question for me, as someone who had worked with the Norwegian Khmer for more than 20 years, in a municipal refugee office, in a clinic, and in voluntary cooperation. My 2007 invitation to participate in a study read as follows:

> This letter is for Cambodian refugees who seem to have managed well even though they had painful experiences in connection with the war in the home country. You are being invited to participate in a research project, which aims to find out more about this, to help other refugees and health workers who work with refugees. Psychosocial Team for Refugees is interested in learning what the refugees themselves think. What has helped you most after exposure to painful experiences? [5].

---

[6] *Parami (Skt/Pali,* "perfection") is a Buddhist technical term for the 10 perfections or virtues, "In a popular reappropriation, … believed to constitute a benevolent form of power" ([21], p. 151)

Except for follow-up questions for clarification, I posed only one question to those who met for interviews: Aaron Antonovsky's simple, "Will you tell me about your life?" [25].

In my qualitative study, I used neither structured nor semi-structured interviews nor leading questions. The biographical interpretive method [26] formed my basis for data collection. I used a modified grounded theory (Corbin and Strauss) to uncover the previously unformulated information and meaning in an Indigenous trajectory—from context to context—viewed from the perspective of those who had lived it.

How Did They Answer and How to Understand Those Answers

The 30 interviewees narrated first-person accounts of their life stories. They chose where they began these biographical narratives, sometimes in childhood, but they usually elected to focus primarily on their experiences of the war and the refugee camp. By 2010, the interview transcripts consisted of about 50,000 words translated into English or Norwegian by an interpreter during the interview. After transcription, a second interpreter back-translated to Khmer to validate the interpretation.[7]

Levels of meaning in the descriptions and explanations of their experiences and behaviour were discovered through various successive forms of analysis:

- NVivo facilitated a microanalysis of the accounts by highlighting and making the themes in the interview transcripts visible and collating subordinate themes under superordinate themes.
- Abductive reinterpretations lifted up the essence of the collected stories in common narratives.
- Retroductive reasoning was a way to find the collected essence—to summarize.[8]

Shared Stories

In the microanalysis, it emerged that informants' narratives clustered around three central themes: *self-reliance, social solidarity,* and *religious worldview*. Surprised by the apparent concurrence, the team returned to the NVivo microanalysis of the 30 interviews and counted. It emerged that more than 85% of the 50,000 words related to three superordinate themes, or strengths: *self-reliance and agency* (subordinate

[7] See also Overland 2011 for more on the translation process.

[8] An additional process of validation was conducted by translating the abductions into Khmer and giving them to 10 informants in Cambodia to read after their interviews (responses: "That's right." "I experienced that." "I agree.")

themes: work hard, escape, struggle, persevere, fight, agency) came up 109 times in the spontaneous life-story accounts. Themes related to *social solidarity* (subordinate themes: gave and received help, tried to find family, caring for others, shared what they had, held family and community together) arose 92 times (107 with the 15 mentions of "lost family" included). Themes related to *religious beliefs and practices* (subordinate themes: good deeds, adaptation, religion, conducting religious rituals and practices, doing ceremonies for the dead, and "understanding the situation") appeared 81 times.

In Their Own Words

Self-Reliance [dto su/prang praeng]

Self-reliance had many aspects, according to context and situation.

> You are given a task, given responsibility. Learn to survive in rain and storm. We were superstitious, so we were afraid of the jungle, but we had to be strong. You get to believe in yourself.

This interviewee, a 69-year-old man, believed that self-reliance developed in the Khmer because the poor in Cambodia had learned to be self-sufficient. In the village, children had to take care of the oxen, carry water for the house, and go out to find food; because of this, he had learned to be self-reliant and self-confident.

There was a striking element of agency and self-reliance in the narratives. This element was so understated that it was not even apparent before the last sample was analyzed, with their tales of soldiering, using the words *dto su* (struggle or fight) in a military sense, in a context perhaps more immediately associated with "agency" in the West. However, once "self-reliance" surfaced as a category, it became clear that this characteristic was also manifest in the quiet persistence of those who served by biding their time, keeping their heads down, and not losing hope in a better future. They could show agency by deliberately taking a chance of sneaking food in the hope of prolonging the lives of those nearest to them. Through the imposition of individual responsibility in early childhood, they had learned to survive in rain and storm. Childhood had taught them how to make use of what they had in nature.

Another informant, 58, attributed his agency to the emphasis on education and knowledge in his family before the Pol Pot coup:

> You must try to find out how to solve a problem—as quickly as possible—that is, we must use our heads. For example, all the other civil servants were forced into the army except me—because I used my head! I said, I can happily work in the defence ministry, I just have one request: that I don't have to wear a uniform. I had a feeling it would be dangerous for me—that it would end in a coup. That's one reason I'm alive today.

Another interviewee, 70 years old, said that during the Khmer Rouge regime:

> They held meetings and they'd ask things and some people would answer, but I *understood the situation* [author's emphasis], so I kept quiet. I adapted myself to the situation to survive

> at a time when it was difficult to survive… I never protested in the meetings. I never said anything. Some teachers were killed because they showed their opinion. I didn't do this… If you volunteered when the Khmer Rouge asked you to go work somewhere—those people were never seen again. Only their clothes....

In Norway, there was work. Word of the Cambodians' incredible industry went round. Farmers vied with one another for their services when they heard that one Khmer had planted 5000 strawberry plants in a day.

> I wanted to be economically independent, and my job meant a lot to me…. The most important for me as a refugee in a big firm was to build bridges. I had to behave myself! I felt like a representative for my homeland. (Man, 63,)

The interviewees did not appear to lose a sense of responsibility for their own lives and destinies. In a socially constructed world, wrote Peter Berger, we can become alienated when the objectified world becomes so separate from us that we forget our part in forming it. Even one's own self can be part of an external, uncontrollable reality. Berger indicated two ways of dealing with this: we can either take back the world and our own responsibility for it; or give up and let everything, including the self, confront us like a fact of nature that we are powerless to control ([27], p. 86). The Khmer struggled (*dto su*) not to succumb or become alienated, and they were able to take back the world. However, modest and unassuming they might seem, the interviewees constructed their lives as they interpreted them, accepting responsibility for the world and the self. They appeared secure, both in their basic trust as individuals and in the ontological security provided by a well-entrenched belief system.

In the absence of a cultural emphasis on individual identity, it may seem paradoxical that self-reliance should emerge as a salient theme in the stories of the Khmer. Yet that was the case for women as well as men, and for civilians as well as combatants. "In the end, it does not matter if we are high class or have a good standard of living," reflected a 54-year-old woman in Norway:

> We still have only one life. So what can we do to make our life meaningful? To make life meaningful: like in Khmer Rouge, I was a victim. But if I think, "I am a victim" I can't get out of the situation. I think, the meaning of life—I always think the meaning of life is that you always can hope… You can wait for support from family, government and so forth or you can choose to face the problem yourself and find a solution.

They did not identify themselves as victims. They held on to their agency by working hard, by not giving up, and by holding fast to their inner independence. They "understood the situation"—understood that *Angka,* the power that was, was a false authority that did not abide by the rules of humanity. They could therefore safely ignore commands, steal food to feed their families, and lie to protect themselves and others, breaking their own codes because they *understood the situation.* They persevered by keeping their behaviour under control, by escaping from the production units, by sneaking out to visit their children in isolated compounds by night, by fighting for Cambodian freedom, and by struggling to survive by any means, however humble. Survival was a responsibility and a duty, not a reason to feel shame or guilt. Despite the value placed on showing respect, they had no respect for the authority of the Khmer Rouge, because *they* were ignorant and they really had *no knowledge* (*ah!k-vi!j-jie [*Skt., *avidya.]*).

Social Solidarity

Another characteristic of the narratives was that they expressed the centrality of family, of extended family, and of general sociability, gatherings, and neighbours, and of the responsibility to care for others. In Durkheim, whose sociology is "mostly about social cohesion" ([28], p. 9), social integration is the source of life energy (Khm. *sah pievet*), while despair, submission, and suicide are aspects of the lack thereof. A woman, 60, spoke of sharing.

> We ate everything that could crawl. Insect, mice—we fried grasshoppers and shared them—one to husband, one to each child, one to me. We held together and showed our love for each other. If I had something to eat, I saved something for husband and children. If the children got something, they saved something for us. We shared our feelings with each other.
>
> I had a sister that was so pessimistic. She just sat like this [*hunches over, as if downcast*]. She died… My sister—her husband didn't show her any love. He went to the *mekonn* and got cooked rice. Only saved the rice water for her.

Many left Phnom Penh and other cities in large groups, but during the Khmer Rouge regime, family members died of hunger and exhaustion or were executed, often until only a few were left. They also experienced concerted attempts on the part of the Khmer Rouge to break the bonds of the nuclear family, but in many cases survivors clung together, comforting each other, finding and stealing whatever could be eaten, and risking their lives to sneak back to their families at night.

In the refugee camps, waiting to be accepted for resettlement, some needed to take chances to hold the family together. A 53-year-old man told his story:

> I took the test for Australia. And was accepted, but because of my child's health—he had a heart problem—I was stopped. They said, "If you want to come to Australia you have to wait until the child dies..." Or Canada. Canada said they couldn't afford to pay for it.
>
> I asked the Canadian embassy what country could save my family—anywhere. They suggested Norway.

That man's child grew up in Norway, and today he works and lives with his own family in his own house.

Many examples of the strength of social bonds, solidarity, and sociality appear in interviewees' tales of their actions after the fall of Pol Pot. Without exception, and sometimes at significant personal risk, their priority was to go to the places where they might meet or hear of the fates of family and friends. A 49-year-old man told this story:

> I walked about two weeks and I met one guy used to stay in my village and he said "Your mother's looking for you!" Just walk back about 15 kilometres… Finally I reached the place and found my mother. Very happy. And she realized I was strong at that time, to carry things back. And we walked from Mong Russei to Pursat, one month. And along the way I

> picked up fruit, mangoes, collected things to sell, saw families, fell into a mass grave—whooh, crazy. But we didn't—we were not scared at that time.

These stories are often told in "we" form. In the *abductive reinterpretation* below, they fuse together naturally into a common story. This one about social cohesion has been translated to Khmer for verification.

> We have always held together. The family is crucial for us, and close neighbours and friends. Some of us grew up without parents, and we loved and respected the old people of the village, who took care of us. During Khmer Rouge, we tried to help each other by sneaking food. Even some of the Khmer Rouge were kind and helped us. Some of us were alone after Khmer Rouge, survived alone, but tried to follow what we had learned from our parents. Most of all, we must not do anything wrong to any person. Especially not look down on anyone. If there's anyone who has difficulties, we must help them. The first thing we thought about after the Khmer Rouge fell was to try to find our families. When we came back, the houses were empty, but we were happy because we knew each other. It was a sign of stability for the whole village. We who went to the camps and later came to Norway, we all lost someone, but we *dto su* (struggled) to keep what was left of our families, together. We *dto su,* to get accepted for resettlement. Afterwards, we *dto su* to find those who were lost and bring them to Norway. Gatherings when we go to the temple, make a ceremony in someone's house—this feels good, brings peace. We must remember the others and, with the thought of those who died or live in poverty, we must do our best help to others in Cambodia.

In a sense, the interviewees could self-reflexively see through these social codes during the Khmer Rouge regime, recognizing them as social codes. They knew that the regime in power would punish people for observing them and that the codes were hard to uphold with a broken heart: "We had no feelings, no sensitive feelings," said one. However, the interviewees had struggled to keep some semblance of solidarity alive in secret, within the family, between trusted friends. The attempt to remember solidarity and trust was part of the struggle for stability and morality in a destabilized state.

Religious Worldview: Beliefs and Practices

> If you sit by the river long enough, your enemy's corpse will float down it. (Japanese proverb quoted by man, 48)

Although the explanations referring explicitly to religious beliefs were fewer than those referring to self-reliance and social cohesion, "to be Khmer is to be Buddhist." Khmer Buddhism was endemic in Cambodia up to the time of the Pol Pot regime, and many researchers find it to be so again (Ledgerwood et al. op cit). In fact, although there were three themes, religious beliefs lay at the root of the other two strengths, the "virtues" of self-reliance and social solidarity.

Asked "Where did your strength come from?" a woman, 52, replied:

> If we think that we are Buddhists, and we have merit, like that, and we were lucky and we're alive...
>
> *You think that you must have earned merit [kosål] from good deeds in the past?*

> *[She laughs.]* Yes, I think so—believe so. Because we earned merit before, that's why we survived. If we hadn't earned merit, we wouldn't have survived.
>
> My parents taught me to do good, behave myself in society, and work hard to earn my living.

The term "theodicy" refers to doctrines and beliefs about how a worldview resolves the problem of evil and reconciles the divine with the imperfections of this world. Buddhist theodicy is, in essence, a belief in the consequences of actions, of *Karma* (see, for example, [27, 29]).

The worldview present in the described behaviour, explanations, and ways of speaking of the Khmer was an implied, rather than stated, Khmer Buddhism. Only a few of the interviewees used words like "karma" in the sense of religious doctrine. As Berger notes, one must distinguish between the Buddhism of the monastic intellectuals and the syncretic Buddhism of the masses ([27], p. 60.). In the childhood contexts of the interviewees, they did not think, "this is Khmer Buddhism": it was simply the way life was. The way life was appears to have been permeated with Khmer Buddhism. As one man, 70, described it:

> Through the experience I learned to do good. To do good always wins. I believe in *kosal* (good deeds). Pol Pot regime was a regime that killed people, but if we did good deeds, it could keep us alive. Buddhist dharma is right.... So I did good deeds. When I came back and it was over, I continued to do good deeds. So I got my good deeds paid back. They didn't want to kill us, because of our good deeds... I survived because they knew my background. I survived because I hadn't harmed anyone.

The worldview surfaced in expressions like "if we do good deeds, we hope we will get a good life." In a world understood as a system of moral retribution, good deeds are rewarded and evil deeds punished. The Khmer strove to live up to the "Six Perfections"—generosity, diligence, patience, endeavour, and so forth—in Norway as well. A 59-year-old man said:

> We cultivate it. In the association we talk about it, about trying to help our homeland – both in fellowship and individually.... We have tried to cultivate a sense of generosity to our homeland. If we do good deeds, we hope we'll have a good life.
>
> Some interviewees, like this woman, 53, were rather shy about their merit.
>
> *Can you explain how you have managed so well?*
>
> It's hard to answer. [She looks down.] But... we're Buddhists, isn't it—maybe we've done good deeds? Maybe it can be like that, we've done good deeds in the past, and in the future we hope we will do only good deeds.

The abductive reinterpretation below is a retelling of the shared explanations and attitudes found in the narratives that related to Religious Worldview:

> We were driven into the street at gunpoint. We were driven out of the city. We didn't understand what was happening or what was expected of us. We were shocked and bewildered by the behaviour of the Khmer Rouge soldiers. We had never seen anything like it before, although we had been living with war for a long time. They took everything that was dear to us and tried to destroy it. We say tried, because they could not destroy that which is always true and that we know in our hearts. We knew what they were doing was wrong, therefore we were freed from some of the rules of behaviour we have, such as always telling the truth. We just followed what our parents and the monks had taught us, always showing respect and humility outwardly and working as hard as we could. One of the hardest parts

> was that no matter how hard we tried, we could not get enough to eat. We had to stand and humbly look on while they killed people we knew, people who were dear to us. We had a duty to persevere and survive *(prang praeng)* and just keep on fighting for our lives *(dto so)*, because this is the life we have got. But we shouldn't do harm to any other person while we fight to live. We should try to help each other survive because that is the key, the way to advance up the chain of being. We managed well because we tried to follow these rules. Others who did the same died. We were lucky, we were no better than them—perhaps it was *kamma* from an earlier life, but we owe it to them to go on fighting for life *(dto so)* and doing the right thing *(kosal)* because it will be repaid in the end, maybe not tomorrow or in this life, but in 1,000 years.
>
> We have never worked to get the Khmer Rouge punished. They will get reborn as dogs or hungry ghosts. If someone else wants to punish them, that's fine. It's up to them. In the end you are responsible for your own outcome and the only way to make it better is by following the good rules of behaviour and helping others. ([5], p. 217)

The reinterpretation above provides new insight that is not immediately apparent in the individual stories. What they did and how they behaved were culturally acceptable: letting oneself be led, feeling shock and confusion, but continuing to observe and to try to understand the situation and to adapt; holding to the worldview, trying to go forward without pride, not comparing oneself to others, remaining conscious of karma, attempting to do good deeds, and leaving the guilty to the self-regulating mechanisms of karma. All of these were culturally accepted virtues. In the end, their explanations of their strengths can be summed up by the sentence "I tried to do what's right."

Retroduction

In a sense, a triple-hermeneutical process took place: the interpretations of the interviewees, as I interpreted them, were then subjected to abductive reinterpretation. Through retroduction, I set out to find the essential, what was "basically characteristic and constitutive" ([30], p. 96). In this study, retroductive reasoning was a way of reducing the results to a more unified understanding and interpretation of these successful survivals.

How is it possible to survive the kinds of extreme traumas experienced by the Khmer war cohort and still be doing well and still define oneself as doing well? How do the three themes interrelate? Here the essences of the three abductive reconceptualizations combine to form a simple retroduction, as follows:

The behaviour and explanations in the data suggest that two essential factors, agency and social integration, were held together by a third: a remarkably tenacious religious worldview with a central karma theodicy.

Social solidarity, family cohesion, holding together, caring for each other, and mutual assistance were central for physical and mental survival. Another critical factor was a sense of agency, autonomy, individual responsibility, and self-reliance. The informants did not appear to have lost the consciousness of their participation or their responsibility. They refused to become victims; instead, they reaffirmed their agency by working, by fighting, and by struggling not to give up. They had an assuredness or confidence in their values that appeared to be related to an individual sense of autonomy. Together, these beliefs and attitudes formed an integrated wall of strength. Holding the wall together was the karma-based theodicy, the conviction that the world was a moral universe, and the only thing one had to watch out for, and be accountable for, was one's *own* behaviour.

The essence of this collective interpretation of the three themes is that a karma theodicy held together the supportive structure of the worldview, of what was acceptable as "knowledge" in that society, which in turn held the person together.

How Do They Guard and Maintain Their Mental Health Today? Present Contexts for Indigenous Practices in Norway

The Khmer in Norway have consciously attempted to recreate the communitarian culture, religion, and ethics that formed such a central a part of the Indigenous Khmer context. Because they were all resettled in a handful of neighbouring towns, they experienced extensive social contact through organizations, meetings, house-to-house fundraising in support of private aid projects in Cambodia, New Year's celebrations, religious gatherings, and high attendance at weddings and funerals. Their social and cultural opportunities expanded with the influx of the 150 or so new refugees who arrived after 2000, after new rounds of political persecution at home. The cultural context in which the Khmer people in Norway pass their everyday lives is still, however, undeniably different from that of a Cambodian village.

Refugees from traditional agricultural societies who end up in post-industrial societies on the other side of the globe often lose their access to rituals, elders, and other resources used in healing, as well as their social networks. The older Khmer refugees, who would traditionally have been ethics-bearers, had traversed centuries in 30 years: from Mead's post-figurative culture to the exponentially developing complexity of a modern Western society, where there appeared to be not much use for what the Elders can teach [31]. What did it mean for these Elders? How have their ethics and cultural practices fared in Norway?

The older Norwegian Cambodians have used visits to the homeland to acquire the equipment necessary for the practice of rituals. They attend, as well as initiating, many religious ceremonies, services of gratitude to parents, and ceremonies for the dead (field notes, 1994–1998). They have brought back clothing, musical instruments, platters, booklets, and recorded instructions from their first visits to Cambodia, and used them to recreate ceremonies in Norway, including weddings and funerals. Sometimes, there has even been a Khmer tape playing in the background, reading the steps of the ritual for the benefit of those who might have forgotten.

A system of values can be contingent and lose its meaning when de-ontologized or uprooted. The Norwegian interviewees, the Elders, might easily have lost their values after the radically changing contexts they had traversed. Yet they appeared to have at their fingertips the norms of the traditional codes for everyday behaviour. It seemed as though they believed absolutely in these norms (see also [32]). Participant observation at religious gatherings in Norway also revealed that those over the age of 45 knew by heart the rather long chants, movements, and gestures used in common rituals, such as the frequently held memorial services, marriages, water-blessings, thanksgivings, funerals, Cambodian New Year, Buddha's birthday, and so on.

After many trials, the Khmer Buddhist Association found a way of getting a visa for and bringing a monk to Norway for their religious holidays in April and May.

> … A table covered with silk and flowers, incense, candles, a bowl of water and a bunch of twigs. Each person rose from the floor and went up to lay a donation on a golden platter. The monk blessed them by shaking a few drops of water on their heads. Teenagers in training clothes were held by the arms, their hands lifted to make a *sompeah* amid laughter and teasing.[9]

A woman cried as she knelt in front of the monk; a young father guided his daughter as they put a spoonful of rice in each of the three bowls in front of the monk: "One for the Buddha, one for the Dharma, and one for the Sangha." Before the monk ate his meal he called the congregation forward and counted, "One, two, three…," so they could chant in unison (field note, May 9, 2009) (see Fig. 1).

Although they expressed gratitude to Norway, Khmer interviewees described their survival and present satisfaction with life as something they had done, rather

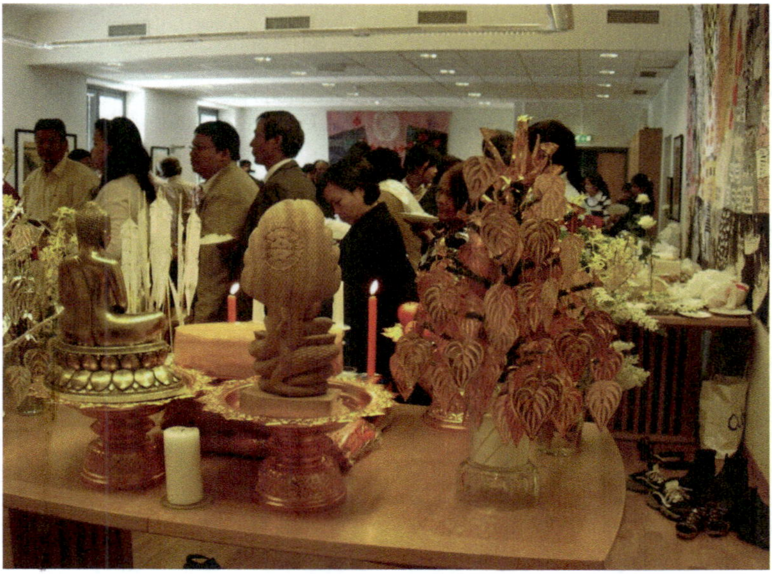

Fig. 1 Offering rice at a Buddha's birthday celebration, Norway. [Photo provided by author]

[9] Field note, Lillesand, June 1, 2003.

than something that had been done for them. Deep down, they had always known how to do it, how to be good and to survive; they had learned it as children. Parameters and explanations for proper behaviour, for how to go on, were supplied by the deep structures of a language imbued with a code of moral conduct, rather like the voice of a grandfather, the bearer of the tradition saying, "It's good that you survived—you did well." The Khmer seem to have learned to regard survival as a seal of virtue, and are thus generally spared the torments of survivor guilt. But as one said, "We who have survived must open our hearts a little bit, for those who died under Pol Pot—they didn't get anything along with them" (Virak Yenn, personal communication, November 11, 2005).

Berger says, "When the known world begins to shake," a person loses his moral bearings, with disastrous psychological consequences, and becomes uncertain of his cognitive bearings. This leads to the ultimate danger of meaninglessness ([27], p. 22). Yet this is what did *not* seem to happen to these resilient informants. Berger appears to underestimate the power of internalized values. Perhaps he is upholding a scholarly methodological atheism, unwilling to extend the suspension of disbelief, the final prerequisite for accepting that everyday habits of belief can keep believers afloat in the stormiest waters imaginable ([33], p. 199).

References

1. Ebihara M, Ledgerwood J, Mortland C. Cambodian culture since 1975: homeland and exile. Ithaca, NY: Cornell University Press; 1994.
2. Geertz C. The interpretation of culture. New York: Basic Books; 1973.
3. Erikson EH. Identity, youth, and crisis. New York: Norton; 1978.
4. Øverland, G. Culture and survival: the continuity of cultural practices among Cambodian refugees in Norway. Unpublished Master's dissertation, University of Oslo; 1998.
5. Øverland, G. Post traumatic survival: the resilience of Cambodian survivors. Unpublished Doctoral thesis, University of Agder, Norway; 2012.
6. Ebihara M. Return to a Khmer village. Cult Surviv Q. 1990;14
7. Him C. When broken glass floats. New York: Norton; 2001.
8. Ngor, H. (2003/1987). Survival in the killing fields (A Cambodian odyssey). New York: MacMillan.
9. Pin, Y. (1987). Stay alive my son. Chiang Mai: Silkworm Books.
10. Pran, D. & DePaul, K. (1987). Children of Cambodia´s killing fields Memoirs by survivors. Chiang Mai: Silkworm Books.
11. Van, N. (1998). A Cambodian prison portrait: One year in the Khmer Rouge´s S-21. Bangkok: White Lotus.
12. Sonn, M. (2007). Prisoner of the Khmer Rouge. Funan: Phnom Penh.
13. French L. The political economy of injury and compassion: amputees on the Thai–Cambodia border. In: Csordas T, editor. Embodiment and experience. The existential ground of culture and self. Cambridge: Cambridge University Press; 2000.
14. Mollica RF. Repatriation and disability: a community study of health, mental health and social functioning of the Khmer residents of site two. Volume I: Khmer adults. Boston, MA: Harvard Program in Refugee Trauma, Harvard School of Public Health; 1989.
15. Mollica RF. Healing invisible wounds: paths to hope and recovery in a violent world. New York: Harcourt; 2006.

16. Kiernan, B. (1996). The Pol Pot regime: race, power, and genocide in Cambodia under the Khmer Rouge, 1975-1979. New Haven Ct. Yale University Press.
17. Ledgerwood, J., Ebihara, M., & Mortland, C. (1994). Cambodian culture since 1975: homeland and exile. Ithaca, NY: Cornell University Press.
18. Williams, CL & Berry, JW. (1991). Primary prevention of acculturative stress among refugees: Application of psychological theory and practice. American Psychologist, 46(6), 632–641.
19. Turner, V. (1995/1969). The ritual process. New York: Aldine de Gruyter.
20. Cohen, R. (ed.), (1997). The Cambridge Survey of World Migration. NY, Cambridge University Press.
21. Bertrand D. A medium possession practice and its relationship with Cambodian Buddhism. In: Marston J, Guthrie E, editors. History, Buddhism and new religious movements in Cambodia. Honolulu: University of Hawaii Press; 2004.
22. Marston J, Guthrie E. History, Buddhism, and new religious movements in Cambodia. Honolulu, HI: University of Hawaii Press; 2004.
23. Keyes CF. Communist revolution and the Buddhist past in Cambodia. In: Keyes C, Kendall L, Hardacre H, editors. Asian visions of authority: religion and the modern states of East and Southeast Asia. Honolulu, HI: University of Hawaii Press; 1994.
24. Mead M. Cultura y compromiso [Culture and commitment]. Barcelona: Granica; 1978/1970.
25. Antonovsky A. Unravelling the mystery of health: how people manage stress and stay well. San Francisco, CA: Jossey-Bass; 1987.
26. Denzin, N. (1989). Interpretive biography. Thousand Oaks, CAL: Sage.
27. Berger P. The sacred canopy. Elements of a sociological theory of religion. New York: Anchor Books; 1990.
28. Durkheim E. Selvmordet (Le Suicide, transl. Dag Østerberg). Oslo: Gyldendal; 1991.
29. Weber, M. The Sociology of Religion. (Translated by E. Fischoff). From Gesammelte Aufsätze zur Wissenschaftslehre; 1993. (Original 1922). Boston, MA: Beacon Press.
30. Danermark B. Explaining society: critical realism in the social sciences. London: Routledge; 2002.
31. Klausen AM. Det fellesmenneskelige og det kulturrelative et sosial-antropologisk perspektiv. In: Østnor, editor. Mange religioner én etikk? Oslo: Universitetsforlaget; 2006.
32. Overland G, Yenn V. Generosity and resilience: transnational activity among the Khmer of Norway. Refuge. 2007;24(1):129–34.
33. Øverland G. Post traumatic survival: the lessons of Cambodian resilience. Newcastle: Cambridge Scholars Publishing; 2013.

Gwynyth Overland holds a PhD in clinical sociology and the sociology of religion. She has been consultant at the Psychosocial team for refugees and special adviser at Southern Norway Regional Trauma Competency Centre (RVTS Sor). In addition to articles on the meaning of culture for vulnerable populations and refugees' experience of psychiatric treatment, she has published *Post Traumatic Survival: The Lessons of Cambodian Resilience* (2013) and edited the anthologies *Nordic Work with Traumatised Refugees: Do We Really Care* (2014) and *Violent Extremism in the Twenty-First Century. International Perspectives* (2018). She has been Secretary of the International Society for Health and Human Rights (ISHHR) since 2017.

The Psychology of Mussar: Cultural Safety as a Verb

Silvia Tenenbaum

For my sister Nora, with much gratitude, and a home in the Middle East.

Cultural Framework

Uruguay shares with the rest of Latin America its colonial legacy and post-colonial institutionalized corruption. Only eight Indigenous families survived through nineteenth-century racism and twentieth-century militarism although their uncanny resilience has permeated vast sectors of present-day society. Uruguay is now well-recognized for its advanced human rights victories: it was the first Latin American country to have granted women's vote in the continent; the third in the world to legalize gay marriage, and most recently, one of the few to legalize marijuana use. Uruguay's recent president, José (Pepe) Mujica—a former Tupamaro revolutionary who lives in poverty and gives most of his salary to social causes—has become somewhat of a celebrity. Because Uruguay used to be part of Brazil, its black history remains alive in contemporary art, music, dance, and politics. This provides a framework of insight and assertiveness that clearly differentiates Uruguayan awareness from other regions of the continent, as Uruguay has been home to an unusual percentage of Eastern European communities with an extensive history of trauma that could have cemented the generational trauma legacy witnessed during the ferocious military dictatorship during the 1970s and 1980s. During the Second World War, as both Jews and Nazis fled to the same areas in Latin America, Montevideo witnessed the genesis of a mixed-society of both oppressors and oppressed, which, according to some sociological analyses, contributed to the ferocious fascist dictatorship that plagued both the 1970s and 1980s. Mediaeval clandestine texts in both Arabic and Hebrew language formed a corpus whose ideology of "inner liberation" remains a dominant ethos in some intellectual elites, and mid-twentieth-century immigration of Italian anarchists

S. Tenenbaum (✉)
Dalla Lana School of Public Health, University of Toronto, Toronto, ON, Canada
e-mail: silvia.tenenbaum@utoronto.ca

D. Danto, M. Zangeneh (eds.), *Indigenous Knowledge and Mental Health*,
https://doi.org/10.1007/978-3-030-71346-1_3

and Eastern Europe refugees contributed to further diversification and a new wave of political awareness. These apparently heterogeneous communities merged with Indigenous survivors to create the unique positionality of Uruguay within the Latin American continent, given Uruguay's unique sociological composition.

In terms of the complex clinical work in Toronto with Uruguayan exiles, it implies a deep cultural understanding of the many layers of its ideological framework. Several population traits are observed: mediaeval Spanish thought, through the cultural mindset of Mussar in all its texts of Aljamiado literature in Spain and Portugal, added to former Black Brazilian slaves in Uruguay, and coupled with newly arrived Slavic refugees, are the alma mater of the fire that ignites the Uruguayan soul both in land and in diaspora. The praxis of cultural safety is at once an art and a science because it has to integrate traditional healing on the one hand, and the psychology of exile on another.

Rationale

This chapter is the result of several decades of clinical practice and my own healing experience. I was born in Montevideo in 1960, in a politically transitional period from the dream of democracy to the nightmare of military dictatorship. In between, we lived through a civil war with the Tupamaro revolution it did not end well. A fierce repression followed, and my family and I ended up seeking refugee status in Canada, which was granted in 1988. This history of exile is shared by many Uruguayan-Canadians.

For this chapter, I have combined the personal accounts of 32 Uruguayan families, as well as the narratives of psychotherapy and healing of a group of Uruguayan Indigenous individuals engaged in culturally safe psychotherapy. I hope to provide a guidepost for non-traditional, effective, anti-oppressive psychotherapy, and also to give voice and texture to the narratives of individuals who did not survive the exile, were deported, or have chosen not to give their name but only their testimonials, as part of the collective process. I am honouring them by adding their ideas while preserving their identity by modifying any potential identifier. I have lived and worked in Toronto long enough to have completed clinical work for Uruguayans who went into exile from Uruguay to Sweden in the 1970s, returned to Uruguay or moved to Canada, and died in Toronto in the 2000s, as many of the Tupamaro fighters did. History and geography intersect in these narratives in ways that break transgenerational cycles of secrecy and validate the healing practices of Uruguayan Indigenous exiles in Toronto.

I tend to vacation in Seville and am fortunate to work yearly with refugees who arrive in Andalusia through various entry points in the Mediterranean. As my clinical practice expanded, I began to see more clearly how my experience as a young adult both resembled and differed from the experiences of those who attended my practice. While writing has been a crucial aspect of my own healing experience, I continue to work on generating more encompassing social change through developing college and university level curricula and through expanding training programme frameworks geared at incoming clinicians and which advocate for culturally safe spaces and practices that are truly inclusive.

Psychology of Exile

Exile is a never-ending story. It is both a burden and a blessing. It feels like a curse because not living in one's land means to live in an indeterminate threshold. Although this in-between space does not provide much-needed grounding, it is true that it affords us the freedom of not having to conform to post-colonial or even colonial values. It is far easier to reject a land of exile than it is to accept the political betrayal of one's land, even though to recognize the twists and turns of history can assuage one's alienation. As I have published recently about the exile within as a concept, I will not expand of this concept here, but suffice to say that exile is a post-colonial, patriarchal imposition that solidifies a condition of otherness, of profound discomfort that is augmented, not diminished, in the host land, as issues of jealousy and hostility run subtle currents in the potential transformation among the host country populations, as well as the cultural and value clashes between first- and second-generation exiles, a psychological construct frequently treated in clinical work.

A limited right to live a full life: In terms of the relationship between exile and the provision of culturally safe psychotherapy/healing work, it is important to remember the prophetic words of Hannah Arendt, reminding us that the fundamental human right is to actually have human rights, a fact still denied to many Indigenous groups living in Canada when they seek support in their psychological claims. Arendt wrote of refugees: "The calamity of the rightless is not that they are deprived of life, liberty and the pursuit of happiness, or of equality before the law and freedom of opinion, but that they no longer belonged to any community whatsoever." The loss of community has the consequence of expelling a people from humanity itself. Appeals to abstract human rights are meaningless unless there are effective institutions to guarantee these rights. The most fundamental right is the right to have rights. Although exiles do have limited rights, such as not having the right of history, the right of having a political opinion in the land they live, and the right to have relevant psychological work.

Exile as a different register of analysis: By the same token, by acknowledging the first inhabitants of lands, both patients and therapists honour where one is coming from, as well as accepting a respectful compass of the work ahead, meaning that the cultural framework has generated a lens through which psychological issues are viewed. Culture is a psychological reality, and as such, needs to guide the healing process. One heals from history as well as from others: that should be the compass to guide respectful treatment. History and geography live in both silence and words, in actions and omissions in both sides of the therapy room, meaning both clinician and patient. In this chapter, I show the measures I have taken to reduce my patients' dis-ease by taking a decolonizing approach, something not yet taught in academic programmes. I see this as a clinical application of Indigenous reconciliation, considering all cultural needs according to the Indigenous roots of my patients' family of origin that endured multiple historical cycles of geographic dislocation, from Uruguay, Syria, Brazil, and Spain.

Aljamiado Literature in Tenth-Century Spain as Über Text?

Mussar can be seen as a road to insomnia.[1] One of the sources of cultural resilience for oppressed Jews in Spain[2] is the idea that creative practice is essential to the liberation of the soul. From the Mussar[3] Jewish code of conduct (sometimes written

[1] I owe this title to Rabbi Ira Stone, who offers it as an explanation of the motivation behind the need to accept Mussar in our lives, that I found full of awe: "Care for ourselves, care for those closest to us, care for the world itself. Despite our possession of a record of Divine and human encounters which have expressed these obligations, and sometimes because of it, we tend to 'fall asleep' rather than face the full demands of these obligations. Mussar can be characterized as a road to insomnia: A way of staying awake to these obligations" ("Musar in the climate of Judaism and the teaching of Emanuel Lévinas," cf. website). Needless to say, the idea of illumination is central to both Kabbalah and Mussar thought, as it resonates with the precept to expand one's humanity, in order to complete God's project after seeing the crooked Golam, imperfect Adam, and less imperfect Eve, according to Gnostic interpretations of the Genesis. For more information concerning the topic of illumination, see Levi [1].

[2] Spain offers an arcane history of imposed multicultural co-existence that might offer some insights about the poly-varied psychosocial development of the human soul under unique circumstances. A detailed yet pertinent account is provided by Yair Davidy: "An area on the West Coast of Spain is referred to in the Bible as Tarshish. King Solomon together with the Phoenician King Hiram of Tyre sent ships to Tarshish. After ca. 700 BCE a population of people of Phoenician culture came to Spain. They bore Hebraic-like names, and Irish legends and other factors suggest that they may have been of Israelite descent. After the Phoenicians, invasions of groups such as the Carthaginians from North Africa arrived. The Carthaginians believed themselves to be descended from the ancient Canaanites whom the Israelites had driven out of the Promised Land. The presence of this element in Spain could partly explain the vicious anti-Semitism and outright sadism later displayed by a portion of the Spanish population. In the north and west of Spain there later emerged a people of Celtic culture. The Romans entered Spain in 218 BCE, and in 409 CE the Vandals, Suebi, and Alans invaded Spain. They were followed by the Goths or Visigoths who subdued the country by 585 CE...." Davidy also writes, "the Goths also ruled over southeast France in which area as well as in Spain the terms 'Goth' and 'Jew' were for a time interchangeable." In terms of the configuration of Spain in the Bible and the Descendants of David, Davidy says that Spain is mentioned in the Biblical book of Obadiah 1:20: "The exiled of Jerusalem who are in Sepharad: Targum Yehonathan translates 'Sepharad' as 'Aspamiah,' meaning Spain in Spanish (España). The Abarbanel says that whole settlements in Spain were founded by exiles from Jerusalem who included families descendants from King David." For more information concerning this unique and fascinating chronicle, please consult *Spain and the Jews,* by Yair Davidiy or its summary at http://britam.org/spain.html. Perhaps the long-seated history of the multiple oppressions Jews have faced through history has made us more aware of the notion of "availability" in terms of self-knowledge and a forced rapid integration of the categories of feeling, thinking, and intuiting, to be comfortable with the Jungian fourth dimension, as called a phenomenology of the body, as Mussar could also be understood. Basically, the idea that because Jewish communities experience ongoing cycles of exile, they became "experts" in its inner works. As a consequence, rather than taking the other out, according to some authors, oppressed Jews have been experts in creating a flexible space for the other in.

[3] *Mussar* is a Hebrew word with a dual meaning. It might mean both "light" and "darkness," depending on which side of the mirror we see it (in life or as a soul), as represented by the letters *rehah, sah-mekh,* and *mem,* and *seen, feh,* and *nun.* Hence, its meaning lies in the juxtaposition of "light within darkness," which encompasses that paradoxical aspect of the soul in its unequivocal journey.

Musar) we learn that one does not "have" a soul: one *is* a soul, and that soul has and is given a body. In that sense, Mussar can be seen as an Über text as a precursor to later views. It refers to the soul before the body, and the origins of Spanish identities before Latin American ones, and original Jewish ethics before Kabbalah and before Judaism as a defined corpus of philosophy. The only prerequisite to study the Musar is to "have experienced the human condition" (cf. Morinis). Spanish Jews created an esoteric literary corpus that in hermeneutic traditions is known as *literatura aljamiada*, the artistic and creative product of the *aljama*, which means, in Arabic language, "the city transgressing and/or beyond itself" (my translation).

Although some Aljamiado[4] stories have Muslim origins, the majority are Jewish, and most of the Aljamiado texts are written in the Arabic alphabet, though some are written in Hebrew script. All Aljamiado texts use Arabic or Hebrew script to articulate stories told in phonetic Spanish, which adds an extra difficulty to the reader. It is thought that their orality reveals their true meaning, however framed in either an Arabic and Hebrew cosmovision. It is written in a language about another language, and in one culture about the other culture, and because it is the mark of cultural unsafety, its ideas are masked through symbols and cues to other texts, which adds to the hermeneutic, or science of its interpretation. Thus, reading and interpreting an Aljamiado text is a complex linguistic, literary, and psychological task that requires extraordinary endurance. In their written recovered versions, Aljamiado texts chronicle superstitions, healing practices, and oracular expectations, and they usually include ethical and philosophical reflections concerning death (typically of the father, or any other male figure of authority), love, and longing (dialogues of suffering between a mother and a young daughter are common), as well as symbolic representations of the mutilated cultural body.

The most famous Aljamiado text—which transliterates in Arabic script oral stories told in Spanish—is called *Duties of the Heart,* written in 933 by Rabbi Bachaya Ibn Pakuda. Rabbi Bachaya travelled from Babylon to Spain, and lived in Muslim Spain, probably in Saragossa, while serving as a judge. *Duties of the Heart (Chovot HaLevovot)*, as indicated by its title, focuses on the moral obligations of the Jew. It is a sentimental education that teaches the duties of feeling, as "one must plummet

[4]*Aljama* is an Arabic term usually interpreted as "the enclosed city," or "the city surrounded by itself." Some have simply defined the *aljama* as "the Muslim and Jewish ghetto in medieval Spain." That term also refers to an interior place in one's soul, a sort of a hidden attic where one preserves untouched parts of the self. Many of most reputable Aljamiado studies have been done by Catalonian scholars, as Catalonia has a long and still unresolved dispute with Spain over the politics of their shared identity. Aljamiado studies are regularly published in Catalan, and sometimes translated in Spanish. It seems that in order to fully understand Catalan phonetics, one need to have a good grasp of medieval French. However, any serious student of this type of literature needs to be well versed in the Romance language archetype. (The Spanish department in the University of Toronto used to offer Medieval Catalan Phonetics to their PhD students, which I have had the honour to take in 1997, with the only Aljamiadist in Canada. When Professor Heigy retired, that course and literature were taken permanently out of the curriculum, so presently it is impossible to study Aljamiado literature in Canada. This shows how little interest Western psychology has in non-traditional techniques, outside the post-colonial, academic agenda of treatment.)

its depths because of the greatness of its inwardness and refinement" (*Judaism* 1). Sephardic Jewry continued the study of his magnum opus to discern ethical issues, accompanied by the influential *Guide to the Perplexed,* written by Maimonides (1135–1204) in Spain. I understand "perplexity" in this context as an act of intellectual resistance and grounding into one's journey, when the mere act of posing questions becomes the answer. In present times, Byung-Chul Han reframes the issue by exploring the issue of otherness (and its dialectical of negativity concerning minorities) by stating that "the tourist is a consumer" ([2], p. 2), while the minority occupies the land and rights, therefore, resisting its otherness.

Mussar as Literature, Philosophy, Spiritual Movement, and Practice

As a literary corpus, Mussar invites us to move beyond a mere hermeneutical exercise and into the endless process of recreating one's existence. As practised by many individuals in contemporary times, Mussar is a set of guiding principles, based on oral stories and popular practices and beliefs that advocate taking a different path toward the understanding the meaning of one's present life. In fact, Mussar is taught to children in a Jewish school in Montreal, with great receptivity by them, in a cultural attempt to capitalize on old ideas about integrity and cultural ethos.

As a philosophy, Mussar elucidates its relation to and departure from Kabbalistic practices. Although both philosophies represent aspects of Jewish moral thought, the Kabbalah dictates specific forms of behaviour, whereas Mussar asks for the exploration of inner desires, which is a much more attainable aim through one's work and will. The Kabbalah's focus on the regulation of conduct might explain why its study seems to have gained popularity nowadays, whereas Mussar has kept its almost cryptical quality, as it teaches private, silent, and daily practices. I find this quotidian and ordinary aspect of Mussar similar to the humble meaning-making process of an existential approach, as conceived by the early work of Frankl with its emphasis on immediacy, exposure, and relationality.

As a spiritual practice, Mussar presents healing in the form of the interpretation of sacred writings for those individuals seeking support, as Rabbi Stone's essay exemplifies. Mussar is an interpretation of a sacred text as related to much-needed help for those suffering. As a hermeneutic practice, it aims at negotiating textual meanings and reading between the lines, a practice which originated among the non-Hasidic Lithuanian Jews circa1850,[5] and which, according to some, greatly

[5] The founding of Mussar as a written rigorous ethical discipline of study is attributed to Rabbi Yisrael Lipkin Salanter (1810–1883), who was inspired greatly by the teachings of Reb Zundel Salant, although the roots of the movement can be traced to earlier developments and rabbinic personalities and their writings. According to Mussar, the roots of all our actions and thoughts can be traced to the depths of the soul, beyond the reach of the light of consciousness, and so the methods Mussar provides include meditations, guided contemplations, exercises, and chants that are all

influenced Freud's and Charcot's treatment innovations. (Although some Jewish scholars value and even admire Freud, they do see him as a talented heir to a millenary tradition of exquisite thought that he had accessed through the privilege of being born in an Orthodox Jewish family, where his mother used to call him "my golden child.") Freud was able to reframe, synthesize, and remarkably resist the critique of his time, in order to negotiate a connection between inner pulsations, dream interpretations, and female manifestations of a wounded uterus wandering—maybe even trapped, in the female body, as hysteria was known at the time.

Freud's systematic analysis generated infinite questions that Mussar techniques have addressed since its inception, such as the imposed role of motherhood to placate women's desire for erotic freedom, as well as the traumatic memory in the body, manifested in the female organs. This level of female oppression manifests through symptoms. These symptoms have been historically given different names and explanations such as hysteria in psychoanalysis, hysteria meaning the uterus wandering through the body in pain and loss. Psychoanalysis originated perhaps as the by-product of the embodiment of human suffering, where each layer/level/*koshar* is indeed a manifestation of human suffering that, in our Western view, does not have its own properties. Mussar speaks of koshars, psychoanalysis of complexes, and modern social psychology of inner conflicts. When living in exile, I believe that one has to counterattack, cancel, integrate, or surrender to historically embedded human suffering the best one can, according to the present circumstances of time and space. I have witnessed in my work many Uruguayan patients acting under these parameters, even after a few decades living in Toronto, or even after coming back from another, first place of exile. In India, a person in exile might work by advancing to the superior level or, as Frankl described it, to start with the most basic one: the will to live. However, in this postmodern, multicomplex life of ours in Toronto, a global, eclectic, and integrative approach might be necessary, in order to resonate in the daily chaos and profound lack of harmony of our patients, since the texture of illness is culturally embedded.

Mussar is path of contemplative exercises that have evolved over the past thousand years to help an individual soul pinpoint and then break through the barriers that surround and obstruct the flow of inner light in our lives. Mussar is a treasury of techniques. Mussar is a guide to daily practice and, as such, it emphasizes the application of its framing principles as well as the virtues of the Healer. For instance, I have been using in my clinical work, as follow-up exercises between sessions, part of the curriculum of Alan Morinis's "Pathfinders" course as an example. Its main focus is on quotidian, mundane tasks—such as brushing one's teeth in the morning, or tying one's shoelaces,[6] and keeping a journal every night about what one

intended to penetrate the darkness of the subconscious, to bring about change at the door of our nature. From its origins in the tenth century, Mussar was a practice of the solitary seeker, until in the nineteenth century, when it became the basis for a popular social and spiritual movement.

[6]In a classic Jewish story, a student tells his friend that he is going to study with a teacher. "What do you learn?" his friend asks him. "I want to see how he ties his shoe." This apparently innocent question provides a full intertextual frame to the Mussar reader, in terms of the relational capabili-

accomplished or not in following a particular practice. Mussar is based on tradition and appeals to a better future, but works in the present as an immanent practice in and of the world. For instance, if we are working on the values of gratitude and compassion, we must be vigilant of our tendency to be judgmental, and monitor our thoughts and responses to others' set of values and inclinations, even and especially when they contradict our own.[7]

It is believed that the Mussar movement originated in Spain during the Middle Ages as a literary and philosophical tradition, which is now being revitalized by some young scholars, not necessarily of Jewish ancestry. Its philosophical vein emphasizes the issues of internalization and resistance of the "wandering Jew" (cf. Potok). This is a historical construct; however, after 80 generations in exile, it became part of the cultural subgroup of Uruguayans in Toronto, according to my observations. In Orthodox Eastern Europe during the nineteenth century, Mussar appears from the time of persecution of minorities in Spain ([4], p. 178) as an affirmation of Jewish life in times of pogroms, perhaps as an(other) balancing act between history and geography, with all its pull and push. Finally, when practised on a daily basis, the Mussar teachings ensure the progressive evolution of its 13 precepts to become fully human, our most important existential project, as Viktor Frankl strongly advocated throughout his provocative psychiatric work after the Second World War.

Two healing approaches follow the precepts of Mussar. One, called "Jacob's intrigue," is a logotherapeutic approach elaborated on in an elegant essay by North American Rabbi David Wolpe. The second, which presents a psycho-educational perspective, is "The Gate of Starting Out" (excerpt from *Climbing Jacob's Ladder),* written by Canadian philosopher and teacher Alan Morinis. Both texts provoke a clear purpose in one's life although their actual application might be limited to a client that mirrors its cultural origins, such as a Spanish Jewish person with a penchant for ethical dilemmas in a love of learning, engagement in elegant arguments, multileveled articulation of one's ideas, and the like. Or they might work for a patient who can appreciate these two approaches by sharing cultural parameters.

---

ties of transmutation/transformation that the student needs to compromise between his/her inner world and existential reality of multiple forms of oppression. That is the cryptic meaning of the metaphor of wanting to see "how he ties his shoe," mentioned in the excerpt "The Gate of Starting Out" from *Climbing Jacob's Ladder.* This is also related to the old German saying: "God provides the strings, and human beings are responsible for threading them" (Eco 43, my translation), which was prevalent in seventeenth-century Germany, when Yiddish emerged as a clandestine language of oral traditions.

[7] This idea is clarified in the introduction of the website for the Mussar Institute, a Canadian institute for basic, beginner training in Mussar. "Our greatest struggle, you and me, is to become good. God set up our lives to do just that by giving us all the tools we need to be and do good, and an inner compass to guide us as well. But being good is not easy. There are obstacles to overcome. *Nisyionos*, the Mussar teachers call them. Tests. We face them every day, you and me, some large, some small. We are constantly being tested to choose the good" [3]. Another relevant teaching of Alan Morinis is the precept to "make the heart feel what the intellect understands" (Path of the Soul, 1). For further information about Mussar training in Toronto, contact the facilitator Modya at modya@mussaratwork.com, or Rachel Melzer at (416) 323–3383.

These characteristics are beautiful traits in a human being; nevertheless, they encompass a certain privilege in terms of intellectual development, cultural upbringing, and perhaps a proper and comfortable navigation toward one's race, gender, and sexual orientations. As a result, Mussar is a remarkable approach, yet limited to a certain type of patient, an exile, politically aware, and psychologically minded, which means not so fragmented culturally that they have to accept contradictory ways of living at the same time. Academics, clinicians and patients who take on the task of cultural integration without losing one's psychological roots usually find themselves unsuccessful. This issue is seen both in clinicians and patients. Academics and clinicians can maintain patients' psychological roots only if they have worked on themselves on a successful integration first. We basically require from exiles what many Indigenous individuals could not accomplish. And that is a blunt reality that non-exiles would rather not face.

Jacob's story in the Old Testament remains a conundrum in Jewish theology, which continues to grapple with two unanswerable questions: "Was Jacob wresting all night against his own shadow?" and "Am I my brother's keeper?" The answers one gives to these questions, even as they change over time, frame our approach to existence as they prompt us to consider fundamental issues such as our role in society, the significance of caring and solidarity, and how one wrestles with seemingly unsurmountable moral dilemmas.

Case Study with a Mussar Application: Alpha and Omega

Is Mussar's meditative approach to living relevant to contemporary psychotherapeutic practice? What are its advantages and its application challenges? I decided to explore these questions in my practice, allowing enough flexibility to accept failure as a potential outcome and a learning opportunity.

A well-known family doctor in the Latin American community who knows about my psychotherapeutic practice with Syrian refugees through Health Canada sent me a referral last year. The doctor also disclosed that I was "her last resort," and that she had heard that I had been successful at working with extremely resistant clients. A proud Syrian/Uruguayan woman in her 50s came to see me at the end of November 2017. She complained about recurring nightmares, which began with her decision to stop seeing her son, who became HIV-infected through needle-sharing during a period in his youth.

At first I saw her differences—in a name written in a foreign alphabet, her accent, her war and trauma experiences, and other forms of distinctiveness. Although I expect patients to be different, it is always a point of significance when somebody is different from their group, or their subgroup among the main group, as in this case. Instead of hiding them, I acknowledged and honoured them, for they made the whole person I had in front of me. By naming her distinctness, I empowered her difference. Paradoxically, that laying up of the groundwork acted as a strong foundation based on various forms of distinction. Perhaps because of them, I also pointed out our commonalities in the interest of facilitating the therapeutic encounter. She was born in Uruguay from an Indigenous father and a Syrian mother, both claiming international ancestry, her father's Brazilian roots coming from his own father, and she was a survivor of those eight First Nations Indigenous groups that had claimed Uruguayan land since the sixteenth century.

This woman acted in a way that was culturally expected and even desirable, as she believed at that juncture that she betrayed her culture of origin by seeking safety in Canada, given her former political activities, which were totally against Western democracies. I did not challenge her perceptions, as they formed the uniqueness of her reality. Her son was her only child and, in the client's words, "very much like my father's personality." She felt uneasy with herself, and was not sure if she was mourning the healthy, young man she thought and wanted her son to be, or her actual son, who was perhaps at risk of dying soon.

After having established a strong therapeutic alliance, I tried sand therapy, but to no avail. Using Western techniques, tools, and tips was simply not working, as this patient did not engage. Using healing techniques, however, clearly did. I had assumed that my client was willing to symbolize the past and imagine the future, without considering that she had done that work by herself before coming to see me. It turned out that she had been doing daily meditations and visualizations that work in similar ways to the sand-therapy work. Later on, my client revealed that she perceived sand therapy as "child's play done by Western counsellors," and she was quite surprised when I admitted it frankly. I explained that I had received all my formal training at the University of Toronto, and that despite being a registered clinical psychologist in Ontario, I was aware of the limitations of my training and of mainstream frames of clinical practice in Canada. I also disclosed having had many experiences with non-traditional, Indigenous forms of healing, and that I was both willing and able to share and implement those techniques with her. I sensed that a heavy burden was lifted and that she felt that she could trust me. During the year-end break, and since this client asked me not to engage in any form of traditional (talk) therapy, I had begun to re-evaluate my own capabilities as a Healer. Disclosing my mother's roots in a nomadic family of storytellers in Lebanon, I decided to employ a storytelling framework that would allow this client to narrate and re-author her own life. I also enlisted the support of a well-respected Elder in rural Uruguay who was willing to consult with me and engage with her via Skype on a monthly basis.

The more I disclosed about my bi-ethnic (Jewish and Arabic) and bicultural upbringing (Catholic Montevideo until I was 28 years of age, then Montreal and Protestant Toronto for 30 years), the more credibility I gained. I shared myself as a student of life, still looking for ways to expand my humanness, which is Mussar in essence, and that worked by opening up inner doors that were closed before. This was my most successful attempt to integrate some Gestaltic (two-chair techniques) body work and soul-searching according to historical and geographical parameters of the mind instead of through pure Western clinical techniques.

Since 2018, I have opted to work on some of the *middots* (engaging one's cultural ethos in daily spiritual practices) to further this client's introspective abilities.

I devoted one session to prayer and some basic invocations to learn my client's sources of comfort. Then I asked for sources of suffering to inform my search for ways to increase her coping mechanisms: Was it shame? Guilt? Intergenerational trauma, which for this person seeking healing for her ancestors was still present somehow in every session? I engaged in disclosing some of my personal work toward healing experiences of trauma and my recovery process from a spiritual point of view, which increased this client's interest in healing as a potentially viable choice. Then I sensed that the terrain was fertile enough to explain the Mussar practice with a focus on the three precepts of cultural safety I asked her to help me plan six sessions with three traits, its aims, and homework assigned. The traits were survivor's guilt, inability to love the host country, and the hostility of non-successful inhabitants toward this person. The more I validated and empowered this patient's feelings and perceptions, the more her motivation and commitment flourished. This became a cross-referential learning process to both of us, as I discovered toward the end of those six first sessions. In general, while working with exiles, I have found that attendance in itself is a sign of motivation and commitment. Avoidance can be a safety mechanism, at least historically (pre-exile), then reenacted for post-traumatic trauma growth. Uruguayan exiles were able to manage their anger, rage, and hatred into a more articulated position of acceptance in the grey area, without some binary sources of differences. The original resentment might have transformed into a creative exilic process that acknowledges historical wounds while managing and generating different present situations according to updated needs and wants.

Conflicted Cultural Values

Although mass media imposes the concept of the present world as a global village, at least for those who define and enjoy the term, it is inevitable that someone living under the psychology of exile will have at one point or another cultural clashes that might bring turmoil, either internally with oneself, or with a second-generation child, or when going back "home" to confront oneself in the past. As I need to move patients into a healthy present, I started with daily work toward silence, humility, and presence. Silence provided me a roadmap to this client's "here and now," in terms of her specific sources of suffering, which can be seen as an ethical decision, or cultural values that sharply contrasted to her mother's instincts; possible changes, as for instance either acceptance or rebelliousness toward one's culturally instilled values; and finally, aspects of the past that could inform my plan of action, as, for example, letting go, some attachment complexities, or other residual or vicarious traumas of my own. Some traits that were used pre-exile needed to have a different use and definition in the new land. The new application of those traits is the vehicle used to move from post-traumatic stress disorder into post-traumatic stress growth, where the exiled person has an increased sense of agency, power, and control, both internal and external.

These are complex human traits, but I sensed that the situation deemed this appropriate, as did my client' s openness to a non-traditional approach to curing/healing/Indigenous ways in what has strictly been (trans)formed or integrated into some of our postmodern terms. The idea is to work on a dual frame of work: both similarities and differences are acknowledged and worked on, from both a traditional and Western cosmovision. To integrate and heal is based upon all elements in a person's life.

I probed with a universal experience: contact with oneself, such as praying, and it got good results. Either the divinity within, or full humanity, or whatever gives an individual strength. One can pray to a divinity in oneself or to our own humanity, or whatever sources our strength. The choices of praying and aromatherapy are classic preparation healing journey techniques in Uruguay, so they are familiar and culturally relevant. Then the patient tried aromatherapy with healing herbs from Brazil used by an experienced Uruguayan *chamán* in Brampton, a city close to Toronto, whom I reached out to. This made the client aware of her shallow breathing patterns, and then open to my teaching of diaphragmatic breathing, touching her stomach when she was lying on my couch, which amazed me at first, for the level of comfort and trust it entails. After 12 sessions, the client began to incorporate the habits of silence, humility, and presence in her work of repairing her relationship with her son. She took the initiative to draw some of her nightmares and to "make a story" about herself and her son in their present relationship.

Duties of the Heart in Healing Clinical Work

What worked with Mussar was its general axiom of our "being" a soul. Thus, I searched for this client's soul in order to touch it with mine. What did not work, paradoxically, was my desire to apply techniques beforehand, maybe pushing my own clinical frames of references. Healing work does not obey the laws of science; so much subjectivity is acknowledged in the sense of healing, both subjectivity of the patients, and the clinician as well, healing is nevertheless, valid and culturally safe. Some individuals—and many therapists—need clarity of dialogue, transparency of assessments, diagnosis, and prognosis, and a clear sense of leadership on the head of the clinician. Others seem to be able to navigate their murky waters, only by the hand of the "other." To this type of patient, the therapist is one who lends a heart—and those are the real "duties," sharing one's own soul in the process, which is obscured by one's labyrinthical approach to well-being. In my own experience within this type of clinical practice, Indigenous women claiming multiple geographically displaced roots tend to be more prone to need a variety of healing practices and Indigenous tools, and immigrants, or people with at least a dual (if not multiple) cultural coexistences provoke a richer cognizance of the sources of their troubles, as well as their alleviation. This opening of "Pandora's box" with all the mystery contained in it gave life after being opened and realizing all the evils in the world and some hope, could indeed be managed with some culturally relevant and safe tools that seemed to be able to provoke intimate moments with certain clients. First, patients need to be ready to the opening of their own fears contained in a box, both negative and positive elements (fear and hope, for instance). Then comes naming, categorizing, and prioritizing the work, accepting agency, and taking chances and change, as well as revisiting what works and what still needs to be modified. This process allows the invisible to be visible and the unnamed to have a name; it allows a sense of agency in one's life. This was especially true of Uruguayan individuals with Middle Eastern ancestry, as perhaps an eerie recognition from other previously lived lives of mine, if I may attempt to disclose an explanation of those innate talents that everybody has, but few dare to develop, such as intuition, that arcane way of knowing, propitiated an opening, discovery, and illumination to occur, only to close again after that fateful instant of Grace in its full radiance.

Obviously, some movement has been precipitated by my risk of engaging through Mussar elements in our sessions. Today I wonder if I had a resistant client, or if she got an initially resistant therapist, who because of being experienced, wanted to impose instead of co-create a viable cure for this client's soul (and mine too, for sure). I am learning quite a lot from this client and her simultaneous relational processes, the various changes in relationship she is living through. I am still seeing her once a month for 6 months, as she is now facing the imminent death of her son, and anticipatory grief is permeating all aspects of her life, including her relationship with her community and other members of her family. This client gave me written permission to disclose the general characteristics of her case, but asked me out of respect, not to change but omit her name, yet to mention her country of origin. Only last week, I learned that for a few years she was following the Muslim faith, and that as a result of a tragic event in her life as a teen while visiting Syria and Jordan, she had decided to abandon that religion. I feel privileged to have earned the right to get to know her deep-seated reason for walking away from Allah. When disclosing that specific event, I sensed a moment of Grace. Perhaps that was God's way of saying how sorry he/she was for being imperfect at times.

In this chapter, I used a healing approach because it allowed the cultural elements to dictate the treatment, both historically and culturally embedded, as well as the geographic context of community Healers. By using a healing approach in my work, as described in this chapter, and allowing historical and culturally embedded elements to dictate a grand part of the treatment, with the inclusion of community leaders, my healing approach took into account where my patients were coming from in pre-exilic life (Montevideo, for instance) and post-exilic life (Brampton, in Ontario), I engaged them in the full circle of their existence—not in a partial way, but in a complete cycle. By acknowledging the context of the early Aljamiado texts, as well as the values of Mussar in Spanish ethos, and present-day cultural constructs of Uruguayan mentality, present-day Uruguayan exiles' families in Toronto could access what they perceive as culturally safe psychotherapeutic practices.

References

1. Levi E. The book of splendours. The inner mysteries of qabalism. Maine: Aquarian Press; 1984.
2. Han B-C, Butler E. The burnout society. Standford, CA: Standford University Press; 2015.
3. Morinis, A. (Morinis, www.mussarinstitute.org). Path of the soul, p. 1.
4. Oz A, Salzberger-Oz F. Jews and words. USA: Yale University Press; 2012.

Silvia Tenenbaum is an applied social researcher and registered clinical psychologist trained at the University of Toronto in the scientist-practitioner model, as well as a postdoctoral fellow at the Dalla Lana School of Public Health. At present, Dr. Tenenbaum enjoys focusing on the exploration of complex ethical dilemmas and traumatic memories across generations in diaspora, applied to writing a textbook on the psychology of exile and its long-term effects, including issues of the perpetual search for one's land (both internal and external). Oftentimes, she shares her lived experience across several continents and cultural parameters as a presenter across the globe. Silvia lives in downtown Toronto with her family, cat, plants, and music, and is both an avid yoga practitioner and a foreign films festival buff.

Part II
The Land and Healing

Healing Practices and Rituals of the Forest-Dwelling Rabha Community in Assam, India

Chinmayi Sarma

The structural–functional, or organismic, model of studying society assumes that changes in any part of the social system will have important consequences for other parts of the social system as a whole. In this chapter, I present the forest as an inseparable part of life and livelihood of the Indigenous Rabha community, where the people dwell and from which they draw food, medicine, and well-being. The Rabhas of Assam share a symbiotic relationship with the forest ecosystem. For them, ethnomedicine means more than meticulous gathering and mixing the products of the forest; rather, it is a complete, environment-centred belief system, one which each member of the community must follow. Besides giving identity to the Rabhas as forest dwellers, the forest has a social role in promoting well-being and health. The Indian Constitution gives protection to the forest-dwelling Rabha community of Assam as a Scheduled Tribe because of their unique relatedness to the ecosystem. Kinship identity is determined by the grove which the clan looks after. They derive both food and occupation from the products of the forest and are directly dependent on it for medicinal herbs and invoking the forest deity for protection.

But today the forest is undergoing a transition that is threatening the symbiosis shared between the community and the groves, and leading to an instability in practices that sustain well-being. This chapter attempts to set forth a few narratives delineating this relationship and its transition, which were collected as part of an ethnographic study to understand Indigenous practices of the forest communities of Assam.

Banamali, the forest deity, is considered omnipresent and supreme. He is called upon by the community for health and harmony but also for death and disease. The

---

C. Sarma (✉)
Centre for North East Studies and Policy Research, Jamia Millia Islamia, New Delhi, India
e-mail: csarma@jmi.ac.in

D. Danto, M. Zangeneh (eds.), *Indigenous Knowledge and Mental Health*,
https://doi.org/10.1007/978-3-030-71346-1_4

Rabhas invoke him during festivals and in ceremonies to bless occasions of celebration and, in times of despair and death, to undo the misery. Banamali is intrinsically tied to every ritual of the forest people. The deity resides in the sacred canopies of the forest, mostly in the Indian smilax tree.

For the Rabhas, health is a psychic state of well-being that is made possible by physical access to trees and herbs often found in the sacred groves. The Indian smilax tree is revered among the Rabhas as sacred for its roots, berries, and leaves, used in traditional medicine to treat rheumatism, anaemia, and skin aliments. By 1870, however, as the Imperial Forest Department understood the revenue potential of the forests of Assam, realizing their commercial exploitation became the predominant agenda of colonial forest policy ([1], p. 146). Soon Indian smilax grew sparse in number and the spiritual and medicinal dependence of the Rabhas on the species began to suffer. While, as part of colonial forest policy, exotic species of trees were introduced to the forest, the concepts of sacred groves, the resident deity, and belief in ethno-medicinal practices metamorphosed.

In this context, the role of Ojha, the forest priest, who administered healing through rituals, was also transformed. As colonial influence has seeped in to the sacred groves, however, in the form of forest department officials, university-trained doctors, and medicinal plant contractors, the symbiosis of the Rabhas with their environment has eroded. This has increased the flow of money into the once autonomous forest tracts of Assam, replacing the former barter system and thereby exposing the Rabhas to several forms of vulnerability. The fragile balance the community maintains with nature has been stressed. Today, the resistance of the Rabhas to illness is weakened by the intermittent use of allopathic medicine even while they still depend on Indigenous herbs. The community has not been able to accept either of the systems fully, yet by intermittently using both they are making themselves vulnerable.

In the first part of this chapter, I introduce the community in the context of the forest as a sacred entity but also an entity that is in the midst of a dynamic resistance to colonial forces. Then, to provide deeper insight into what make the forest and its people part of an interrelated system, I focus on two aspects, namely spirituality and Indigenous medicine. These two areas are undergoing significant changes in the present era.

The Forest-Dwelling Rabha Community

The Rabhas are one of the Indigenous tribes of Assam, extending to the adjoining states of West Bengal and Meghalaya. Under the constitution of India, they are categorized as "Scheduled Tribes—Plains," that is, living in the plains. The Rabhas are a culturally diverse group and their plurality is increased by their ongoing assimilation with the neighbouring Hindu population of the Brahmaputra Valley. The material and cultural heritage of Rabhas is rich with diverse oral narratives. The community does not have a written history of its own. The construction of history is governed by community memory, which has been passed down generationally, and depends on archival sources that include reports made by colonial ethnographers. Various such reports claim the Rabha people are offshoots of other tribes such as the Bodo, Kacharis, and Garos [2], based on their dialect and Mongolid features, but the Rabhas consider themselves unique. The Rabhas are internally classified into seven groups, which were originally stratified by occupation, each group having its own dialect and specific territory. For instance, the oral history of the Hana Rabha suggests that this subgroup specialized in singing songs to make horses dance.

The oral history gathered from the community tells of how the Rabha traversed from the Tibetan region, moving across the Garo Hills, and finally reaching the Assam Plain. Today, the Rabha population is distributed along the Duar (also Dooar) region, which is covered with semi-tropical forest and undergrowth and has a rugged topography. Falling between the fertile plains of Assam and the Eastern Himalayas, this region experiences heavy rains, often making the location humid and steamy. The deepest cores of the forests abound in wild animals and their fringes are dotted with tribal hamlets.

Rabha hamlets are clan based; these clans, commonly referred to as *husuks,* are totemic in nature and animistic in faith. For example, the vulture is a totem for some *husuks* of Kamrup district in Assam. Due to rapid industrialization and the use of diclofenac for cattle as painkillers, vultures, being scavengers, are in danger of extinction. For the clan members, each dead vulture is given a ritualistic burial and mourned. The totemic value of the vulture comes from the belief that the soul of a dead man takes the shape of a vulture before escaping to heaven. Thus, the death of a vulture is understood as the completion of a life cycle, but a rapid increase in the number of carcasses is a cause for concern among the Rabhas.

Even today, many Rabhas continue to reside in the forest hamlets and lead a traditional socio-economic life, depending mostly upon the forest resources and practising age-old slash-and-burn methods of cultivation. *Hamzar*[1] songs, which are sung during weeding and sowing, depict the forest that once was and the Rabhas as its ultimate protector.

The tribe has been relatively reclusive, yet recent technology has left its mark. Today, local activists speak about a diluted Rabha identity [3]. Issues such as assimilation and the simultaneous loss of Indigenous knowledge have been at the fore of these discussions. In this chapter, I explore only a few sides of this multidimensional issue.

The economic interdependence between village-based agricultural caste groups and forest tribes is a historic fact. However, with the government's intervention, forests began to be classified as isolated entities, and the communities living in them began to migrate outside of them to the plains of Assam. Those migrant Rabhas began to work mostly as agricultural labourers and, with the passage of time, became absorbed into caste-based Hindu society. Thus a transition ensued, from

[1] *Hamzar* are folk songs in the Rabha dialect sung at the time of shifting cultivation, that is, during tilling of the land and burning the forest. The etymological root of the term *hamzar* lies in two words: *ha* means earth and *mazar* means middle of the forest.

tribalism to Hinduism, which diminished their former self-sufficiency, but was described by western-trained, American anthropologist Robert Redfield as moving from a *little* to a *great* tradition [4]. This transition also affected their belief system: leaving behind a largely matrilineal animistic community, they started imbibing the mainstream patriarchal values.

The ecological and social crisis of the forest-dwelling communities began in the British era and with the coming of forest department, when the customary rights of local communities were ignored.[2] Those rights disappeared as forests were categorically declared protected areas, beyond the reach of communities who traditionally depended on them for basic needs such as food, medicine, and religion. The exclusionary model of forest conservation, through the creation of people-free zones, displaced the traditional forest dwellers from their lives and livelihoods.

The historical wrong committed against the forest dwellers was supposed to have been amended and undone by the *Scheduled Tribes and Other Traditional Forest Dwellers (Recognition of Forest Rights) Act,* 2006. Legislation entitled forest dwellers who had lived in a hamlet for 75 years or up to three generations, until December 13, 2005, with residence rights as well as "bona fide livelihood needs," meaning the right to produce and sell produce resulting from self-cultivation of the forest in order to fulfil the sustenance needs of themselves and their families [5]. Although the *Forest Rights Act* made limited provisions for land and resources within the forest for the traditional forest-dwelling communities, its practical implementation has led to several irregularities, such as reluctance of the forest bureaucracy to give up control, and the requirement for intensive documentation of communities' claims, which makes the process harrowing for communities challenged to communicate with the dominant culture [6]. It is today, in this socio-legal setting, that the claims of the Rabhas are being represented, but an unmistakable degeneration of cultural capital prevails.

The Forest as Community Space Meets Modernization

Forest has always been central to Indian civilization, representing the feminine principle of *prakriti,* or nature. The Vedic literature depicts the forest as the primary source of life and fertility, a heaven for wanderers and seekers, and a model for societal and civilizational evolution. The Vedas were written by sages living in the forest who saw it as their home and a source of revelation, exaltation, and creativity. These sages also composed the Forest Books, referred to as the Aranyakas, which

---

[2]The Imperial Forest Department was established in 1864. Subsequently, three Indian Forest Acts of 1865, 1894 and 1927 curtailed century-old customary use rights of local communities. Such governance continued even after independence in 1947 and, only in 2006, with the passing of the Schedule Tribe and Other Traditional Forest Dwellers (recognition of Forest Rights) Act, 2006, recognized the rights of any community to protect, regenerate, conserve, or manage forest resources, which it has been traditionally protecting and conserving for sustainable use.

consisted of chants, hymns, and remedies. The texts also tell of an elusive goddess, Aranyani, who is fond of solitude yet fearless. Ancient Sanskrit texts also make mention of forest tribes, who were referred to as *nishadhas,* and strategic marriage alliances conducted with them by ruling dynasties. In subsequent literature, the unfamiliar forest tribes began to be referred to as *rakshasa*. The word *rakshasa* comes from the Sanskrit root word *raksha*, which means to guard, protect, and preserve. These forest tribes were the inhabitants and protectors of the forest, who opposed the expanding settlements that were destroying the forest [7]. According to Hindu scriptures, the forest assumes an important role in greater Indian tradition and falls within the realm of sacred geography.

The forest is not a source of material to serve the biological needs of hunger or the economic need for timber, but instead a sacred place with multiple levels of meaning for an Indigenous culture. The forest-dwelling Rabha population of Assam see their ecosystem as replete with traditional stories and oral narratives, and with spirits who receive physical manifestation in the form of sacred groves, sacred water, and totems. The religious experiences and rituals bind members of Rabha community into one cohesive unit. Similarly, the traditions of Indigenous medicine emerged in the particular context of living in the forest and depending on it for all utilitarian purposes such as livelihood, food, fuel, and medicines. For instance, soil is considered sacred by the forest dwellers, and traditionally they have abstained from plowing. The forest dwellers resort to collecting the products of the forest, such as fallen fruits, roots, and tubers from the surrounding habitat. They also undertake slash-and-burn cultivation, often referred to as *jhum kheti*. The Rabhas believe that ploughing would amount to tearing across the breast of Mother Earth. The traditional saying is that Earth produces enough to satiate everyone's needs, but not for everyone's greed.

Even though shifting cultivation may sometimes become counterproductive, the Rabhas hold on to their belief that Mother Earth needs to be taken care of from time to time and that *jhumming* increases her fertility to regenerate. Scientific research has also highlighted that post-shifting cultivation, the forest recovers at a faster rate, in spite of its obvious drawbacks such as soil erosion. Given the geographical context and topography in which the community lives—the semi-tropical forest ecosystem, rugged topography, and limited population—shifting cultivation is entirely appropriate. First, during heavy monsoon spells, the need for drainage is taken care of and, second, rotation the land for cultivation keeps the soil richness intact. As noted, there are folk songs referred to as *hamzar,* which are specially sung during *jhumming*. This pattern, however, was diverted by the arrival of the *Forest Rights Act* in 2006.

Members of the community who were undertaking some form of cultivation at that time are, since 2006, now entitled to up to 4 hectares of land. The *Act* gave great impetus to settled cultivation, thereby confining nomadic forest Rabhas into semi-agricultural villages. Today one finds small villages of about 20 households instead of tiny hamlets of three or four households. This has made the villages bigger and more cohesive. The *Act* has also led to a clear-cut demarcation of spaces, thereby separating the forest from the homestead. Forest tribes who had been living in the forest were slowly becoming alienated from their ecosystem. This process of physical removal has also led to a mental gulf, in which the people are becoming spiritually removed from the forest to which they previously offered prayers. The community also depended upon the forest to cure ailments and diseases. The products of the forest ensured the well-being of the people and healed them both physically and mentally. But now there was a distance between many of the people and the forest.

Alterations in patterns of livelihood have also had a domino effect. First, the social structure of the group is slowly being altered. Previously scattered settlement is becoming more and more nucleated. This means that a divide between forest and homestead has occurred, reducing the forest to being of utilitarian service only. The people of the forest were intimately connected to it in many ways, from offering oblation (in the form of ritualistic sacrifices of small animals) to the spirit of ancestors residing in sal trees (*Shorea robusta*) to consumption of swartz (*Diplazium esculentum*) for medicine. But those connections are now in decline. The community was considered unique because its members were capable of adapting themselves to the forest and regenerating symbiotically. The forces of industrialization, however, seem to have ignored such Indigenous epistemology. In this transition, kinship-based ties are also becoming complex. Members of the community are today migrating outside for better livelihood opportunities. There has also been a steady decline in the barter economy, which is having an impact on existing societal relations. An elderly Rabha candidly reported that "life is becoming more certain and more comfortable, but the past ethos is lost beyond repair" (personal communication, February 28, 2016). According to him, this is creating a gulf between man and nature.

Today, the settled villages are provided with medically trained health professionals sent by the government. Under the developmental drive of the government, more and more households are coming into the fold of settled agricultural villages. The youth are increasingly out-migrating and thereby becoming alienated from the rich biosphere. The knowledge of bark, herbs, and wild plants, which was once essential to survival, has become a matter of choice. Sarukanta, a village Elder, lamented how in the olden days it was considered auspicious to serve as the Ojha's apprentice, but today's heirs to this role would not be able to identify simple herbs (personal communication, March 16, 2016). This, in his opinion, is an indicator of the loss of cultural capital of the Rabha nation, as roles have become more symbolic, losing significance and meaning.

A *hamzar* verse depicts the step-by-step process by which a patch of forest must be cleared and seeds sown. It is interesting to note that before clearing and burning the forest, there is a designated step for collecting both herbs and weeds for medicinal use. But today such ritualistic picking, storing, and extraction is no more. Sugandh Mantri *(Homalomena aromatica),* a rhizomatous aromatic herb, is found in the forest of this region. Rabha tradition suggests that the community has long been using it to cure pain, inflammation, and infection. However, as ethnobotanists made inroads in studying this region, the herb's other pharmacological properties became better known, such as its analgesic, antidepressant, and antifungal benefits

[8]. The scientific studies of Sugandh Mantri opened doors for its commercial exploitation. Today, this herb is systematically planted in the region and the harvest from these plantations is sold to multinational companies; this has had the effect of reducing the Rabha people to being merely suppliers of raw materials.

In the past, before clearing the forest for jhum, the Bejas (apprentices to the Ojha, the principal Medicine Man) used to pick an essential herb, meticulously extract its oil, and then mix the oil with sawdust and wrap that mixture around a bamboo stick. Traditional incense was made out of this composite mixture and offered to honour deities and heal the diseased. Today, the practice is no more. The Rabha people buy incense sticks from the weekly market and burn them. The commercially sold incense has little healing property; neither does it serve as antidepressant or sedative. Today, large corporations use sophisticated technology to separate the herb's aromatic property from its pharmacological properties. With the decline of shifting cultivation (slash-and-burn), the collection of locally available medicinal herbs is also being affected. As a whole, the Indigenous healing practices of forest communities are in decline, now at a crossroads between the law and the marketplace, as unregulated pharmaceutical companies venture into forest villages without standard operating procedures or laws to monitor their exploration.

Spirituality and Medicinal Practices

The system of healing among the forest communities is not merely confined to extracting forest resources for preparation of medicine; beyond that, it embraces the forest as a living entity with metaphysical manifestations.

In this context, allopathic medicine is very reductionist because it is restricted by its medical gaze. The simple categorization of an ill person as patient with a set of ill-functioning organs is grossly inadequate. The "medical gaze," as described by Foucault, does also probe into the elements causing the disease and the environment propelling it [9]. Yet in spite of that, the modern medical system fails to see disease as a part of the whole system in which people and environments interact with one another.

According to traditional forest communities, humans interact with their environments and such interactions are value laden. Not all kinds of trees and fruits are seen as accessible at all times. Every tree is supposed to have a guardian spirit, and disturbing the guardian spirit at an inappropriate time calls up the spirit's wrath. For instance, people are prohibited from visiting the *ouu tenga* (elephant apple) tree at midday. The elephant apple tree (*Dillenia indica*) is customarily visited during morning hours only, and upsetting the norms amounts to upsetting the residing spirit's will, thereby causing the trespasser to become possessed [10]. Each of these spirits has a particular name and dedicated rituals for appeasement.

In the context of Rabha society, possession by a spirit is not uncommon. When possessed, the body of a person becomes inhabited by a formless forest being, which leads the host to be tormented by pain, irrational behaviour, convulsions, and hallucination leading to identity displacement. In this part of the world, medical doctors have failed to interpret such spirit possession and trance phenomena. Instead, allopathic practitioners have dismissed these cultural maladies as superstition and Healers as fanatics. Regardless of the failure to recognize it, possession by forest spirits is a reality, and the ritualistic expulsion of such spirits symbolically demonstrates the relationship between matter and ether as mediated by the Ojha. The practice of liberating the possessed is beyond positivist examination and its execution is ritualistic alchemy. Healing the possessed is a complex process which interferes with the senses of the possessed and also of the audience of the rituals, who report hearing shrill sounds or experiencing gusts of wind.

Bira is a malevolent spirit that resides in bamboo groves or elephant apple trees. It possesses unlucky travellers. The afflicted usually demonstrates abnormal behaviour, thereby making it necessary for the Ojha to intervene. The possessed person is taken to community ground and tied there, where the expulsion ritual goes on until the afflicted is relieved of the invading spirit. Throughout the entire process, the afflicted begs mercy of the possessing spirit to free it while simultaneously, in another voice through the afflicted, the invading spirit denies those requests. This may appear almost like a dialogue between Doctor Jekyll and Mr. Hyde except the physical attributes of the afflicted person remain unaltered. The Ojha begins the rituals by playing the cymbal and other Indigenous percussion instruments, assisted by two apprentices, the Bej (male) and Beja (female). The village people gather to observe the ritual. Attendance is mandatory, as the ritual performs two organic roles. First, watching the spirit afflicted being tormented by pain is a lesson for other community members not to venture into the forest at inappropriate hours while the fauna rests; and second, the spiritual and medicinal ritual instils in the people a sense of cohesion and of reverence for the forest and the spirits residing in it.

After the initial ceremony, the main ritual begins, in which a pair of pigeons and a cock are sacrificed and offered along with rice beer to the principal forest deity, Longa Deo. Longa Deo, a benevolent spirit, is invoked with ceremonial recitals. The arrival of the benevolent spirit is marked when the primary Healer, Ojha, in whose body the benevolent spirit enters, assumes a trance-like state. What ensues is a battle between the good and the evil, represented by Longa Deo and Bira. After the duel is over, the Bira stands vanquished and recedes to the forest, and the victorious deity is offered tobacco. Then the community joins together in a ritual smoking of marijuana to mark the triumph of benevolent over malevolent spirit and also to celebrate that the afflicted has been relieved of his malady. The afflicted is prescribed specific doses of Sugandh Mantri, pigeon meat, and water from the sacred pond for healing. The formerly possessed person is banned from venturing into the forest for two full moons.

The entire community becomes involved in the act of curing and also in the process of healing. Unlike in modern medicine, where clinics are seen as a safe haven for the diseased, Indigenous healing practice exposes the ailing to the other members of the community, making it a social affair. There is no categorical opposition between the disease-free and the ailing, as both are connected by one process of healing. Another interesting Indigenous perspective regarding health is that being possessed is not merely a state of disease from which one needs to be cured; instead, it is a state in which the possessed individual exhibits human limits to reason by transcending to a metaphysical realm. Thus the possessed person, representing the embodiment of the metaphysical element, provides insights into the world of the spirits during its trances and convulsions. In spite of its malevolent nature, the spirit, speaking through the individual, reveals information about herbs, their locations, and the manner of cure. Thus, possession is not seen as essentially barbaric but instead as an episodic revelation of wisdom.

Sacred Geography and Indigenous Medicine

Forest is sacred geography for the Rabha people, for many reasons. Forest is not merely a place of refuge for ascetics but also a source of medicinal plants [11].

The Rabha tribal community is animistic in faith and worships their sacred groves. Such groves, which are known as *thaan* and are often located around a water body, must have at least five sal (*Shorea robusta*) trees. The community holds the fauna found in the forest in great reverence. The vulture, a critically endangered species in India, thrives in these forests, and the Rabha people offer ritualistic offerings to these birds. In the Loharghat forest range, for instance, vultures are a common sight and protected by the people. The nesting of vultures atop sal trees is considered sacred by the locals, as interaction between the flora and fauna is an indicator of its health. The bird is also the clan totem for Pati Rabhas of Loharghat.

It is believed that the *thaan,* or grove, is a place where the spirit of the great ancestress resides. Annually, *Marei puja*, a ceremony seeking blessing against famine and serpents (personal communication, April 3, 2016), is conducted by clearing the space around the grove for the community gathering. The Ojha makes a ceremonial offering to the deity and the spirit, and it is during this that *Deodhani* dancers perform. It is believed that the recitals made by the Ojha are so powerful that the spirit of the great ancestress emanates out of the groves and possesses young maidens with long hair.

The sacred geography of a grove, beyond its ecological component, comes from its spiritual character, which is connected to the myths and memories of the people. The rich biodiversity of a grove is enhanced by its esoteric dimensions. The shared spiritual connection the people have with the grove socializes them for the preservation, care, and nurture of the forest. The sustainability of the groves depends upon the belief system, which engrains in the community a respect for common property resources. The apprentices of the primary Healer, the Bej and Beja, male and female respectively, perform binding roles. They recite verse in couplets to connect man and nature, and every community ceremony begins in the groves with such recitals. These designated roles help to sustain the people–forest relationship.

The practice of traditional medicine is a hereditary one, in which the Ojha, or Healer, passes the knowledge to selected members of his or her family. The Healer enjoys a special place in the society. The role of the community Healer includes everything from spiritual treatments of hallucination and delirium, to providing birth control and abortions. The traditional knowledge is carefully guarded and methods of preparing special herbal mixtures are not shared. For instance, spiny amaranth (*Amaranthus spinosus*), in its paste form, is used in the hilly jungle tracts as effective birth control.[3] It is also mixed with the juice of the root of *Musa paradisiaca* (a kind of banana) for the purpose of abortion. For cultural reasons, it is the female Beja who administers these kinds of medicine. Although the Ojha does not reveal this traditional knowledge, ethnobotanical researchers have made such information available in the public domain.

Even today, for cultural reasons, many people rely on the Ojha for medicine and the Bej and Bejas to administer it. There are a number of reasons why modern medicine is still only supplementary to ethnomedicine for many of the Rabhas.

First, ethnomedicine is holistic in nature because it caters to regaining health as well as mental well-being. Further, when the community makes use of various aromatic plants, their by-products are segregated judiciously. While some parts of a plant are kept for consumption, the other parts are retained for essential oils. The residue is also used for feeding livestock and other animals. Second, the community is interwoven with the ecosystem. People depend upon the flora and fauna for daily sustenance. The cycle of mutual dependence is complete as people depend on the ecosystem for health and healing. Third, the administering and receiving of medicine does not simply mean the consumption of a particular product but goes far beyond that to include performing and participating in rituals.

The process of identifying and collecting leaves from the trees of the sacred groves is entrusted to a particular group of Rabhas. As noted, occupational classification occurs among the Rabhas, dividing them into various subgroups within the forest economy. These occupational categories are clan endogamous and traits of work are inherited. This system aptly represents their organismic view of society. The Pati Rabhas are designated, according to occupational stratification, to collect the leaves which are offered to the deities and thereafter processed for preparing medicine. In the Rabha language, *patra tang* means "leaf cutter" and it is believed that the name of the subgroup Pati Rabha is derived from it.

However, with present-day acculturation, such etymology is being compromised. This has affected the occupational diversification and also the forest economy. The traditional knowledge possessed by the Pati Rabhas, which guided them to collect the leaves appropriate in age, size, colour, and texture, appears to be in gradual decline. The collection of fruit, flowers, roots, and tubers is also learned through traditional knowledge systems passed on inter-generationally and in oral form. But with the passage of time, this traditional transmission of information is declining.

First, the younger generations are migrating outside the forest economy or taking up other pursuits, thereby reducing the number of individuals actually putting the forest products to medicinal use and increasing the likelihood of such knowledge being lost to future generations.

[3] *Abrus precatorius* and *Ricinus communis* are other ethnomedicines used as birth control.

Second, the nature of the forest itself is transforming with the introduction of commercial cropping, monoculture, by laws enforced by the forest department, and climate change. The Pati Rabhas, who used to provide the raw material to Ojha, Bej, and Beja of the village for preparation in ethnic medicine and ritual offerings, do not consider their traditional occupational classification to be sacrosanct any longer. Today, it is only during religious festivals such as Baikho, when traditional goddesses are honoured, that these occupational classifications are closely followed. Thus, former occupational roles are becoming merely ritualistic.

Third, the symbiosis between the forest and its people is being weakened by globalization. Globalization is a logical consequence of modernity, and the science of medicine is a by-product of modernity, which "knows no borders; its technology transcends territorial boundaries; its politico- cultural aspirations—democratization of society, and the autonomy of the individual—tend to become our shared aspirations" [12]. Among the Rabhas of the Loharghat Reserve Forest, modern medicine has percolated across the valley and the hills. Today, allopathic drugs are supplied free of cost by governmental agencies, and large-scale health camps are organized for treatment and generating awareness. This service, however, has had a mixed impact. The prevalence of infectious diseases, mainly malaria, and other ophthalmologic ailments such as cataract, has declined, but jaundice, in its overwhelming prevalence, has continued unabated.

Regarding jaundice, it is believed that Sheetala Devi, a cold female spirit, enters the body of a living being, thereby turning it yellow. Those afflicted are provided with careful treatment and dietary restrictions such as avoiding meat or fish are recommended. The rationale behind this remedy is that the power equation with the possessing spirit must not be challenged. Dokha khamflai (*Hatsiatum hypericum*) and dudhali bindog (*Argyreia roxburghii arnnott ex choisy*) along with the tuber dibauli bidat (*Stephania glabra miers*) are tied in the form of a garland around the patent's neck for a period of 7 days. Kharo khandai (*Oroxylum indicum*) is mixed with one hen's egg and common salt and then fried and given to the diseased to eat. In addition to these treatments, recitations are made to appease the deity. Although allopathic cures for jaundice are available, for forest folks, these seem to be either inaccessible or unaffordable. Moreover, there is an issue of trust, which places the Indigenous medicinal practices on a higher pedestal in the community's consciousness.

The prevalence of Indigenous medicine is a reality; however, the wide social acceptance of its use encourages one to ask why it is still so favoured. One important component of traditional medicinal system is that its influence expands much beyond treatment. Healing is a cultural act embedded in the community consciousness and influenced by what is available in the environment, the accessibility of Indigenous Knowledge and the carrying out of that knowledge, the social status of the diseased and his or her attitude toward accepting Indigenous or modern medicinal treatment. The socialization of the Rabha community is such that there is an inclination toward internal resources. An outsider bias is also prevalent, because the forest tribe is often looked at differently by the valley people. There is little or no representation of the Rabha people in the modern medical profession. Thus, the gap between the two worlds has not been bridged.

When colonialism beckoned, it offered objectivity and measurement as its greatest weapons. The modern concept of health began to be identified with tangible indicators. But for Indigenous communities, well-being, not health, is the ultimate indicator of prosperity. Well-being is an umbrella term spanning physical, mental, and emotional prosperity. Health is understood in terms of disease, from which one may be cured by undergoing medical treatment. But well-being cannot be measured or achieved. It has to be felt and it is fluid.

An Ojha from Jaramukhuriya hamlet explained well-being in this way: "*Ne-rogi* is a state of diseaselessness but *nirapod* is freedom from harm" (personal communication, April 4, 2016). When the Ojha undertakes mass rituals and ceremonies, he usually asks blessings for to the community to remain *nirapoda*. *Nirapod* is considered to carry greater weight because disease is understood to be something already embedded in the environment and spirits therein. Remaining free from harm entails keeping benevolent and malevolent spirits in check. It is believed that with every breach to the sacred nature of the forest, the chance of well-being for its people is reduced.

Allopathic medicine is seen as value neutral, devoid of environmental and subjective biases. The approach to the provision of such medicine is very impersonal in nature, and generally ends with targeting the disease. The aim of such medicine is to cure the person. But for the Rabha people of Loharghat, a thriving health system is much more than the objective execution of modern medicine.

Moreover, there is a lack of trust among people who see the products of modern medicine as an alien imposition. Especially for the older generation, who regard the cartons of allopathic medicine with suspicion, it is difficult to adjust. Further, emerging with this modernization is a "medical gaze," through which people are seen as healthy or non-healthy. This perception clearly dismisses instances where context-specific issues emerge, such as spirit possession through animistic magico-medicinal rituals. In these situations, the medical gaze is supposed to be empirically verifiable and replicable, a characteristic often missing in traditional healing practices, because such methods can suggest an aggregate of effects which may not be exactly measurable and therefore not considered scientific enough [9].

And finally, traditional healers are disgruntled by the coming of allopathic medicine since it has interfered with their practice and institution. More of the younger members of the community are now consulting government-supplied doctors and visiting Ojhas for secondary cures only. This widespread trend has slowly eroded the traditional authority of Healers, and the knowledge of these Healers is also being affected. It is not uncommon for the Ojhas to be described as "quacks"—a characterization that reflecting their declining legitimacy.

Conclusion

In this chapter, I introduce a number of variable elements within the larger framework of modernity and change, including the forest-dwelling Rabha tribe, the forest as a living entity, and Indigenous medicinal knowledge and practice. I have argued and illustrated that environment-specific belief systems are prevalent, along with cultural manifestations of those systems in the form of social roles performed by the Ojha and Bejas. People are socialized into a particular way of understanding health, not merely as freedom from disease but as all-round well-being. The community and the forest are participants in the process. At the same time, government and commercial interventions are alienating the people from their traditional ways.

In this chapter, I also demonstrate that here are multiple perspectives, beyond the modern medical gaze, from which disease can be understood, just as there are culture-specific modes in which it can be healed. Although some in the dominant culture may reject possession by forest spirit as superstition, for the Rabhas tribe it is a perpetual threat. Unlike medical doctors, the Ojha, or community Healer, is also a priest, thereby providing a link between spirituality and prosperity. One interesting consequence of this environment-centred belief system is the prevalence of community altruism, where other members of the society must participate in the process of well-being for all other members.

I have also touched on the challenges posed to the community by the opening up of the forest economy. There is much to understand about this forest-dwelling community and their system of well-being, which is suffering from an erosion of Indigenous Knowledge, loss of identity, and the devaluing of their roles as guardians of the forest. Thus, an exploration of the traditional healing practices and ethnomedicine used in the Indigenous Rabha community reveals their dependence on the forest ecosystem, and the imperative need for a policy for the protection of the community and the forest in our times.

References

1. Saikia A. Forest and Ecological History of Assam, 1826–2000. New Delhi: Oxford; 2011.
2. Basumatary P. The Rabha Tribe of North East India-Bengal and Bangladesh. New Delhi: Mittal Publication; 2010.
3. Sarkar SR. Jungle Rabha Masks and Mask Dance. New Delhi: GIAN Publishing House; 2015.
4. Redfield R. Peasant society and culture: an anthropological approach to civilization. Chicago: Chicago University Press; 1956.
5. TRI-GOI & UNDP-India. Forest Rights Act 2006—act, rules and guidelines. 2014. Retrieved from tribal.nic.in: https://tribal.nic.in/FRA/data/FRARulesBook.pdf
6. Shrivastav, K.S. Forest Rights Act under scrutiny. 2015. Retrieved 28 October, 2019, from Down To Earth: https://www.downtoearth.org.in/news/forests/forest-rights-act-under-scrutiny-32957.
7. Vannucci M. Ecological reading in the Vedas: Matter Energy, Life (Reconstructing Indian History and Culture). New Delhi: D.K. Print World Ltd.; 1994.

8. Raomai S, Kumaria S, Tandon P. In vitro propagation of Homalomena aromatica Schott., an endangered aromatic medicinal herb of Northeast India. Physiol Mol Biol Plants. 2013;19(2):297–300.
9. Davenport BA. Witnessing and the Medical Gaze: how medical students learn at a free clinics for the homeless. Med Anthropol Q. 2000:310–27.
10. Sarma J. Rabha Folk Tales. New Delhi: Sahitya Akademi; 2017.
11. Tamuli P, Ghosal A. Ethnomedicinal plant used by major ethnic groups of Assam (India) for curing skin disease. Int J Herbal Med. 2017;5(4):140–4.
12. Pathak A. Modernity globalization and identity: towards a reflexive quest. New Delhi: Aakar Books; 2011.

Chinmayi Sarma completed her Ph.D. on Socio-Cultural Context of Earthquake and Indigenous Communities at the Centre for the Study of Social Systems, Jawaharlal Nehru University, New Delhi, India. Presently, she is working as Assistant Professor at the Centre for North East Studies and Policy Research, Jamia Millia Islamia, New Delhi, India. She is keen on Social Anthropology and Ethnography in the Indian context. Her areas of interest include Disaster Studies, Indigenous Knowledge Systems, Ecology and Development Discourses. One of her recently concluded studies includes "Indigenous Women in Assam: Bearing Burden of Nature, Culture and Market" for Heinrich Boll Stiftung, Germany. Another related work is "Indigenous Practices and Sustainability," in the *Indian Journal of Sustainable Development*, (2016).

Learning from Those Who Do: Land-Based Healing in a Mushkegowuk Community

David Danto, Russ Walsh, and Jocelyn Sommerfeld

Within Canada, there are three distinct Indigenous groups: First Nations, Inuit, and Métis [1]. As per a recent federal government survey, "There are more than 630 First Nation communities in Canada, which represent more than 50 Nations and 50 Indigenous languages" ([2], para. 3). Inuit live in 53 communities across four regions of Canada, with each region speaking its own dialect [3], and Métis are spread out across all provinces and territories of the country [4]. Despite this diversity, Indigenous People are often referred to as a single group. However, just as "Caucasians" or "Westerners" do not represent a homogenous group, Indigenous People are also highly diverse.

There are broad experiences that Indigenous People share, including marginalization, displacement, and loss of culture [5]. In fact, Indigenous People have faced persecution and colonization around the globe [6]. Nevertheless, two communities located in geographical proximity will also have distinct experiences—even families in the same community may have unique experiences within the context of their

A previous version of this chapter was published in the International Journal of Mental Health and Addiction, May 2020.
The Authors express their appreciation for the hospitality and participation of the participants and the community in Mushkegowuk Territory. We acknowledge the contributions of the University of Guelph-Humber Psychology Students: Sara Mancuso and Marlena Williams.

D. Danto (✉)
Psychology Department, University of Guelph-Humber, Toronto, ON, Canada
e-mail: David.danto@guelphhumber.ca

R. Walsh
Psychology Department, Duquesne University, Pittsburgh, PA, USA
e-mail: walshr@duq.edu

J. Sommerfeld
Department of Psychology, Trent University, Peterborough, ON, Canada
e-mail: : jocelynsommerfeld@trentu.ca

D. Danto, M. Zangeneh (eds.), *Indigenous Knowledge and Mental Health*,
https://doi.org/10.1007/978-3-030-71346-1_5

community and history. Indigenous People both share experiences and are also distinct in many ways and on many levels [6].

The purpose of this study is to better understand features of healing that are shared across communities, as well as those that are distinct. This is not so that one strategy is held above others, but for the purpose of enriching knowledge transmission to future generations and identifying important practices and traditions for those involved in providing mental health services for Indigenous People.

Research suggests that more traditional, holistic forms of treatment have exhibited positive effects on mental health within Indigenous communities, as more conventional Western approaches do not typically involve the beliefs and practices of many Indigenous People. For example, a significant component of Indigenous well-being comes from a connection to the land [7]. As Wildcat and colleagues [8] discuss, "...if colonization is fundamentally about dispossessing Indigenous peoples from their land, decolonization must involve forms of education that reconnect Indigenous peoples to land and the social relations, knowledges and languages that arise from the land" [Abstract].

These types of programs are aptly named "land-based interventions," and generally involve the teaching of culture, participation in traditional activities, transfer of intergenerational knowledge, and reconnection with the land [9]. For instance, in an effort to address the intergenerational wounds of residential schools, Elders are returning to the land with Indigenous youth in order to "...transmit their culture and knowledge, not only to the generation of their children, but also to that of their grandchildren" ([10], p. 16). At present, there are many such programs being developed in and for Indigenous communities across Canada [7].

The authors have previously conducted studies on land-based interventions with two different communities in northern Ontario [7, 11]. In 2017, Danto and Walsh studied the self-identified strengths of one particular Indigenous community, and found that a sense of connection to the land was a major contributor to maintaining physical, spiritual, mental, and emotional health. Furthermore, the land was implicated in bridging diverse spiritual beliefs among community members and facilitating community cohesion. As such, the authors suggested that connecting with the land should be a central aspect of future mental health interventions. These discoveries prompted a later study which focused on the application of a land-based intervention within a different community, including the program's background, components, advantages, and challenges [7].

In line with similar programs across Canada, renewing connection to the land and traditional culture, fostering intergenerational connection, and developing relationships between participants were cited as key features of this land-based intervention. In order to illuminate the implications of these findings, particularly with regard to the relevance of the land to non-Western approaches to mental health treatment, the current study serves as a follow-up to the authors' 2020 study, with the goal of articulating similarities and differences that may exist in relation to providing land-based interventions within divergent Indigenous communities in Canada.

Method

Introduction to the Method

The purpose of this introduction is to situate the method of the current study within Indigenous methodology, which typically involves the entire community and includes "…peoples' views, feelings, and experiences with nature, culture, and spirit" ([12], p. 3). Indigenous research methods may include: conversation, journaling, research-sharing circles, and storytelling [13]. For instance, stories are "a legitimate tool for relating with others, sharing knowledge across generations, analyzing life circumstances, and seeking solutions for the future" ([14], p. 65). According to Bishop, "…story telling is a useful and culturally appropriate way of representing the 'diversities of truth' within which the story teller rather than the researcher retains control" (as cited in [15], p. 146). In addition, Kovach [13] cites the growing trend of using research-sharing circles as a method of gathering information, which are "…meant to provide space, time, and an environment for participants to share their story in a manner that they can direct" (p. 124). These types of flexible, open-ended methods are more appropriate for use with people who have strong oral traditions and are highly relational in nature, as opposed to more structured research methods (e.g., interviews) [13].

Furthermore, Kovach [13] differentiates between Indigenous and Western forms of data interpretation. More conventional, Western methods involve coding data according to certain themes, and then analyzing these themes in a way that generalizes people's experiences. On the other hand, Indigenous methods involve individual stories, which are condensed and checked by the storyteller, that the researcher reflects upon to find meaning. Therefore, the goal of interpretation is not to "…fragment or decontextualize the knowledge [that stories] hold…" ([13], p. 131).

In terms of the present study, the authors incorporated aspects of both methods. While the typically Western approach of identifying and analyzing certain themes was used, the authors also checked all initial findings with the participants themselves, and revised and elaborated the results in light of these conversations. Ensuring that the community checks and approves of all interpretations is necessary to ensure participants are accurately represented, especially "…because of the misrepresentation of Indigenous cultures and communities within research…" ([13], p. 100). In so far as this method integrates Indigenous and Western approaches, it may be identified as a two-eyed seeing approach. According to Mi'kmaw Elder Albert Marshall, two-eyed seeing acknowledges the strengths of both Indigenous and Western knowledges and involves learning to use both together (as cited in [16]). The goal of this approach is "…to bridge the divide of power and understanding between Indigenous and Western researchers and processes" ([17], p. 5), and as such constitutes an important part of decolonizing methodology [12].

Historically, Indigenous communities have had to endure research conducted by "people who have had limited knowledge about Indigenous peoples, worldviews, or communities" ([18], p. 1). As a result of these experiences, several protocols have been put in place to aid Indigenous People in having greater control over their own information. For instance, The First Nations Principles of OCAP (Ownership, Control, Access, and Possession) are "a set of principles that reflect First Nation commitments to use and share information in a way that brings benefit to the community while minimizing harm" ([19], p. 4–5). These principles assert that First Nations communities have collective ownership of their knowledge, control over how this information is managed, easy access to data concerning themselves, and the ability to physically control this information [19].

In addition, Chapter 9 of the Tri-Council Policy Statement on Ethical Conduct for Research Involving Humans [20] presents ethical guidelines for research with First Nations, Inuit, and Métis peoples in Canada. For example, researchers should identify and respect Indigenous customs and practices, ensure the research addresses relevant community needs and produces valuable results, include Elders and other knowledge keepers in the design and implementation of research projects, involve the community in reviewing and interpreting data, and respect the community's privacy and confidentiality [20].

In carrying out research with Indigenous populations, it is important to keep in mind for whose sake the research is conducted. As stated previously, research has often benefitted the investigators themselves rather than the community, leading "...Indigenous peoples [to] continue to regard research, particularly research originating outside their communities, with a certain apprehension or mistrust" ([20], p. 107). Consequently, researchers need to ensure that information gained from research with Indigenous People should be useful to and easily accessible by community members. After all, according to Graham Smith, "At the end of the day it belongs to the community..." (as cited in [13], p. 149). This goal of ensuring "...that traditional indigenous knowledge...remains connected intimately to indigenous people..." ([15], p. 226) is at the heart of decolonizing research. The present study is a two-eyed approach incorporating Indigenous research methodology, though "...some have used the term 'Indigenous science' to capture the rigorous aspect of this knowledge" ([21], p. 14).

Procedures

The authors invited the three participants, all known to each other within the same community, to take part in a conversation regarding the land-based intervention with which they are involved. In attendance was the first author (facilitator) and two research assistants. Following a territorial acknowledgment and opening words, an overview of the meeting was provided by the facilitator. Following this introduction, the facilitator posed three open-ended questions for conversation:

1. What are the key components of land-based interventions?
2. What are the challenges in offering land-based interventions?

3. What are the main steps in transferring knowledge about land-based interventions?

The facilitator posed brief follow-up questions (e.g., "Can you tell me more about that?"), and the conversation was audio recorded. The resulting conversation lasted approximately 2 h. Following this meeting, the research assistants transcribed the audio recording and the transcriptions were analyzed qualitatively in order to find apparent themes within the conversation.

Transcribed interviews were subjected to the following stages of qualitative analysis: The second author, an expert in hermeneutic research, highlighted keywords and phrases pertaining to the following categories: (1) referents to key components of land-based interventions, (2) referents to challenges in offering land-based interventions, (3) referents to the transfer of knowledge regarding land-based interventions. These initial categorized data were then reviewed by the first author, and refinements were made until consensus was obtained. Once a list of common themes was articulated, participants were invited back for a second meeting.

The categorized data were brought back to the participants and reviewed for inconsistencies, omissions, or alternative interpretations, and were then edited in light of participants' elaborations. At this second meeting, participants were presented with the themes and asked: "In trying to understand what was said at our last meeting, we have come up with the following list of themes. Please let me know if you have anything to add, or if we have misunderstood anything." At this meeting, participants verified, adjusted, and expanded upon themes. These additional comments were recorded and once again transcribed in order to further clarify the list of themes.

Results

Our two-stage process of interviews and analyses yielded the following broad themes:

1. Land-based work aims to heal disconnections from: language (a gap between the youth and traditional ways), culture (specific skills, practices, and a sense of history), spirituality (a sense of connection with the land and the Creator), and Elders (wise and knowledgeable, often older members of the community). It seeks to foster connections to the land, to the Elders and the community, and to a fuller sense of self (understood as four dimensions: spirit, mind, emotions, and body). Land-based practices include working together (and sharing while doing so), talking circles, teaching and talking, and learning traditional skills and songs.
2. The challenges of doing land-based interventions include costs and funding, liability concerns and restrictions, the language gap between youth and Elders, and the need for collaboration between natural healers and mental health/addiction professionals.

3. Transferring knowledge about land-based interventions, or "training the trainers," requires training by demonstration and working together, as well as fostering leadership skills to bridge the gap between young people and Elders.

In the following paragraphs, we will elaborate these categories.

What Are the Key Features of Land-Based Work?

Participants described how land-based work helps to bridge the "gap between youth and the Elders" by inviting them to "reconnect to their language to communicate … effectively with the Elders." The gap is evident in the young people's lack of familiarity with traditional language, through which the Elders' teachings are typically communicated. Because this "old language" is "very descriptive" and "pertains to nature," engagement with nature facilitates learning:

"our language is more nature. Like those Elders that told you, if you wanna learn your language go back to the land. If you wanna learn, same thing with your culture. Go back to the land. That's where you feel more connected, more comfortable. 'Cause it talks your language. It speaks your culture."

Traditional land-based practices, such as gathering around a fire, also facilitate connection and openness:

"we take our young ones (onto the land) and they're more open, for some reason they start to open up. Ready to talk, they start to talk. They start to open up a little about their troubles and their dreams"

> "First, physically, how to make that fire. How to fashion tools… And then they will start to open up and then that's where that conversation comes. When you work with those kids they start open up to you and trust you."

> "we sat the kids out in a teepee. And something about that fire brought them in there and it made it easier for them to open up. And in a teepee, you're almost like inclined to sit in a circle. It's so important to sit in a circle. In a circle there's nobody in front of you, you know, you sit beside each other. And it's symbolic at that. You know, so we believe in the Creator being in a circle, it's a whole."

> "So that's what that fire does. It makes us open up and warm up to each other. And there's always a connection with nature with us because we come from nature, we were made from nature."

Learning the skills for living in nature (hunting, chopping wood, building shelter, and a fire) help to connect young people to traditional ways and their historical and cultural connection to the land. This also allows for the teaching of moral lessons based in nature:

> "there's teachings to fire too. It can either save you, or it can kill you. There's two sides to it, you know. And you can never make the same fire no matter how many times you try. It's unique."

> "There was a story of a young hunter killing more than what he needed... And it finally came where the moose was scarce... So one of the Elders was a Shaman. So the Shaman went into a ceremony and they contacted the moose spirit. Said, 'moose how come you're not coming around our area anymore? We're going hungry here, we can't find you'. The moose spirit told him, 'well my bones are scattered all over, you're disrespecting me. You're not taking care of me'.

> "You know but all those things that were done, there was always teachings to them. You know you gotta be patient. Patience was really important. You know when you go hunting you gotta be patient when you fish you gotta be patient. You gotta sit there. You know when you go goose hunting you gotta sit in the blind all day. But they don't fly you gotta be patient. You know and patience it sometimes really teaches you to pray."

This connection to the land and traditional practices also affirms Indigenous spirituality and identity, both individual and communal:

> "Cause our culture is based on the land, on nature. It kinda makes it easier for us to connect to each other. It kinda brings the spirit back. It kinda makes the emotions good emotions. Back to us and were able to feel gonna use the land or take those kids out, teach them."

> "if you take care of the land, and respect the land, the land will take care of you. This is where you came from, this is where, you know, that part of you is connected to. And I remember my grandmother teaching us this as little kids, she used to say and used to tell us stories how this survived on the land. And she always knew, and you get this when you go out, when you see the sunset or when you see the sunrise, God is there. You just know, you just know that the great spirit is there. The one that watches over everything. He's there. You feel it, you just know it. And you see that."

"People that lived on the land, they prayed a lot...because they knew who was watching them, they knew who was taking care of them. They knew who was - who to rely to. So this is where spirituality came in. Knowing that you have that being that watches over you, you know. You rely on the sun, you rely on the wind, you rely on the rain."

Land-based practices include working together (and sharing while doing so), teepee circles as well as teaching and talking lodges (which foster connection and closeness), and learning traditional skills and songs. They also allow for the release of emotions:

> "When you go in a teaching lodge they would sing those teaching songs that explains how we came to be... There's a talking lodge, so people would discuss their problems there. I guess for us to know people like us, like myself, need those things. We need our talking lodge, our teaching lodge... so we can reconnect and be whole again."

> "when you're in the land you can shout and cry all you want without being judged for nobody. Get your emotions out."

Land-based interventions aim to foster connections to nature, via the experiences of (a) observing and learning the wisdom of nature and what it can teach (e.g., how animals care for their little ones; the uniqueness of each fire); (b) being part of nature (rather than being cut off from it, for example through reliance on technology); and (c) recognizing one's reciprocal relationship with nature (and interdependence). Connections to the Elders and the community are also sought via (a) recognizing the importance of relationships and extended family; and (b) learning traditional language and culture through shared activities. Connection to spirituality is also a goal, in that (a) the Indigenous creation story underscores being of the land; (b) connection to the land is a means of connection to the Creator; (c) the beauty of nature shows that "we are taken care of"; and (d) patience in nature is a form of prayer. Lastly, land-based work aims to foster a fuller connection to oneself, through (a) allowing the expression, sharing and letting go of difficult emotions; (b) allowing for patience and stillness; and (c) emphasizing the four dimensions of being: spirit, mind, emotions, and body:

> "to describe a person, we say "Inninu". They interpret it as "people" but it really means a four dimensional being - I don't know how you say that in English - 'cause this person that has four areas to his life. He has a spirit, a mind, emotions and body… and this person has to work to balance those things in his life."

What Are the Challenges of Doing Land-Based Work?

The challenges of doing land-based interventions include costs and funding, liability concerns and limitations, the language gap between youth and Elders, and the need for collaboration between natural healers and mental health/addiction professionals. The costs of land-based programs include transportation, equipment, and accommodations as well as those needed to bring in "holders of knowledge" to facilitate teaching lodges.

> "You know we have some natural healers up here. We have some natural counsellors that know how to connect with people. How to bring out the best in people. We have those, but cost of living is also a challenge up here… you know, to buy what we need. Cause it limits you, the length of time you want to stay out on the land."

> "We need those people to teach us, about whatever we need to learn. Ceremonies, songs and everything… and then they can pass it on to us or they can pass in on to their people, and then pass it on to their next generation."

> "We need money to bring those people that have- those teachings. To re-introduce those things we forgot. It takes money to bring them. To, relearn those things."

Regarding liability concerns, facilitators of land-based programs must grapple with restrictions that they feel are imposed on them:

> "…like policies, the western policies, the liability. We never used to have that. We just take the kids out on the land, you know and didn't have to write down, waivers… so this new way of things now are kinda like challenging us with taking youth out on the land. 'Oh make sure you sign a waiver okay?'. You know, it's kinda- I understand why but it kinda just sometimes you know, kinda holds you back of doing. You gotta follow the policy. But where did the policy come from? It came from outside, but we have to follow it."

The language gap between youth and Elders, while to some degree ameliorated through the shared activities of land-based work, remains a challenge for both for communicating the wisdom of Elders and collaborating on land-based activities:

> "Language, I find it becomes a burden for some Elders that created frustration- they think kids don't listen to them. When they speak to them in their language, and they get frustrated. This kid doesn't listen to me.... but the others were persistent. They kept gathering kids at bedtime. They say, you have to listen, you know, and they start explaining the words to them."

> "And just simple things like cast the boat away from shore in Cree..., we say it "ni mi ta bwah, ni mi ta bwah". They're looking at me like they didn't know. So it was that language barrier like with our youth you know so when you're in the rapids, when you're trying to navigate, your boat through the rapids... it becomes a safety issue."

The need for collaboration between mental health professionals and land-based healers is also important, as individuals actively abusing substances are not good candidates for land-based activities:

> "This young man was out in the bush once and... withdrawal symptoms kicked in... he ran away into the bush. Search team were looking for him, and they couldn't find him... so this is why he's saying we need professionals to make that assertion if this guy is still struggling with post-acute withdrawal symptoms. Or has an active addiction. That it's dangerous for them to be on the land... without the necessary supports."

> "There's a safety concern there. When people have withdrawals they might turn on you and hurt you. There's gotta be some kind of steps to bringing people. Maybe send them out. Maybe to like a detox and then the lodges, healing lodges, and then they get to further their healing... so that's why we need professionals like you to work to work together with the natural healers"

How Do You Transfer the Knowledge of Doing Land-Based Work to Others?

Transferring knowledge about land-based interventions, or "training the trainers," requires training by demonstration and working together, as well as fostering leadership skills to bridge the gap between young people and Elders.

> "So you work along and train... people. Teach people how to lead. How to work with other people that need help. What was it? Yeah pretty much like I said, people know how to go about- to live off the land. They know. But they have to learn, the other thing you have to learn is how to work with people with addictions."

> "Yeah teach them leadership skills, the one's they're gonna train to take over. How to handle, how to socialize with the young people... not only do you have to let em learn what you have learned, but you also gotta learn their habit, learn their new language, their new way of connecting."

Participants also discussed the potential benefits and pitfalls of having facilitators with prior histories of substance abuse, and together suggested that perhaps the ideal composition of group leaders would include individuals who have overcome substance use problems and others with some degree of training in the area of mental health.

Discussion

In Mushkegowuk Territory, along the James and Hudson Bay Coast of northern Ontario, lies a small number of communities with many cultural bonds and similarities that have shared the trauma of colonization. Each community is also unique and has developed its own identity in many ways. Unfortunately, each community also struggles with its own challenges, and sadly, regardless of the community in the region, the topics of suicide and substance abuse are never irrelevant or distant. In this specific community, as in others in the region, a number of "natural helpers" have responded to the needs, primarily of the youth, in the community by stepping forward and offering their own cultural knowledge and skills. They invite those community members who are considered at-risk to both study the sources of strength of their people and develop those same strengths within themselves. Those who take youth out on the land demonstrate great knowledge and skill, but also resilience as they cope with inadequate government support and a variety of hurdles as they continue to offer this crucial service.

Challenges include: the cost of fuel, groceries and transportation, insurance policies that are ill-equipped to meet the cultural needs of land-based programming, working with addicted youth who may be at-risk on the land without additional professional supports, and language gaps between youth and Elders. This language gap, which is in some ways a challenge, is also one of the rifts that these interventions can mend; among the group that we interviewed, this was one of the key features of the program. Much of the culture that has been lost by youth can be captured in the language, and familiarizing youth with their language not only connects them to their history and identity but also concretely teaches them about their relation to the land, as much of the terminology is descriptive and functional. If one attains Cree language, then one will better understand one's place in creation.

Generally, from our meetings we learned that land-based approaches heal disconnections, including those from one's history, the land, tradition, culture, spirituality, family, and community, including Elders. This healing is fostered by lessons that are learned from nature and experiencing oneself as part of nature. Learning language from Elders fosters a recognition of the broader familial bonds beyond one's nuclear family and a care and respect for surrounding community members, as well as humility among participants who learn to see the familiar through the "new" lens of traditional knowledge. This knowledge, however, is not foreign, and therefore can strengthen one's sense of identity, agency, meaning, and purpose.

A theme that arose repeatedly was the value placed on practical experience—physically being out on the land, building a fire, sharing stories, and engaging with nature, for example. Importantly, the transfer of knowledge is experiential. Great value is placed on lived experience, so that Elders or knowledge keepers, those who spend large amounts of time in the bush, those who have histories of addiction, and even potentially those who have training and experience in mental health, share their time, experience, and knowledge with youth or those who are struggling at present. Those who work through their struggles and gain knowledge through this experience may become the helpers, leaders, and Elders of the future.

Consistent with our prior research in the region are the larger themes, such as the broad significance of the role of nature, the value of culture and language, the role of Elders, the need for care and shared responsibility for a community and its members, as well as the importance of traditional knowledge and the risks associated with its loss. Specifically, there were some similarities that arose between the land-based intervention in this study and the one from the authors' previous study [7]. For example, both programs included the transfer of traditional skills and knowledge related to living on the land (e.g., hunting and camping), largely taught through demonstration and collaborative work, which enhanced participants' sense of identity. Another important goal for each program was to bring together youth and Elders in the community, thereby fostering a sense of intergenerational connection. Participants in both programs were also given the opportunity to work together through shared activities, which helped facilitate relationships not only between each other, but with family, the wider community, and the land as well.

On the other hand, a few differences were found between these two land-based programs. For instance, the level of Elders' involvement was described differently: whereas participants in the prior study emphasized the importance of the mere presence of Elders for land-based interventions [7], the present participants emphasized the role of Elders in teaching traditional language to the youth through engagement in land-based activities. The present participants also emphasized moral lessons that can be learned through engagement with nature. For example, a participant spoke of there being two sides to every fire: it can both give life and take it away. Also, being wasteful and taking more than is needed was described as being disrespectful to nature and having negative consequences (e.g., scarcity of food). Finally, a reported focus of the present program involved enhancing participants' sense of spirituality and facilitating a deeper connection to the Creator through prayer and respect of the land.

Of course, in each community distinctive narratives arise in relation to unique histories of oppression and resilience, specific knowledges about nature and medicines, knowledge of the land specific to the region, and traditions, beliefs, and customs that are local. Similarly, the Cree language itself has broad features that allow members from one community to communicate with members from other nearby communities, yet there is also significant diversity between the five dialects of the language [22].

Whether described as the four dimensions [23], the medicine wheel [24], or the biopsychosocial model [25], for example, healing is often described as requiring a holistic approach. According to many participants, what amounts to a two-eyed seeing approach can be a useful perspective in efforts to heal the whole person. The authors encourage Western funding agencies and organizations including provincial, territorial, and federal bodies to meet the broader needs of these grassroots efforts. Community members who help local people by taking them out on the land are often minimally funded and may have difficulty accessing practical financial support for their operations. These individuals, therefore, often volunteer their own time and resources to address crises in their own communities, such as high rates of suicide and substance abuse. As pillars of strength within their communities, they may potentially lack social and emotional supports such as peer counseling and debriefing services.

Further effort is needed to train Western-educated mental health professionals in Indigenous cultural literacy and build links whereby mental health staff can be of greater support to natural helpers in the community. Appropriately trained mental health professionals may facilitate community-led initiatives to better support the work being done, including, for example, assisting in detox programming and stabilizing individuals at high risk of suicide or acute withdrawal so that they can safely participate in healing on the land. For example, as noted in the Canadian Psychological Association and Psychology Foundation of Canada's Response to the Truth and Reconciliation Commission of Canada Report [21]:

> By working with and within communities, psychologists should discover how Indigenous Peoples in a particular place have addressed their needs and how they were able to use their traditional knowledge to deal with hardships for generations. As such, mental health programs should be strength-based, in that they acknowledge the identity and culture of that Indigenous group and recognize the pre-existing values, traditions, and resources that contributed to and supported the strength and resilience of that community for many generations. Psychologists who have a role in the development of programs should make them explicitly for specific Indigenous communities. Psychologists may then take on the role of facilitating Indigenous visions of programs for a current situation or challenge. (p. 29)

Ultimately, an important aspect of healing common across a number of Cree communities in northern Ontario involves providing land-based programming. While the specific content and form of the program will certainly vary, a number of challenges are shared. Western trained health professions as well as funding agencies and government bodies may have important roles to play in the facilitation of these approaches that are intrinsic to a particular community and manifest a specific Indigenous identity and locally grounded resilience.

References

1. Government of Canada. Indigenous peoples and communities. 2017b. https://www.rcaanc-cirnac.gc.ca/eng/1100100013785/1529102490303
2. Government of Canada. First Nations. 2017a. https://www.rcaanc-cirnac.gc.ca/eng/1100100013791/1535470872302

3. Government of Canada. Inuit. 2019. https://www.rcaanc-cirnac.gc.ca/eng/1100100014187/1534785248701
4. Government of Canada. Métis. 2017c. https://www.rcaanc-cirnac.gc.ca/eng/1100100014427/1535467913043
5. George J, MacLeod M, Graham K, Plain S, Bernards S, Wells S. Use of traditional healing practices in two Ontario First Nations. J Community Health. 2018;43:227–37.
6. Browne AJ, Varcoe C, Lavoie J, Smye V, Wong ST, Krause M, Tu D, Khan K, Fridkin A. Enhancing health care equity with Indigenous populations: evidence-based strategies from an ethnographic study. BMC Health Serv Res. 2016;16:544. https://doi.org/10.1186/s12913-016-1707-9.
7. Walsh R, Danto D, Sommerfeld J. Land-based intervention: a qualitative study of the knowledge and practices associated with one approach to mental health in a Cree community. Int J Mental Health Addict. 2020;18(1):207–21.
8. Wildcat, M., McDonald, M., Irlbacher-Fox, S., & Coulthard, G. (2014). Learning from the land: Indigenous land based pedagogy and decolonization. Decolonization: Indigeneity, Education & Society, 3(3), I–XV.
9. Sommerfeld J, Danto D, Walsh R. Indigenous land-based interventions and nature-oriented wellness programs: commonalities and important differences. J Concurrent Disorders. 2019;1(3):37–5.
10. Roué, M. (2006). Healing the wounds of school by returning to the land: Cree elders come to the rescue of a lost generation. International Social Science Journal 58(187), 15–24.
11. Danto D, Walsh R. Mental health perceptions and practices of a Cree community in northern Ontario: a qualitative study. Int J Ment Heal Addict. 2017;15(4):725–37.
12. Marsh TN, Cote-Meek S, Toulouse P, Najavits LM, Young NL. The application of two-eyed seeing decolonizing methodology in qualitative and quantitative research for the treatment of intergenerational trauma and substance use disorders. Int J Qual Methods. 2015;14(5):1–13.
13. Kovach M. Indigenous methodologies: characters, conversations, and contexts. University of Toronto Press; 2009.
14. Minthorn RS, Shotton HJ. Reclaiming Indigenous research in higher education. Rutgers University Press; 2018.
15. Smith LT. Decolonizing methodologies. 2nd ed. Zed Books Ltd.; 2012.
16. Bartlett C, Marshall M, Marshall A. Two-eyed seeing and other lessons learned within a co-learning journey of bringing together Indigenous and mainstream knowledges and ways of knowing. J Environ Stud Sci. 2012;2:331–40. https://doi.org/10.1007/s13412-012-0086-8.
17. Hall L, Dell CA, Fornssler B, Hopkins C, Mushquash C, Rowan M. Research as cultural renewal: applying two-eyed seeing in a research project about cultural interventions in First Nations addictions treatment. Int Indig Policy J. 2015;6(2):1–15.
18. Peltier C. An application of two-eyed seeing: Indigenous research methods with participatory action research. Int J Qual Methods. 2018;17:1–12.
19. The First Nations Information Governance Sector. Ownership, Control, Access and Possession (OCAP™): the path to First Nations information governance. 2014. https://fnigc.ca/sites/default/files/docs/ocap_path_to_fn_information_governance_en_final.pdf
20. Canadian Institutes of Health Research, Natural Sciences and Engineering Research Council of Canada, & Social Sciences and Humanities Research Council. Tri-Council Policy Statement: Ethical Conduct for Research Involving Humans. 2018. https://ethics.gc.ca/eng/policy-politique_tcps2-eptc2_2018.html
21. Canadian Psychological Association & The Psychology Foundation of Canada. Psychology's response to the Truth and Reconciliation Commission of Canada's Report. 2018. https://cpa.ca/docs/File/Task_Forces/TRC%20Task%20Force%20Report_FINAL.pdf
22. Alberta Education. Cree language and culture: 12-year program guide to implementation. 2009. https://education.alberta.ca/media/563938/cree-12y-guide-to-implementation-k-3.pdf
23. Reading, C., Wien, F. Health inequalities and the social determinants of Aboriginal peoples' health. National Collaborating Centre for Indigenous Health; 2013. https://www.nccih.

ca/495/Health_inequalities_and_the_social_determinants_of_Aboriginal_peoples__health_.nccih?id=46
24. Verwoord R, Mitchell A, Machado J. Supporting Indigenous students through a culturally relevant assessment model based on the medicine wheel. Can J Nativ Educ. 2011;34(1):49–66.
25. Lehman BJ, David DM, Gruber JA. Rethinking the biopsychosocial model of health: understanding health as a dynamic system. Soc Personal Psychol Compass. 2017;11(8):e12328.

David Danto is a clinical psychologist, registered in Ontario, Canada. He is the Head of Psychology at the University of Guelph-Humber. Dr. Danto serves on the Board of Directors of the Canadian Psychological Association (CPA), is Board Liaison to the CPA Committee on Ethics, and is a Trustee for the Psychology Foundation of Canada (PFC). He recently chaired the CPA and PFC Task Force on Responding to the Truth and Reconciliation Commission Report, and he currently Chairs the CPA Standing Committee on Reconciliation. Dr. Danto has worked in psychiatric hospitals, university counseling centers, private practice, and correctional facilities in Canada and the United States. In partnership with Indigenous Knowledge Keepers, Dr. Danto developed a field course on Indigenous Mental Health, which he has delivered in Mushkegowuk Territory along the James and Hudson Bay coast for the last 9 years. Dr. Danto researches the role of the land in healing the impacts of colonialism and trauma within Indigenous communities.

Russ Walsh is an Associate Professor at Duquesne University, where he has at various points served as department chairperson, director of clinical training, and psychology clinic director. His scholarship has focused on qualitative research methodology, and he has conducted and supervised hermeneutic and phenomenological research for over 25 years. He is also a licensed clinical psychologist.

Jocelyn Sommerfeld is pursuing a Master's of Psychology at Trent University, with an interest in the connections between nature and health. She has an Honors Bachelor of Applied Science in Psychology from the University of Guelph-Humber, where she received numerous recognitions for academic excellence. Jocelyn is also a member of the Canadian Psychological Association.

Part III
Culture, Identity and Resilience

Mental Health and the San of Southern Africa

Christopher Low and Joram |Useb

This chapter brings together Joram |Useb, a Hai||om San, or Bushmen,[1] Elders from Namibia, with Chris Low, a physician and anthropologist who has worked on health and healing among southern African San for more than 19 years. Having worked as a long-term employee and subsequent director of the leading San advocacy organization, Working Group of Indigenous Minorities in Southern Africa (WIMSA), Joram provides this review with exceptional insight into day-to-day life of many San communities and of wider government and non-governmental organization health initiatives.

Our analysis is a broad account of San mental health which identifies problems and response strategies from beyond and within San communities. Our findings are based on the limited government and academic research that has been undertaken, our mutual insights, and a series of recent informal conversations initiated by us with a range of diverse San. The lack of research data available for this review reflects a longstanding neglect of mental health issues and, even more so, San mental health issues, within overstretched southern African government health services.

It is unfortunate that we have not been able to draw directly on San health workers for our data, but this brings us to a more fundamental reality about San lack of access to and success in education. It is only in very recent times that San have been

[1] The names "San" and "Bushmen" refer to the same people. Bushmen is the older, colonial name. Both names are potentially problematic but continue to be used. Different individuals or groups often prefer one name over the other. Each group will also have their own name for themselves, and these endonyms are always preferred.

C. Low (✉)
!Khwa ttu San Heritage Centre, Research Affiliate, Pitt Rivers Museum, University of Oxford, London, UK
e-mail: Chris@thinkingthreads.com

J. |Useb
!Khwa ttu San Heritage Centre, Grootwater Farm, Yzerfontein, South Africa
e-mail: development@khwattu.org

D. Danto, M. Zangeneh (eds.), *Indigenous Knowledge and Mental Health*,
https://doi.org/10.1007/978-3-030-71346-1_6

able to engage with higher education and had access to skilled jobs. Currently, there are no more than a handful of San with research and health-related qualifications although the situation is improving as governments increasingly recognize and respond to issues of San marginalization, dependency, and disenfranchisement.

It is significant to San mental health that discrimination has characterized the colonial life of all Africans, but many San feel particularly let down by the failed promises and lack of development of their respective African governments. A 2014 report on Namibian San observed that many southern Africans face significant challenges, ranging from high unemployment, dependency, poverty, food insecurity, and political alienation to low levels of education and lack of access to secure land, resources, and services—with associated alcohol abuse, violence, and social conflict. What is, however, exceptional is that, unlike other African groups, these challenges are faced by virtually all San regardless of where they live in southern Africa ([1], pp. xiii–xv).

Our theoretical approach for this study is underpinned by research conclusions from different Indigenous and non-Indigenous mental health contexts. A foundation to our approach is well represented by the medical philosopher Seedhouse. In pursuit of better psychiatric treatment, Seedhouse [2] emphasized a need to move away from conventional Western medical notions that brain dysfunction is the primary key to mental health. In ways pertinent to San, Seedhouse recognized that Indigenous Peoples are often in a better starting position to address mental illness because they do not associate problems of thoughts just with the brain but also with the body. This holds true for the San, among whom it is impossible to understand many mental health problems without understanding San ontology, or the nature of being, and consequently how feelings and internal voices may enter, sit within, or leave a person. Many San treatments for mental health problems work simultaneously at a community level and on an individual's body and mind.

A second relevant observation from Seedhouse is his belief that psychiatrists should place mental health more firmly within personal and group experience and social and historical context ([2], pp. 55–56). This latter point lies, of course, at the hub of Indigenous mental health concerns—what is it in Indigenous experiences and worldviews that relates to manifestations of mental health problems, or how are mental health issues different among Indigenous Peoples and how does this relate to their particular historical experiences? For the San, like the vast majority of Indigenous Peoples, a key to addressing their mental health issues lies in better understanding of their particular worldviews and their particular experiences, which are shaped profoundly by colonialism.

Seedhouse's observations alert us to the mismatch between Western ideas and experiences and Indigenous ideas and experiences. This is a situation well recognized in Indigenous mental health literature. In a report on how to support mental health among Aboriginal and Torres Strait Islanders, for instance, the authors stressed that implementing effective treatment strategies requires recognizing that "social and emotional wellbeing" has a much broader scope in their Indigenous context than it does in Western contexts [3]. For Australian Aboriginals and Torres Strait Islanders, just like the San, social and emotional well-being encompasses "the importance of connection to land, culture, spirituality, ancestry, family and community" (2014, p. 4). This mismatch presents us with the challenge of choosing what to discuss—which Indigenous concepts and practices fit within the Western mental health category.

But the problem does not rest simply with a mismatch of ideas. To really understand San mental health requires grappling with a more fundamental problem—the root terms of this discussion come from a very un-San position. As Joram observed, the Western idea of mental health casts a net over a diverse range of San behaviours, illness categories, and treatment strategies, including some phenomena which are neither clearly recognized nor talked about. In the process of trying to pin down San ways of understanding mental health, we risk misrepresenting the reality that San ideas and responses come from a different orientation to the world and are characteristically flexible and inchoate ([4], p. 216) and not a good fit with Western categories or analysis. In a small way, what we are really recognizing here is something of the existential crisis post-colonial Africans have to negotiate every day, as a "new" world unravels in which ideas and practices Africans know as traditional smack head on into Western medical "realities" and social and economic structures. We will meet a concrete example of this when we consider census questions in a Namibian mental health survey report.

Given the importance of the colonial legacy to understanding San mental health, we open our discussion with a brief background to San history including a summary of who the San are today. This we follow with a baseline review of government health concerns, leading into San perspectives on mental health. Having identified what San recognize as problems among themselves, we are then in a position to discuss San strategies of treatment both traditional and emerging.

Background

An estimated 130,000 San live in southern Africa, of whom 34,000 live in Namibia and 48,000 in Botswana ([5], p. 4). Small San populations of a few thousand each live in South Africa, Zimbabwe, Angola, and Zambia. Currently between 300 and 600 San are thought to live predominantly by hunting and gathering (Hitchcock, personal communication, n.d.). Most San now pursue mixed economic strategies including manual labour, working with tourists, craft making, and subsistence farming. Despite their move away from traditional hunter-gatherer life, many San continue to live in deeply rural areas, on the very margins of society, with poor access to resources and opportunities. In these contexts, hunting and gathering persists to supplement both foods and medicines.

Like many other Indigenous People, San names for themselves reveal a traditional orientation that roots them in their home regions and in relationship to others. San endonyms reveal either a belonging to place, such as Gllanakhwe, sip well people, or, by referring to themselves as "people" (Khwe, Jul'hoansi) or a person

(!Xun), the uniqueness each community feels, the importance of knowing who they are, and the importance of ideas of relationship.

San leaders frequently encourage San to recognize themselves as Indigenous People and First People. They do so both for political reasons and because the status sits well with their traditional origins stories and academic accounts of the past.

In other post-colonial contexts, it is often relatively unproblematic to self-identity as a First Person because clear distinctions exist between people who inhabited particular regions and people who then came into those regions, the latter typically being colonial immigrants. In Africa, however, the situation is more complex because African governments consider all Africans to be Indigenous and they are reluctant to recognize San ancestors as the original inhabitants of lands that they, as other Africans, have historically moved into and dominated. Not all San leaders promote the First People status perspective, but many do, as they fight for land rights, land redistribution, benefit sharing, and development. "We San are Africa's First People" has become a powerful message across many communities. Regardless of the legitimacy of this claim, the politicizing of identity within San communities that are challenged by limited natural resources and high unemployment often has the unfortunate effect of pitting community members against one another, as people strategically pursue the opportunities they perceive.

The second way in which San are First People comes out of academic research that links the San to the origins of modern humans and historically locates them in southern Africa before other African groups. Because of the complex effects it has at a community level, it is valuable to briefly sketch this background. At its most extreme, this thinking buttresses certain radical "Khoisan" groups' political claims of indigeneity and land rights. More broadly, it adds to the complication San experience as they negotiate their identity in a fast-changing world.

Western scholars have linked the San to accounts of human origins since early colonial times. In recent decades, new research has emerged that rekindles old links but does so in new ways, based principally on new findings in archaeology and genetics. One particularly influential example of how the San fit into these human origins accounts lies in the work of the archaeologist Curtis Marean. Marean proposed that early modern humans emerged across Africa before 195,000 years ago, but between 195,000 and 123,000 years ago a challenging glacial period brought a radical reduction in human population numbers. Marean suggested that during this time and over proceeding years the southern African coastal region provided a refuge where people could thrive while others populations succumbed to the harsh environment [6]. The argument then runs that as environmental conditions later improved and populations recovered, some people left southern Africa to populate the rest of the world and some remained. Those who remained are the ancestors of the San.

Archaeologists analyzing evidence from Border Cave, South Africa, trace San culture as far back as 44,000 years [7]. But evidence from other South African archaeological sites, particularly including Pinnacle Point and Klasies River, reveals that the geographical ancestors of the San lived persistently in South Africa since around 164,000 years ago [8, 9]. This means that the San have an exceptionally long ancestral connection to their land.

Around 2000 years ago, African herders moved into the regions of the San and merged with many San groups, bringing a new herding dimension to San hunting and gathering ways of life. The mixed groups that emerged became known as Khoekhoen [10]. The term Khoisan (Khoe-San) is sometimes used as a way of referring to San. The term is an amalgamation of the two names, Khoekhoen and San. It was originally introduced by scholars in the early 1900s to refer to people who looked the same to Europeans. Over time the phrase has become popular as a way of referring to the "click-speaking" peoples of southern Africa whose histories have been intertwined for so long. Many San, however, are keen not to be referred to as Khoisan.

Bantu-speaking Black farmers moved into landscapes inhabited by San and Khoekhoen between around 1800 years and only a few hundred years ago or less [11, 12]. Europeans began to arrive and settle in significant numbers after the establishment of Cape Town as a Dutch colonial refreshment and supply station in 1652.

Evidence suggests that early relationships between African farmers and San varied considerably, ranging from living together and employment of San as trackers, spies, soldiers, and stock herders to violent conflict ([13], pp. 136–185).

By contrast, European relationships were far more one-sided. The popular understanding of Europeans from the 1600s through to the 1800s was that the Bushmen were on the lowest rung of what it meant to be human. From the 1730s, Cape settlers characteristically cast Bushmen as cattle-thieving "vermin" and groups of armed and mounted colonists frequently set out on "commandos" to hunt down the men and capture or kill the women and children. Many settlers believed it was legitimate to wipe out Bushmen in the name of progress. In the 1800s, an old persistent idea of Bushmen as romantic, exotic, primitive relics from the dawn of humankind became more prominent. With the expansion of the colonies, settlers and colonists argued for the study and preservation of Bushmen before these "living fossils" disappeared forever. Some colonists argued for reserves where Bushmen could live with some measure of protection. Others believed Bushmen could live in game reserves, where they might be an attraction for visitors alongside the animals.

After years of extreme violence in the Cape Colony, the last independent San hunter-gatherer groups finally disappeared in the 1880s. Scholars have only recently recognized that what happened to the San in the Cape constitutes genocide. Despite the overwhelming violence, San nonetheless survived in what is now South Africa, but to do so required losing their identity and language as they became "Coloured" colonial farm workers or lived on the margins of Black African or Coloured villages.

Elsewhere in southern Africa, colonialism was brutal to the San but not as devastating as it was in the Cape. From the 1800s onward, San communities throughout southern Africa were universally dislocated and traditional life drastically transformed by factors including starvation, land dispossession, relocation, farm and mine labour markets, missionaries, and war. Yet despite this wholesale disruption, a considerable numbers of San were still living predominantly hunting and gathering lifestyles in the central and northern Kalahari basin into the 1950s and beyond.

In summary, contact with Africans brought significant changes to the San but nothing like the overwhelming attack on their lives, livelihoods, and identities that came with European colonization. For hundreds of years, generations of San have faced enormous challenges.

San Mental Health Baseline

Despite extraordinary and prolonged interest in the San, it is only in very recent years that any studies have explicitly addressed mental health. The earliest significant research came with psychologist Richard Katz's work of the San healing dance. In *Boiling Energy* [14] and *Healing Makes our Hearts Happy* [15], undertaken with anthropologists Megan Biesele and Verna St. Dennis, Katz focused on the dance as both a physical healing treatment and a social healing and coping strategy. Katz's contributions emphasized the possibilities the dance holds as a strategy for San to cope with the radical changes besetting their communities ([15], pp. 52, 131–144). Katz did not, however, broach mental health head on. From the 1990s, psychotherapist Bradford Keeney also began publishing extensively on the healing dance, but Keeney has focused more on the dance as an exceptional channel of divine healing energy rather than a strategy for treating specific social and individual health problems [16].

In the 1990s, work emerged on conflict resolution and witchcraft [17–19], which is again relevant but addressed mental health only in an oblique manner. By 2003, however, studies began to emerge with explicit relevance to the topic, notably McCall and Resick published on post-traumatic stress disorder among Ju/'hoansi [20], and Mollema [21] on conflict avoidance in a !Xun and Khwe South African San community at Platfontein.

The most thorough study of San mental health to date again features the Platfontein community. This was undertaken recently by den Hertog, a Dutch PhD candidate examining the role of context in understanding mental health, issues of depression, and the nature of informal care strategies for San with chronic psychotic symptoms ([22, 23], personal communication). We will return to this work as a way of fleshing out broader San perspectives on mental health.

In terms of government research reports on mental health among the San, we are restricted to very broad national health reviews. Although these studies give us little direct detail regarding the San, they do provide an important background to the problems San and other Africans face and the states' engagement with these problems. As this is not the main focus of this study, the following health review draws only on reports from Namibia to serve as a guide to the background of San welfare across the region. While the regional national health policies are differently conceived and resourced, the interwoven environments and histories of these countries are sufficiently similar to warrant one of the major San countries speaking broadly for the wider situation.

In 2004, the Namibian government approved a National Policy for Mental Health (NPMH) which emphasized that the need for mental health intervention was very great, but effort was not yet sufficient to reduce the burden [24]. Evidence suggests this situation still stands many years later.

This 2004 report outlined how Namibia suffers from the same issues that affect populations the world over, while emphasizing that the Namibian situation is worse than that of many other countries because of Namibia's history. The report observed that the colonial political system and the apartheid policy of discrimination and oppression has had a negative impact on Namibia's population. Years of liberation struggle and accompanying psychological stress contributed to the poor state of the nation's health. This 2004 report emphasizes that the situation is exacerbated by high unemployment and associated substance abuse and violence. In 2004, rising suicide rates were also a particular concern ([24], p. 4).

A Namibian national health report for 2013 flagged "the double burden" of Namibia, as a developed and developing society. The critical health concerns singled out by the report were HIV/AIDS, STIs, malaria, and tuberculosis. Close behind these problems came non-communicable diseases including cancer, diabetes, obesity, high-blood pressure, and an endemic issue of domestic violence ([25], pp. 253, 259).

It is an indication of the low priority attributed to mental health within the Namibian health services that it only appears in a brief subsection of "Other Health Issues," where it sits alongside fruit and vegetable consumption, wearing seatbelts, and use of tobacco and alcohol. Revealing as this is, the report then continues to include the census that informed the report. It is this census that takes us back to our core mismatch conundrum. The census involved four questions. The first of these asked if people had ever "seen or heard things that are actually not there" ([25], p. 272). The following three questions then asked if people had ever experienced feelings of worthlessness, lack of interest and pleasure, suicidal feelings, and prolonged bad or sad moods.

The latter three census questions carry across multi-cultural divides pretty well because they relate to feelings that translate well across cultures, and do so regardless of what might lie behind these feelings. However, this first question completely blindsides Indigenous conceptions of the world by asking interviewees to be complicit in a scientific rationalized world that has no room for day-to-day African life, including interaction with dead people, divinities, spirits, and personified communicating life forces.

San Perspectives on Mental Health

To present a well-rounded account of San mental health, this section begins with my colleague Joram's understanding of the phenomenon and then proceeds to a specific example of mental health research undertaken in the San community of Platfontein, South Africa.

My discussion with Joram revolved around our core conundrum—that the idea of mental health does not translate readily into San worldviews. Joram observed that San ideas are "quite different compared to Western ideas of mental health because we have very few cases of mentally ill people." Then he clarified, "but simply, the disease is not understood in our society." Joram expanded: "It is more or less seen as a curse person, someone who has been cursed." The point that Joram opened is that most San view symptomatic presentation of mental illness as an indication that someone has been bewitched for doing something bad. Alternatively, they might recognize a San illness which they might try and treat in accordance with their wider knowledge of traditional problems and cures, probably using animal or plant parts as the basis of the treatment.

Joram explained that it is only in very recent times that San have heard of "mental health" and the sorts of illnesses the category includes, such as depression. Like many other Africans, most San know some traditional healing strategies plus some of the "new," introduced medical ideas. When it comes to treating mental illness, they will probably start by involving a Healer alongside trying their own familiar folk remedies. If these approaches do not work, they will then seek help elsewhere among their San or African neighbours or at hospitals and clinics [26]. Joram emphasized that many San are reluctant to be treated in mental health clinics because they are afraid of being recognized by other San and becoming stigmatized for having done something bad and having consequently been bewitched. Joram contrasted the public exposure of a shared hospital waiting area to the privacy of a San Healer's hut. In the Healer's hut only the Healer and their partner know that a person has visited because of a mental health issue, as opposed to visiting for a "normal illness," which holds no stigma. The normality and discretion of the Healer's hut precludes community conjecture and stigmatization.

If we are looking for traditional San ways of treating mental illness, we must tease out what resonates with and works within San cultures. This raises the questions of what place witchcraft has in San culture and might it hold any clues as to causes of mental illness and means of possible treatment?

In line with wider academic interpretations of Bushman culture, in which the San have long been recognized as fiercely egalitarian and shamanic, Guenther [17] argued that witchcraft ideas and practices are present among the San but they are not traditionally San and have been borrowed from their African neighbours. In the light of this argument, it is tempting to interpret Joram's emphasis on bewitching as representative of this acculturation and not look to witchcraft for insight into core, deep-seated, San relationships in the world. However, understanding San relationships with witchcraft is important, because not only does witchcraft underlie current everyday life for many San, but San ideas of where illness comes from and how it can be treated hold an essential core in common with those of witchcraft—that something enters a person and makes them sick, be it a bad thought from someone, a spirit, a spirit animal like a snake, a wind carrying dead people, a shock, an invisible arrow shot by dead people, or an object like a lump of black "goo" (fat and soot?).

Further still, one of the key characteristics of African witchcraft is the divisive role jealousy plays in African communities, and this again is something present in San communities. Not surprisingly, urbanization has caught up with the San, and this goes some way to explaining the fact that Joram recognizes material inequality and jealousy as causes of mental illness among them. Still, just as the San seem to have had witchcraft-like ideas of illness for a long time, Joram also reminds us that jealousy was a key concern of San communities "in the old days." This is something academics have also noted, and we come to this later in contexts of suicide. I have similarly encountered jealousy when talking to very old San about their past. Numerous San who lived as hunter-gatherers described how jealousy was normally over partners or food and would cause tempers to flare. This sometimes resulted in arguments in which someone grabbed a poisoned arrow and fatally stabbed another community member.

This reminds us that not all the old ways were easy, which is something Joram further highlighted with his explanation of how small communities dealt with people with problems that threatened the group's stability. "In the olden days, community problems were resolved in a very simple manner. Elders would come together to discuss a problem person. If they felt they could not help the person they would ask them to leave the village. If they did not leave, they would just kill them to get the problem out of the way. That is what was done in the old days."

These examples demonstrate that we should not idealize and romanticize the past, but it would be a critical mistake not to engage with past practices and knowledge as a guide to developing future culturally appropriate and familiar health-seeking strategies. For example, Joram's observation that people prefer the privacy of the Healer's hut to the public clinic is a good indicator of appropriate approaches to San mental health treatment. A further insight goes back again to the difference and similarity between San witchcraft and that of their African neighbours. Joram flagged that San Healers will know the causes of someone's sickness just like African witchdoctors ("Black" "Bantu speaking Healers"), but it would be very untypical of a San "doctor" to "point a finger" and name a community person as the cause of someone else's illness, which is something readily done among their neighbours. Joram highlighted that concern with maintaining social harmony is a significant San characteristic, and traditional ways of doing this could be encouraged as a means of accepting and supporting those with mental health problems living with a community.

Joram offered a further example which relates to San relationships with spirit. He began by identifying fear as a primary cause of mental illness: "Fear is the number one thing and people don't really talk about it and it develops as a kind of a sickness." Joram elaborated that many San become involved with "witchdoctors" because they are seeking help in obtaining a particular partner or they want material possessions and to "get rich quick." A non-San witchdoctor will commonly promise a solution to their problem but will demand that the client first commits some deliberately shocking act, including killing their first- or last-born or sleeping with their mother. Faced with this demand, clients often descend into a trough of fear because they are quite rightly horrified by the idea of acting on these demands. At the same time, they are terrified that they must act because they have already made a commitment to the witchdoctor and his spirits. What Joram emphasized, though, is that unlike their African neighbours, San have options:

> You still have free will and it is up to you to decide— do I allow this spirit to attack me? ...there is always the protection of your spirit, it will lead you to a right decision but there will be counter spirits attacking from both sides, so that is why the Healers always tell people, if you wake up in the morning, listen to yourself, early in the morning listen to yourself. The spirit will tell you how the day will go.

What Joram has revealed is a profound San ontological and epistemological orientation to the world that hinges on listening to and trusting your feelings. The idea is cast in many ways in different contexts, but it boils down to San listening to their feelings and prioritizing them as an appropriate way of making decisions. The key is to listen to the right feelings, or voices, and that is something of a gift. To better understand this idea of a gift and the sorts of causal connections lying at the heart of bewitched San, and hence San concepts of mental illness, we need to consider San ontology.

San ideas of the self are rooted in an understanding that the human body is permeable and is born with, or can later take on, special potent connections to animals, plants, people, and other phenomena, notably weather. In one respect, these relationships are something like "owning" a story, which can amount to knowing the story is inside oneself and recognizing it as a substantive thing—and even recognizing that your story can be passed on to someone else. When the story is felt within you, maybe it makes your "gut ache" or your "head whirl"—this is proof that it is there. In a San idiom, because the story is felt and it speaks to you, it becomes a substantive entity living inside you. When it speaks to you it has woken up from being asleep within you.

The basis of these ideas is that every living thing holds the gift of life that was given by God. Different animals, people, and plants hold different life-defining gifts. The gift defines what an organism is. In this sense, the gift is like the essence of a person or animal or plant. In people, this primary gift of life is frequently thought of as the gift of breath or wind from God. In people, animals, and to a lesser degree plants, this gift or essence is also thought of as an organism's specific smell. This essence is also present in urine, faeces, spit, and parts of animals, including hair, hooves, and skin.

Traditional San treatments involve putting the essence of one phenomenon, like a strong eland antelope, into another to transfer the power or characteristics of that source into the host. This entails physically moving the essence into someone by having them smell it, by rubbing it on, blowing it on, shooting it in using an invisible "arrow," having it enter through a "shock" or a cut, or as wind entering a body orifice. It can even be transferred by a stare or a thought. Having received the essence, the host then holds a relationship with the source (person, plant, animal, weather)—the host will have some of the perceived strengths of the source or they may be able to influence the source. In this manner, a Healer may put healing power into another person to make them a Healer, or put their healing power into a patient to heal them. A slightly different example is that a person might "own" the gift of rain or wind, meaning they have, inside them, a relationship with rain or wind which can be woken up and used to affect rain or wind, principally stopping, starting, or moving it.

It is putting in this essence and the ability to take out "bad things" that underlies most San healing, including the San healing dance. Academics have identified the healing dance as a traditional San strategy that could play a particularly important role in San dealing with new health and welfare challenges [15]. In a healing dance, the whole community typically comes together. The women sing and clap while one or more men and women Healers dance vigorously, talk with the ancestors, wake up the healing power within themselves, pull out sickness from the afflicted and put in good Healer power, often described as arrows. Healers will not only treat the afflicted but work their way around everyone gathered, pulling sickness and sharing their God-derived healing power. By involving the whole community, social divisions and quarrels are pacified.

As Joram observed, a healing dance is an important starting point for the treatment of someone who is bewitched. An alternative treatment involves using plants, which, "if they believe in them, they will work." Joram described how San will take a plant and "chew and spit just to chase that spirit of that [bad] person away. That is how they are protected." Using plants in this manner is all about moving potencies, and there are many medicines that work in this way for problems related to mental health, such as Hai||om burning aardwolf dung to drive away "naked witch people," bad spirits, bad winds at night, and bad dreams, or aardwolf dung being used if someone has "taken your footprint" for malevolent means. Ju|'hoansi similarly burn aardwolf dung for protection from dead people. Hai||om and Naro use the kidneys of the bat-eared fox to drive away *g||âuas,* or evil spirits, and ǂKhomani use bat-eared fox or jackal kidneys to stop Tokoloshe, the malign "little people" of Bantu-speaking cultures. Smoke from elephant dung is a similar alternative used by Ju|'hoansi and Hai||om. The Naro will also use ostrich eggshell to stop a foetus from being bewitched.

Ostrich eggshell is a very widely used medicine. San know ostriches are strong and they associate ostrich eggs with strength, growth, life-giving, and cooling water. San believe ostriches are strong because they are seldom seen to be sick. San are also impressed by ostriches living in the harshest conditions, including sitting out on their eggs in extreme heat in the open. San gain strong ostrich potency by wearing ostrich eggshell beads or eating ground and roasted eggshell. The association of ostrich eggshell with cooling relates to the use of ostrich eggshells as water containers. Some Healers wear ostrich eggshell "jewellery" to "cool themselves down" when healing. But as with anything, potent ostrich eggshell also holds dangers. This is particularly true for the Ju|'hoansi, who know that the shell should never be eaten because it can induce madness. A more widely known cause of madness is excessive wind blowing on a woman who has just given birth and the wind moving up into her head. Treatment involves placing something warm on the woman's head to drive the winds back down.

In our discussions, Joram brought up problems he had seen in San communities, plus the incidence of suicide and problems of violence and alcohol abuse endemic in many San communities. As Joram explored the themes, he reminded us again that community life is not all about support and not all traditional solutions are appropriate for current times.

> I think the person starts to forget to take care of himself properly maybe hygienic[ally], meaning not washing. He or she is talking by himself, a lot of the time alone, and or maybe laughing by himself or making funny physical signs… It all depends what kind of condition this person has. Is she most of the time oriented or most of the time she's speaking to himself or herself? So all these things, if it becomes worse, you'll see in the society that this person is rejected from the society. It is a very painful situation because there is no help. The traditional doctors normally do healing dances to understand what might be the causes of the disease, but as I said, we don't see it as a disease, we see it as someone who has been bewitched.

> I think it is very little, the number of San people doing suicide, it is very little, and it is mostly associated with jealousy over girlfriends or boyfriends. [But] I have also seen many, many young people in Platfontein especially, and in Andriesvale, killing themselves because they could not take it any more because of the AIDS. They do this by overdose with the pills they are receiving or some of them use whatever poisons there are locally.

As he reflected on mental health in terms of wider social problems, Joram referred to the terrible consequences of colonialism when San were exposed to new forms of violence, directed at themselves as farmworkers and set within contexts of their employment as soldiers. "Most of the San soldiers have become mentally ill. Even the maids at the household level [show] violent abuse of alcohol…the husband comes back angry, beats up the wife because he was angry because of what is done. It was exactly the same on the farms." Joram-related stories which are commonplace among certain San groups about the extreme physical violence inflicted on San by some colonial farmers. It is commonly said by San that some farmers even murdered workers to avoid paying them.

Joram concluded his thoughts on mental illness with the observation that the colonial and post-colonial imposition of leadership through regional San chiefs, as opposed to village Elders, has been a real problem. The regional chiefs cannot possibly know all the details that lie behind the problems of individuals, and most of the time they are too distant to assist people with their problems. Hence, communities lying far from regional San chiefs cannot easily obtain help from a regional chief and the people suffer. Joram believes it would be better for people to have more control of their affairs at the very local community level.

Platfontein

Platfontein is a community near Kimberley in South Africa's Northern Cape Province. The community consists of around 6200 San who are ex-soldiers and their families from !Xun and Khwe communities of southern Angola and northeast Namibia (SASI, 2010, cited by den Hertog [22], p. 386). The old soldiers living at Platfontein fought alongside the Portuguese in the Angolan War of Independence (1961–1974). They then fought with the South African Defence Force (SADF) in South Africa's war with South West Africa People's Organization (SWAPO), which culminated in Namibia's Independence in 1990. With the end of the wars, these !Xun and Khwe were fearful of retribution from SWAPO and took up South Africa's offer of a home and jobs in the Northern Cape. Once in South Africa, the San were housed in an army tented camp at Schmidtsdrift, about 80 km from Kimberley. In 2003, they began a move to Platfontein, a farm much nearer Kimberly. Although Platfontein has a school, churches, a radio station, and even a community computer centre (with no internet), its infrastructure remains that of a poor township.

Platfontein San live with a variety of difficulties, many of which are typical of other San communities. Quite typically, community members are frustrated with their community leadership, but tension also exists between the two San groups and between the San and their African neighbours. As among virtually all San, poverty is a serious problem and is underscored by extremely high unemployment rates (95% in 2010, [22], p. 387). The community is beset with alcohol abuse, social conflict, and violence. Health workers and community members are very concerned about the incidence of HIV/AIDS and tuberculosis.

The Platfontein San community has attracted unusual interest in mental health research largely because of its military population and its very poor community welfare standards.

Den Hertog has carried out the most extensive mental health research in Platfontein and has particularly focused on depression. Reflecting the sort of medical pluralism identified by Joram, den Hertog's research indicates that community members understand depression in ways which combine biomedical definitions with more traditional San ideas.

Platfontein San talk about depression in familiar terms including "low in energy," "stress," "old age," "sickness," "sadness," and "loneliness." Other terms they use are more idiomatic and include "thinking problems," "thinking too much," "thinking about many things," "bad thoughts," "pain in the heart," and "bad spirit" ([23], p. 5).[2] "Thinking too much" was a problem also highlighted by Joram. Participants in den Hertog's research cited a range of causes and multiple causes, key among which were social and socio-economic problems of poverty, lack of employment, alcohol abuse, "violence, loneliness, lack of support, relationship issues, and losing loved ones" ([23], p. 5).[3] Some also linked suicide to either being ill or being rejected

---

[2] Paper still under review restrictions—to be advised soon.

[3] Paper under restrictions.

by community members because they are ill. This latter point fits with Joram's understanding that there is no shame in being ill in a San community unless that illness is to do with bewitchment or HIV. Joram remarked that San in towns who had contracted HIV often feel isolated. They are too afraid to attend clinics where they will be seen by members of the public as "AIDS patients." At the same time, they have no other community support mechanisms. Joram noted that San in this position are very vulnerable to suicide.

Although statistics are not available, it seems that suicide and suicidal thoughts are not uncommon. Classic studies of the San emphasized the low or non-existent presence of suicide. When identified, suicide tended to concern issues of relationships and jealousy ([27], p. 29; [28], p. 285; [29], p. 171; [30], p. 61). Suicide has also flared in contexts of destabilizing social change, particularly surrounding the alcohol abuse that came with employment of San in the SADF in Tsumkwe in Namibia in the 1980s. Perhaps then we should not be surprised if suicide surfaces again in the later lives of these soldiers and their families in Platfontein.

Further causes of depression included "ancestors," "witchcraft," and "bad spirit." Community members spoke about a range of solutions for depression, including sharing problems and seeking social support; medication, psychological referral, and treatment for clinical problems; exercise and other strategies to divert negative thoughts; and use of traditional Healers to deal with ancestors and witchcraft ([23], p. 6–7).

Platfontein San address depression by using both traditional and Western approaches. Particularly in the light of Joram's insights, I strongly suspect San talking to den Hertog downplayed the presence and role of witchcraft in their health-seeking strategies. Although many other San communities use traditional medicine far more extensively than the Platfontein San seem to, this probably says more about the lack of environmental resources, the lack of animals and plants available for medicines, than any more profound shift away from traditional San practices. Our wider knowledge of Platfontein points to both continuation of old traditions and the making of new in the vein of the old combined with new influences. A particularly strong example of this recreation of tradition is the San cultural performance groups coming out of Platfontein and other communities. As part of their repertoires, many groups perform healing dances.

Authentic San healing dances featuring powerful singers and Healers are now diminishing rapidly and have largely disappeared in the southern Kalahari. This raises the question of whether the dance should be encouraged to continue as a potential way of dealing with change. Many San and development workers seem to recognize a need to encourage the dance, but the fate of the dance as a real mediator of sickness and change is not promising. The current contexts in which the dance is encouraged do not necessarily facilitate the more profound role of healing and conflict resolution that the dance plays in traditional settings.

In the past 20 years, there has been considerable enthusiasm among the San for cultural performance groups. Although San cultural groups play a positive role in terms of fostering skills and pride, providing employment, and supporting heritage, it is not clear that they have encouraged perpetuation of the authentic dance and what it can or might achieve. Further research is needed to clarify this situation. Performance healing dances may be diminishing the power of the dance by pulling it into a performance context. Some of the living museum initiatives might do a better job of retaining authenticity and potency than some of the performance groups because they are located in more rural settings, where traditions are stronger and Elders are involved who still have direct knowledge of the older San hunter-gathering lifestyle.

To supplement his study of San concepts of mental illness in Platfontein, den Hertog also examined strategies of resilience, particularly including "informal care for people with chronic psychotic symptoms." Den Hertog [23] identified that informal care of the mentally unwell by family members and unrelated community members plays an important role but suffers from being uncoordinated and undependable. Informal care is also characterized by caregivers avoiding confrontation, which may or may not help in the long term but keeps things balanced and peaceful in the short term. This brings us back to life within the traditional San camp. Confrontation holds the possibility of violence and stands as a potential threat to the camp. San culture holds a number of strategies for avoiding confrontation, ranging from the healing dance to a rich world of metaphor, joking, and social custom. In older times, when these strategies failed, it was common for one of the parties to withdraw for a time to another camp.

On multiple occasions, I have witnessed confrontational instances when it seems bystanders are keen not to get involved unless things become critical. It feels as if San fuses burn slowly but then things blow very quickly and often very violently. Across the San, lack of confrontation, accompanied by avoidance and withdrawal strategies, continue to be key ways in which people deal with problems (cf. [21]). San have a tendency to come at things obliquely and often mildly to defuse potentially hazardous confrontations. In related ways, they are often reluctant to blame someone and are culturally tolerant of idiosyncrasy and difference, except, it seems, in cases where it involves witchcraft or HIV—and in traditional settings, when an individual's behaviour clearly threatens the survival of the group.

McCall and Resick ([20], p. 449, citing [15]) have identified cultural tendencies to deflect confrontation among the Ju|'hoansi, similar to Mollema's findings on conflict prevention and avoidance in Platfontein. They note that, in cases when someone has performed morally and criminally reprehensible acts under the influence of alcohol, it is culturally disapproved of to blame the perpetrator for any length of time. In such cases, Ju|'hoansi seem to attribute violence not to the perpetrator but to "the fault of the beer." I have observed a similar phenomenon among the ǂKhomani, when someone I know well hacked their friend to death with an axe. There seemed to be some acceptance in the community that it was not even the alcohol within the perpetrator that led him to do this, but the malign "spirit" that entered him. The point is thereby reinforced that community harmony is maintained by blaming outside influences.

The notion of San being accepting of difference is one supported by den Hertog and Gilmoor [31], who note that being different holds little stigma. This San disposition seems to relate back to San ideas of gifts—people are given different gifts by

God and it is not up to them what they receive; it is just how things are. I have encountered numerous people who are patently "not normal" to either their community or to me, but they seem to be given a very natural and supported place in their community. On the other hand, however, as Joram pointed out, communities in the old days readily rejected people from their community if they were thought to be a threat, so we should not overplay simplistic ideas of San tolerance.

Community Initiatives

In this chapter, I have discussed how certain cultural traits and practices of the San have persisted as ways of dealing, more or less well, with pressures of radical social, economic, and lifestyle change. While there is strikingly little evidence of new San initiatives aimed explicitly at tackling mental health problems, in recent years projects have emerged that aim to foster traditional values and knowledge and develop better San self-esteem. The emergence of these initiatives reveals a widespread recognition among San that many of their social problems relate to loss of their identity, and a related belief that building networks to foster traditional values and identity will help them engage far better with their changing world. Whether the celebration of traditional values called for by such initiatives can really deliver effective solutions or whether loss of context and lack of authenticity leave no space for traditional strategies and thinking remains to be seen.

Here, I want to consider three examples of recent development initiatives that tackle welfare problems by juggling the traditional with new dynamic agendas. They all represent an inspiring new era in San development because, particularly in the case of the second two, the initiative, skills, insight, delivery, and energy come from among the San. I will conclude by returning to Joram and ideas he holds about intervention strategies.

The first example was instigated by Braam le Roux of the Kuru Family of Organizations. Working intensively with a team of San, le Roux set out to "rediscover and document traditional values that the San people all treasure and keep in spite of modernization and development" (ǂKhomani San Values, 2014). Their project began by producing *Naro San Values* (2012),[4] a manual to guide and support San Elders and youth in education, representation, and organizational processes. This initial booklet was then followed by a series of booklets with similar aims developed among eight different San language groups. The booklet relating to the ǂKhomani San of the Northern Cape, titled *The Way to Live: Values of the ǂKhomani San* [32] is worth close examination.

The tiny number of San who survived the massacres, displacement, and violent reshaping of South Africa's colonized landscapes did so by hiding their identity and assimilating. Between the 1890s and 1930s, the Northern Cape became the last

[4] Naro San Values, 2012, Kuru Family Organisations (Letloa Trust).

refuge of San still with significant connections to their hunter-gatherer roots, and there they mixed with neighbouring groups who had been pushed into this remote outpost. In the 1990s, a wave of interest developed around these San as scholars recognized that they still maintained a Bushmen identity and that some people still knew a little of their old ways and even some of their old languages.

In 1995, members of the South African Kalahari Bushmen communities worked with outside help to launch a land claim. To satisfy the legal requirement of this claim, a new and subsequently problematic ǂKhomani identity was constructed. Although the land claim was successful in terms of restoring land, local people became deeply divided and their communities were beset with severe problems of substance abuse, and related infectious diseases, violence, and social conflict. On the back of the claim, money poured into the communities with the aim of generating future income streams. Sadly, the majority of these projects failed and only served to exacerbate community difficulties.

This Kuru booklet stands as an acknowledgement by the ǂKhomani and the Kuru workers that money and employment projects were not addressing the root of community problems. The communities had lost their way. People no longer knew who they were or who they were meant to be. They had no clear values and ways of behaving. They had no guiding principles to live well and succeed.

A ǂKhomani reference group for the booklet came up with a number of values that they believed important to remember and encourage. The booklet lists the female initiation ceremony; marriage practices; hunting practices and ways of working with and respecting the environment; respect for property, each other, Elders, the Creator and the environment; responsibility for teaching who they are and how to behave; courage as hunter-gatherers; sharing and caring in relation to each other, healing and the environment; protection of the environment; giving freely to each other; wisdom of knowing one's dependence on God's gifts, including survival skills and knowing what to value and how; trust in each other as hunters, Healers, parents, and sharing members of their groups; and leadership.

The similarity of these values with those deemed important by other San is striking and especially so considering how long it is since there were any Bushmen in this region living primarily as hunters and gatherers. This ǂKhomani booklet reveals people with real memories of what it means to be San as hunter-gatherers, but also of people negotiating a complex identity arena. Both the young and the old seem in agreement that they should be proud of who they are and that building on their traditional knowledge and values will serve them well in their contemporary environment.

The second example concerns ||Ana-Jeh, meaning "New Light" in the language of Namibian !Xun. The organization was founded in 2014 by two young !Xun women, Kileni and Tertu Fernando, both of whom are students in Windhoek, Namibia.

The Legal Assistance Centre (LAC) in Namibia estimates that fewer than 1% of San children enrolled in schools complete tertiary education. The LAC pins debilitating school dropout rates on poverty, bullying, violence, and racial discrimination from learners and teachers. ||Ana-Jeh seeks to support educational attainment and particularly among San girls, for whom the broader problems of education are exacerbated. ǁAna-Jeh's strategy is to work on San self-esteem that is threatened by poverty, denigration of San cultures, loss of traditional strengths, and lack of role models. ǁAna-Jeh seeks to "motivate and inspire the next generation of San learners and students to follow in the footsteps of their role models from various communities in Namibia and Botswana" [33]. So far, ǁAna-Jeh has embarked on an number of impressive tours around San schools in which they present examples of San role models to the San learners and share their firsthand knowledge as young San women of the difficulties achieving an education represent, and regarding some of the solutions and ultimately the benefits that come with perseverance for both individuals and the San as a whole. The organization has also produced and distributes a booklet on education which is being well received. It is early days for the organization, but the enthusiasm and surprise with which children learn about San role models speaks volumes.

The third example is the San Youth Network (SYNet), which was founded by Job Morris and !Xukuri !Xukuri, two impressive Naro graduates based in D'kar, Botswana. The organization was registered in 2017. SYNet is primarily a website platform that aims to bring together San youth in South Africa, Botswana, and Namibia to encourage advocacy and share their experiences, particularly in issues of education and "how they have transitioned as San in their contemporary lives." The common San problems SYNet flags include poverty, marginalization, lack of employment opportunities, high illiteracy, family breakdown, alcohol abuse, and associated illnesses of TB, HIV, and diabetes. The website is a landmark achievement for the San, as it hosts discussion at the higher end of the education spectrum on the hardest issues facing the San and how engagement with these issues is or is not succeeding at local, national, and international levels. Driven by Morris's insightful discussion, the website has so far raised and pursued a number of critical issues, including poverty, gender-based violence, and challenges facing San girls in education and climate change. An underlying theme of the website is recognizing the traditional qualities of the San and applying these to address contemporary problems. In the longer term, the organization aims to implement youth development projects, especially including advocacy [34].

Conclusion

The three initiatives outlined above follow a path in which in the 1980s and 1990s development programs were initiated for the San, and institutions were set up by development workers working with San, with the aim of the organizations eventually being run entirely by the San. These included Working Group of Indigenous Minorities in Southern Africa (WIMSA, founded in 1996), the South African San Institute (SASI, founded in 1996), and the San Councils of South Africa, Namibia, and Botswana. Although these bodies did eventually become San-run organizations, over the years a degree of frustration manifested among younger San that they were not involved in good decision-making processes, and that their leadership hung on to their jobs and power and did not always spread material benefits equitably across their communities. Quite understandably, as these organizations became more San, they wished to stand on their own and increasingly resisted overtures of support from outside development workers and academics.

Now, for the first time, significant numbers of young San are starting to emerge with university-level education and professional skills. Many recognize that things have not gone well for the San despite the considerable resources put into development work. They are keen to change things and they have the ability to do so. Perhaps as testament to both their inherent San culture of respect and their recognition of the fact that something has worked—they do, after all, have new kinds of qualifications, skills, and experience—these San are not seeking to attack the established institutional structures head on but wish to support them and develop them. At the same time, they approach outside development workers and academics on an equal playing field and are happy to join forces against their considerable community challenges.

The name ||Ana-Jeh, or "New Light," and the motto of SYNet, "Because we matter, we make change that matters," capture the spirit in which San development initiatives are emerging. The instigators of these projects recognize that welfare resources are poor in their respective countries and what there is does not function well for the San. They aim to mobilize innate San cultural strengths as a means of encouraging San presence at local, national, and international levels. It is too early to say how successful these organizations might be in helping to address the problems of the San, or the role traditional ideas and strategies may play in future welfare improvement, but the capability, vision, and commitment of the San running these projects suggests a promising future.

> Joram recognizes these emerging organizations as representing a new era for San development, which he finds extremely encouraging because the processes are led by San. But Joram also sees room for a more direct way of tackling San with mental health and welfare problems which explicitly builds on the strengths of San traditions. Particularly in his work for WIMSA, Joram encountered a number of programs to either treat alcoholic San through Alcoholics Anonymous or to treat alcoholics by placing them in San communities. His experience indicates that neither strategy is a good solution. As we talked, Joram reminded me of the desire of Petrus Vaalbooi, traditional leader of the ǂKhomani San, to set up a secluded camp at !Khwa ttu San Heritage Centre where Joram and I both work. Petrus's plan was that Elders from the ǂKhomani community would live at !Khwa ttu for short periods and simply spend time with youth and other troubled persons in the bush, teaching them the old ways and helping them by holding dances and employing traditional remedies. In our dialogue, below, Joram expanded on this proposal.Joram: I think if it is set up, it will be helpful for the San people, then maybe it should be a remote area, far from everything. So maybe the places like Nhoma [near Tsumkwe, Namibia] could be the ideal place because it is very remote, you cannot get alcohol easily, you cannot get tobacco easily—where people can detox and maybe get help from the Elders—maybe take people through a very dedicated program like tracking, learning about the different medicines, learning everything the way it used to be in the past.
>
> Chris: Why do you think that would help?

> Joram: It would help. I think it will help because the areas are remote and there are a lot of activities one can do. You could go looking for game or any other thing.
> Chris: So what would be good about that as opposed to a remote Western clinic?
> Joram: I think it's back in the nature. It's in the village on their traditional land, so even if you're alone, it's still a San land so you know it's ours, you understand. … the Tsumkwe area is well-known, so people still feel they are home there and there is plenty in that remote areas. If people feel down, they will take a walk, and one thing which also helps them is, there are dangerous animals so they're also not going to wander around far, so it will keep them.
> Chris: So it's something to do with still belonging, you are still in your community but just outside your community. Land itself will teach you?
> Joram: Exactly, yes, because you get everything almost there. It's almost like your wilderness on its own.

Joram's plan unfolded into a vision that such a place would involve combining Western style detoxification treatments with traditional activities, especially healing dances, tracking animals, using medicinal remedies, and spending time in nature. The point he made about living within community lands but surrounded by wild animals is interesting; not so much because it is risky, but because it is about reconnection, reminding San that you have to be awake in nature just as traditional San life requires people to be awake in all aspects of their lives, listening to spirit and greeting the world with respect.

Kileni Fernando, who leads the ||Ana Jey project, suggested that a key reason many San lose their connection to nature is that drinking alcohol prevents them from dreaming. She suggested we recognize dreaming as a state of wakefulness and being in a wider than every day connection. Fernando also observed that when !Xun hunters set off into the forest, they ask for help and protection from the ancestors, who are both dead people but are also lions and elephants. The hunters say: "*//e//e yi oa !o yi, !nui eka e sua ||aure hng |a e ke ǂona,*" meaning ancestors or Elders from the forest, "protect us and give us luck on our hunt." It is a reminder of a San way of living that fosters respect and connection. It is a way of living that is becoming increasingly unfamiliar.

Joram's proposed combination of a remote camp which builds community and connection while cutting people off from alcohol is not a radically new idea, but it is a strong one that could be helpful for carefully selected San with appropriate problems. It would not suit all San, but there are many Joram feels would really benefit, especially including the old soldiers who originally come from remote communities. For many young San, such a place could introduce them to aspects of their past that are long gone but still have much to contribute to the present. As Joram suggested, we need to take this idea back to the Elders.

References

1. Dieckmann U, Thiem M, Dirkx E, Hays J, (Eds). 'Scraping the Pot'. San in Namibia two decades after independence. Windhoek: Legal Assistance Centre and Desert Research Foundation; 2014.

2. Seedhouse D. Total health promotion: mental health, rational fields and the quest for autonomy. John Wiley and Sons Ltd.; 2002.
3. Dudgeon, P., Roz, W., Scrine, C., Shepherd C., Calm, T., Ring, I. Effective strategies to strengthen the mental health and wellbeing of Aboriginal and Torres Strait Islander people. Issues paper no. 12, Closing the Gap Clearinghouse, Australian Government; 2014.
4. Guenther M. The Nharo Bushmen of Botswana: tradition and change. Helmut Buske Verlag: Quellen zur Khoisan-Forshung; 1986.
5. Biesele M, Hitchcock R. The Ju|'hoan San of Nyae Nyae and Namibian Independence. Development, democracy, and indigenous voices in Southern Africa. Berghahn Books; 2011.
6. Marean C. When the sea saved humanity. Sci Am. 2010;303(2):54–61.
7. D'Errico F, Backwell L, Villa P, Degano I, Lucejko JJ, et al. Early evidence of San material culture represented by organic artifacts from Border Cave, South Africa. PNAS. 2012;109(33):13214–9.
8. Brown K, Marean C, et al. Fire as an engineering tool of early modern humans. Science. 2009;325(14):859–62.
9. Deacon, H. Guide to Klasies River. 2001. http://academic.sun.ac.za/archaeology/KRguide2001.PDF. Accessed 28 Feb 2019.
10. Orton, J. The introduction of pastoralism to southernmost Africa: thoughts on new contributions to an ongoing debate. Azania: Archaeological Research in Africa. 2015 http://doi.org/10.1080/0067270X.2015.1019262.
11. Huffman T. The Archaeology of the Nguni Past. South Afr Humanit. 2004;16:79–111.
12. Schlebusch C, Prins F, Lombard M, Jakobsson M, Soodyall H. The disappearing San of southeastern Africa and their genetic affinities. Hum Genet. 2016;135:1365–73. https://doi.org/10.1007/s00439-016-1729-8.
13. Jolly, P. Sonqua. Southern San history and art after contact. An illustrated Synthesis. A handmade book; 2014.
14. Katz R. Boiling energy: community healing among the Kalahari !Kung. Harvard University Press; 1982.
15. Katz R, Biesele M, St. Denis V. Healing Makes Our Hearts Happy: Spirituality and Cultural Transformation among the Kalahri Jul'hoansi. Inner Traditions; 1997.
16. Keeney B. Bushman Shaman: awakening the spirit through ecstatic dance. Destiny Books; 2005.
17. Guenther M. Not a Bushman thing: witchcraft among Bushmen and hunter-gatherers. Anthropos. 1992;87:83–107.
18. Vorster L. Towery by die !Xu van Schmidtsdrift: 'n verklaring. South Afr J Ethnol. 1994;17(3):69–82.
19. Vorster L. Konflik en konflikhantering by die !Xu en Khwe van Schmidtsdrift: 'n verkenning. Codicillus. 1996;37(2):4–13.
20. McCall G, Resick P. A pilot study of PTSD symptoms among Kalahari Bushmen. J Trauma Stress. 2003;16(5):445–50.
21. Mollema N. The San values of conflict prevention and avoidance in platfontein. J Transdiscipl Res Southern Africa. 2017;13(1) https://doi.org/10.4102/td.v13i1.429.
22. den Hertog TN, de Jong M, van der Ham AJ, Hinton D, Reis R. "Thinking a Lot" among the Khwe of South Africa: a key idiom of personal and interpersonal distress. Cult Med Psychiatry. 2016;40(3):383–403. https://doi.org/10.1007/s11013-015-9475-2.
23. den Hertog TN, Maassen E, de Jong J, Reis R. Contextualized understanding of depression: a vignette study among the !Xun and Khwe of South Africa. Transcult Psychiatry. 2020;0(0) 1–14.
24. Ministry of Health and Social Services. National Policy for Mental Health [NPMH]. Republic of Namibia; 2005. Windhoek
25. The Namibia Minstry of Health and Social Services (MoHSS) and ICF Interntional. 2014. The Namibia Demographic and Health Survey 2013. Windhoek, Namibia, and Rockville, Maryland, USA: MoHSS and ICF International.
26. Low CH. Khoisan Medicine in History and Practice. 2008.Rüdiger Köppe Verlag, Cologne

27. Marshall L. Nyae Nyae !Kung beliefs and rites. Peabody Museum Monographs. 2004;8
28. Marshall E. The old ways: a story of the first people. Farrar Straus Giroux; 2007.
29. Truswell SA, Hansen DL. Medical research among the !Kung. In: Lee R, Devore I, editors. Kalahari hunter gatherers: studies of the !Kung San and their neighbours; 1998;166–94.
30. Howell N. Demography of the Dobe !Kung. 2nd ed. Naldine de Gruyter; 2000.
31. den Hertog TN, Gilmoor A. Informal care for people with chronic psychotic symptoms: four case studies in a San community in South Africa. Health Social Care Commun. 2017;25(2):538–47. https://doi.org/10.1111/hsc.12339/full.
32. Le Roux E, le Roux W, editors. The way to live. Values of the ǂKhomani San. Letloa Trust: Kuru Family of Organisations, Ghanzi, Botswana; 2014.
33. Fernando K, Fernando T. Education Pamphlet, ||Ana-Djeh San Trust. 2015 Windhoek.
34. SYNet. https://sanyouthnetwork.wordpress.com/about/

Chris Low started his professional life as an osteopath and acupuncturist. Following this he returned to university to study archaeology and history of medicine, which led up to his Oxford University based DPhil on health and healing among the Khoisan of southern Africa (2004). From 2005 to the present, he has held a number of long-term research posts and short teaching contracts at Oxford and other universities. His publications include books and articles in leading journals. He is currently Museum Director, !Khwa ttu San Heritage Centre, Cape Town and an Affiliate Researcher of the Pitt Rivers Museum, University of Oxford.

Joram |Useb is a Hai||om San who grew up the village of Tsintsabis in Namibia's far northern Oshikoto Region. In 1999, following volunteer work at the San's primary advocacy group, Working Group of Indigenous Minorities in Southern Africa (WIMSA), Joram was appointed as Assistant to the WIMSA Coordinator and began to represent WIMSA in national, regional, and international fora. In 2005, he was appointed WIMSA Coordinator. In 2008, he commenced a new job at the Indigenous Peoples of Africa Coordinating Committee (IPACC) as the Southern Africa Programme Officer responsible for the SADC region. In 2016, Joram worked as a consultant for the Namibian Government and United Nations, especially on the Permanent Forum on Indigenous Issues (UNPFII) in Namibia. From 2017 onward Joram has been leading the community curation of a new heritage centre being set up with the San and for the San at !Khwa ttu, near Cape Town, South Africa.

Indonesia's Political Reform: Challenges and Opportunities for the Adat Community's Mental Well-Being

Tody Sasmitha Jiwa Utama, Isnenningtyas Yulianti, and Nurul Saadah Andriani

Abbreviations

AMAN	Aliansi Masyarakat Adat Nusantara (The Indigenous Peoples' Alliance of the Archipelago)
BOS	Borneo Orangutan Survival
BPS	Badan Pusat Statistik (Central Statistical Agency)
Komnas HAM	Komisi Nasional Hak Asasi Manusia (National Commission on Human Rights)
MIFEE	Merauke Integrated Food and Energy Estate
MK	Mahkamah Konstitusi (Constitutional Court of Indonesia)
NGOs	Non-Governmental Organizations
PMHI	Person with Mental Health Issue
RHOI	Restoration of Indonesia Orangutan's Habitat

Introduction

Given that around 50–70 million members of the population of Indonesia are Indigenous ([1], p. 336) and that they are members of more than 1300 tribes ([2], p. 5), the country faces serious problems assessing the mental well-being of the adat

T. S. J. Utama (✉)
Faculty of Law, Universitas Gadjah Mada, D.I. Yogyakarta, Indonesia
e-mail: tody_sasmitha@ugm.ac.id

I. Yulianti
Researcher on Center for Research and Development of Social Welfare Services (B2P3KS), D.I. Yogyakarta, Indonesia

N. S. Andriani
SAPDA Foundation (Yayasan SAPDA), D.I. Yogyakarta, Indonesia
e-mail: direktur@sapda.org

D. Danto, M. Zangeneh (eds.), *Indigenous Knowledge and Mental Health*,
https://doi.org/10.1007/978-3-030-71346-1_7

(Indigenous) community.[1] To date, there have been very limited dedicated studies or official statistics that could be used to understand issues of mental well-being in an Indonesian context. Indigeneity and the socio-cultural differences of the Indigenous community are not yet part of Indonesia's legal and policy framework on mental health.

Official records state that 6 percent (19 million) of Indonesia's total population (250 million) lives with a "mental-emotional disorder" or a mental health condition [4]. However, the country has only 51 psychiatric hospitals located in 27 out of 34 provinces [5]. Worse still, half of these hospitals are located across only four provinces. Moreover, there are only 600–800 psychiatrists across the nation. These numbers imply that one trained psychiatrist has to serve 300,000–400,000 people. As a result, nearly 90 percent of people with mental health issues are unable to access mental health services ([6], p. 4–5). However, those records portray mental health issues only as an individual psychosocial issue. Problems with mental well-being in the broader sense, as well as issues related to Indigenous mental health, remain unidentified.

For decades, the Indigenous community in Indonesia, also known as the adat community, has been oppressed by the New Order regime (1966–1998). Marginalization, land grabbing and dispossession, and a disrespect for human rights often affect the well-being of the adat community. Most of the injustice inflicted by this regime was influenced by the state's developmentalism orientation [7]. In Indonesia, this ideology has been featured as an authoritarian-centralized governance policy that aims to support political stability and economic growth.

The fall of the authoritarian Soeharto regime in 1998 gave rise to discourses on the decentralization of state power and recognition of the adat community as a self-governing group.[2] Adat, which was constructed as a national cultural symbol, now emerges as an influential local power. The so-called revivalism of adat is not merely a cultural resurgence in response to modernization and democratization, but also the political and legal movement of customary groups in Indonesia. From the legal viewpoint, adat revivalism is initiated by the second amendment of Indonesia Constitution in 2000. The amendment recognizes and respects the existence of *masyarakat hukum adat* (adat communities) and their rights. From the political context, the resurgence of adat is manifested through the movement of self-identified minority groups striving for their rights. This resurgence also allows adat communities to channel their voices about injustices that they have experienced and to reclaim their traditional rights over territories and natural resources [8, 9].

The revival of adat in the post-authoritarian Indonesia—along with the continuing state development orientation—has triggered a paradox in the adat community. On the one hand, the constitutional amendment has provided adat communities with

[1] Adat does not necessarily have the identical meaning as Indigenous. Adat means "tradition" or "custom" (*kebiasaan*—Bahasa Indonesia). In the field, adat is a concept loaded with a high variation of meaning. It comprises customary beliefs, practices, and social institutions [3]. In this chapter, the term "adat" is also used to contextualize cultural identity; normative order (adat law); political resurgence (adat revivalism); and Indigenous Communities (Adat Community).

[2] This chapter uses "adat community" as a generic term to refer to hundreds of self-governing indigenous communities in Indonesia. We are aware that identity, tradition, and social structure of the adat communities are highly varied from one another.

a strong basis to be recognized by the state. Using the narrative of "adat rights" as a constitutional right, adat communities contest the state's developmentalism projects and policies. On the other hand, many adat communities are also benefiting from modernization and development narratives. Some of them are actively involved in cooperation and agreements with plantation or mining companies. Some adat territories have been utilized as the company's working site, while the adat members work as a security guard or other low-level employees.

Consequently, this paradox promotes social disruption and disintegration among members of the adat community. Overlapping claims of adat territories, suspicion between adat members, and the exclusion of non-adat groups are more prevalent among the adat community today. The distress that the communities have experienced, and which they continue to suffer, puts them at risk of high rates of neuro-psychiatric and behavioral problems, especially depression and anxiety ([10], p. 3). Structural conflicts experienced by adat communities also bring trauma and grief, substance abuse, domestic violence, poverty, unemployment, assaults on cultural integrity, and the loss of territories or dislocation. These situations have driven the adat communities to re-negotiate their identity and territory with their needs to be involved in the development projects.

Nevertheless, the adat community is a resilient group. Local knowledge and values enhance the community's ability to adapt and overcome stressors. Local community wisdom has become socio-cultural capital which supports their notion of well-being. Adat, which literally means "custom," has been transformed into values, norms, and beliefs, as well as a symbolic power which is able to consolidate factions and harmonize imbalance in the community. Adat is perceived as a communal knot that binds the community through solidarity.

Local notions of harmony can be found in every adat community. In Ambon, the adat have made a significant contribution to resolving conflict using the narrative of Baku Bae.[3] The adat community in Aceh uses Peusijuek as a traditional justice mechanism to finalize a "reconciliation" process. Meanwhile, people in central Sulawesi employ the Motambu Tana ritual to resolve land disputes, by burying a buffalo's head to symbolize the intention to forgive past conflict [13]. The Balinese are bound by the concept of Tri Hita Karana (three causes of happiness), which motivates people to balance their relationship with God, their fellow human beings, and the universe.

This chapter discusses the adat revivalism in post-authoritarian Indonesia from two points of view. First, it examines how some aspects of adat resurgence and the development projects that revivalism is responding to in the present economic and political context, generate challenges to the mental well-being of the adat community. By reviewing the contemporary injustice experienced by the adat community, we found that the development projects and the adat revivalism have affected the community's notion of well-being and their treatment of individuals within the adat

[3] Baku Bae is a peacemaking narrative employed by the reconciliation agency during conflict between Moslem and Christian groups in the interreligious violence of Ambon (1999–2003). This local term was used to replace "peace," as the word itself was perceived as "surrender." The Baku Bae also helped the reconciliation process as it avoided the use of "perpetrator" and "victim" ([11], pp. 85–104; [12]).

community. Second, this chapter also identifies the available opportunities for progress nurtured by the resurgence of adat. We investigate how the adat communities in Indonesia manage the continuing pressures that arise from the impact of development projects, while they are reviving their community as a political-cultural power.

Method and Terminology

Most of the empirical data used in this chapter were collected during field work conducted in West Sumatra, Bali, East Nusa Tenggara, and Toraja from 2014 to 2018. However, that research was not dedicated to studying the mental health issues of the Indigenous community and did not employ Indigenous psychology in its methods. It was conducted to identify the positions of women with disabilities in the *adat* (Indigenous) community and the response of *adat* (customary) mechanisms to that situation from a socio-legal perspective.

Nevertheless, some findings from this previous research remain relevant by providing insights into how the Indigenous concept of well-being and mental health has been constructed in socio-cultural life. These findings also highlight opportunities for the community to be more involved in facilitating mental well-being.

In this chapter, we use the term "adat community" to refer to the historical dynamics and the present condition of the Indigenous Peoples of Indonesia. The term "Indigenous People" is used in a broader context when discussing the adat community's position in international discourse, or to refer to Indigenous groups in a global context.

There are two sub-concepts that are determinant to the notion of Indigenous People. First, there are the characteristics of native and distinct groups which are different from other sections of the national community (see Article 1 of the Convention). Second, Indigenous groups are understood to have a strong historical continuity with pre-invasion and pre-colonial societies [14].

For countries in the Global North, Australia, or Oceania, the International Labor (ILO) Convention 169 concept of Indigenous People is almost uncontested. However, in an African and Asian context, the criteria employed have triggered a heated debate, ranging from concerns about the onset of social disintegration and "intrinsic dissimilarities" between Indigenous People and national or ethnic minorities ([15], p. 10), to a simplification of a variety of historical, cultural, and rights complexities [16].

In Indonesia, the usage of "Indigenous People" to refer to the adat community is problematic. The involvement of the Indonesian government, NGOs, and the adat community alliance in international forums related to Indigenous People has led to some acceptance of this concept. However, this term is not commonly used in the national level. The concept of *Masyarakat Adat* (the adat community) cannot be directly translated to "aboriginal groups" as perceived in the Global North context. *Masyarakat Adat* formed from resistance to colonialism was reshaped during the New Order period and revived with support from democratization policy during the

Reform era.[4] The contemporary position and relationship between these groups and their nation-states are typically different from Indigenous groups in the United States and Canada, for instance.

Changes in Indonesia's Indigenous People: An Overview

Indigenous People in Indonesia are widely known as *Masyarakat Adat* (adat community) or *Masyarakat Hukum Adat* (adat law community).[5] It is not too much to say that past colonialization in Indonesia has formed the understanding of the way the adat community articulate themselves. The last term was initiated from the concept of *rechtsgemeenschap* by Van Vollenhoven, a Dutch legal scholar who believed that natives of the East Indies had to be considered as an autonomous community with self-determination and self-governing capacity. After independence, the *rechtsgemeenschap* were termed the *adat* by Indonesian legal scholars and legislation.

During the New Order regime, adat communities were at a nadir. This regime confined the adat community into a tradition-based ethnic community. Many adat communities were forced to conceal their adat identity [18]. According to Franz and Keebet von Benda-Beckmann ([19], p. 30), under Soeharto's New Order, the state used the same legal and political logic as its colonial predecessor. Through its policies, the regime has uniformed Indigenous villages and institutions to become a lowest unit of the state administration. The manipulation of consent to expropriations and the attenuation of the traditional basis of village organization (in Minangkabau) indicate that a repressive approach was undertaken by this regime. Land grabbing and military intervention in adat territories often occurred during this period.

After the fall of Soeharto, the adat movement was reconceived as "adat revivalism." It was encouraged by the decentralization and democratization processes which continue to this day. The establishment of the Indigenous Peoples' Alliance of the Archipelago (*Aliansi Masyarakat Adat Nusantara*, AMAN) in 1999, with an increase in NGO and international initiatives supporting the adat community's

4 Indonesia's *Reformasi* (Reform era, also known as post-Soeharto era) was marked by the fall of the authoritarian regime of President Soeharto in 1998. It was followed by some fundamental changes such as democratization and decentralization processes. The reform has also transformed the notion of adat from national cultural identity and tourism commodity into a political identity with power to influence local and regional politics [17].

5 Some scholars believe that the difference between these terms is more a linguistic expression rather than socio-legal construction. However, *Masyarakat adat* is more popular in NGOs and the adat community itself. This terminology is also used to connect the struggle of local communities with the global discourse of Indigenous People. Meanwhile, *masyarakat hukum adat* is more common as a legal and academic term. As a legal term, it is constructed by top-down and state-determined indicators.

movement, became a significant stimulus for adat revivalism.[6] State recognition began to flourish after the Reform era and reached a peak after Constitutional Court Decision No 35/PUU-X/2012 (MK 35) in 2012. This decision annulled the state's prolonged claim on adat forests.[7] According to Epistema Institute's 2017 outlook document, 69 local regulations had been promulgated since MK 35 was issued on May 16, 2013. In total, since the Reform era in 1998, 191 local regulations have been enacted [20].

These regulations mostly cover the recognition of the adat community, adat territory, adat rights, adat law, and adat institutions. As Bedner and Huis [21] explained, in most adat revivalism cases, the articulation of rights tended to be more popular than self-government narratives. This agenda was neither well-defined nor consistent, but it was shared by many local groups and actors to urge for recognition and protection of adat rights.

The post-Reform era has also changed the way the state's apparatus (and institutions) interact with adat entity. Some synergies can be noted, such as the collaboration between Traditional Healers and professional healthcare, adat involvement in local politics and local elections, collaboration in dispute settlements between adat and law enforcement agencies, and most recently, the recognition of the adat village as a local government administration [22]. Adat movements also began to showcase sensitivity in gender and disability issues as demonstrated in a dedicated session during the fifth AMAN Congress, in Tanjung Gusta, North Sumatra, in 2017.

Nevertheless, especially in the land and natural resources sector, conflicts between the adat community and the state (along with its corporate allies) remain unresolved. Foreign investment and development projects are still leading to food insecurity, human rights violations, land grabbing, and the dispossession of the adat community. With more political space available to express grievances and new legal channels for exerting native tenure claims, tensions arising from the resurgence of adat are more dynamic than during the previous regime.

Development Projects Bring Injuries and Injustice to Adat Communities

In 2013, the National Commission on Human Rights (Komnas HAM) reported that 1123 of the complaints they received were related to the adat community. These complaints increased to 2483 in 2014. Of those complaints, 20% pertained to agrarian issues and occupied the top complaints received by Komnas HAM over the past

---

[6] AMAN represents 2332 Indigenous communities throughout Indonesia, amounting to about 17 million individual members (http://www.aman.or.id)

[7] In that decision, the Constitutional Court annulled some provisions Forestry Act No. 41of 1999, including the concept of adat forest (*hutan adat*), which considered designated forest located in adat territory as state forest. This concept has been maintained since 1967 by the Basic Forestry Law (Act No. 5 of 1967).

4 years [23]. Before this, 622 cases of land grabbing and confiscation were also recorded by the Commission in 2012 [24].

Komnas HAM also identified those agents who were suspected of committing human rights violations related to agrarian issues. Corporations were cited the most, as the perpetrators of 558 violations. The provincial/district government was involved in 167 cases, while the National Land Agency was involved in 156 cases, the national army in 66, and police in 34. Considering there are 31,957 villages whose territory overlaps with state forest areas and depends on forest resources, this conflict is predicted to continue to grow [24].

As a result, the adat community has suffered many injuries and injustices. Many adat community members have been arrested and have experienced violence during the struggle. This brings fear and trauma to the community, especially among women and children [24]. The uncertainty about rights to Indigenous territory has also frustrated the adat community. Many state regulations negate the adat territories, adat institutions, and authorities, by issuing concession permits in the adat forest. Ironically, military and police forces are often employed to ensure the security of investment and development projects. The state has also limited the community's ability to cultivate forest resources by establishing the so-called conservation forest area. The continuing deforestation on the one hand, and the "fence and fine" approach of conservation programs on the other, have threatened food security, the spiritual balance, and local knowledge practiced by the adat community for generations. This situation can lead to intergenerational trauma and disconnectedness, especially for children whose parents have been arrested when protesting the destruction of the socio-cultural landscape. The recent case in Merauke District, West Papua, shows that development projects run by the government are still threatening the adat community. "Project MIFEE" (Merauke Integrated Food and Energy Estate) is intended to integrate farming and food-based energy generation to replicate the success story of Brazil's large-scale agricultural projects [25]. In its master plan, the government is targeting Merauke and Kalimantan as a site for large-scale rice fields and other basic food crops. It was designated to secure Indonesia's food self-sufficiency in the future and to contribute in global food security. The project uses 1.2 million hectares of land in Merauke District ([26], p. 159). Further, this project is threatening the livelihood and cultural practices of the Malind Anim, one of the adat communities in Merauke. Outsiders have been brought into Merauke to work, while local people have been subjected to arbitrary detainment and violence at the hands of the police [27].

Despite the MIFEE Project's huge ambitions to ensure national and global food security, Papua, ironically, has become the region with the most famine and malnutrition cases in Indonesia. The Ministry of Agriculture and the World Food Program 2015 show that the Province of Papua has the highest poverty levels and is the most vulnerable based on the Composite Food Security Index [28]. Even worse, 973,057 hectares of MIFEE land allocated for food crops has actually been used for tin mining [29].

The Orang Rimba[8] in the Province of Jambi, Sumatra, have also experienced similar threats. This nomadic community lives in the forest area of Sumatra and is very dependent on nature for the availability of food and other resources necessary to support their lives. Since various palm oil industries entered Jambi and encouraged massive land clearing and forest burning, the Orang Rimba have lost their roaming area and their life-supporting essentials. In 2015, 11 Rimba people died from starvation and a lack of clean water. Relocation began to be discussed as a way to resolve the problem [30].

In reality, relocation is not always successful at solving this kind of problem. In 2010, when an earthquake and tsunami hit some of coastal Sumatra, the Mentawai people were one of the most severely affected groups, and the disaster caused the deaths of 124 people. After the tsunami, the people of North Pagai and South Pagai were relocated to the highland area, without consideration of the historical and socio-cultural practices essential to their community. As a result, the Mentawai people have encountered difficulties finding water resources and in farming. They are no longer able to access the river, which has been their key resource to secure their basic needs [31].

Development and government projects using opportunistic and coerced approaches have caused traumatic experiences and depression in the adat community. Prolonged conflict, lack of long-term security, and relocations driven by development programs have all affected community well-being. Various projects have not only been detrimental economically, but have also uprooted the adat community and destroyed their ancestral bonds. At the same time, poverty exhibits a relatively consistent and strong association with common mental health challenges, especially in relation to education, food insecurity, housing, social class, socio-economic status, and financial stress [32].

Nevertheless, the revival of the adat community has also led to their benefiting from development projects and to their urge to be involved. In Muara Wahau, East Kalimantan, the Dayak Wehea have been managing 38,000 hectares of the Hutan Lindung Adat Wehea (Adat Protected Forest of Wehea) since 2005. The Nature Conservation (TNC–Wehea supporting NGO) and local government have provided funding to support adat surveillance in this protected forest.[9] Interestingly, at the same time, seven members of the adat have also been deployed to work as *Petkuq Mehuey* (adat rangers) in the forest area, under the concession of the group Restoration of Indonesia Orangutan's Habitat (RHOI), an independent organization established by the Borneo Orangutan Survival Foundation. Both forms of surveillance of the adat forest and the RHOI's concession are managed by the adat authority of Wehea in the village of Nehas Liah Bing. Several companies whose site

[8] This literally means Forest People.

[9] Recently, the number of *Petkuq Mehuey* who patrol in this area has decreased from 35 to four rangers, as a result of the termination of funding support from TNC and the provincial government. The adat authority itself could not provide sufficient funding for the *Petkuq Mehuey* salary and operations.

projects are located around the adat territory pay fees to the community and support the adat rangers with supplies and vehicles.

Another form of interaction is also evident in the community of Airu Hulu, Papua. In the name of adat, the community conducted a protest to reject the intervention of Greenpeace (the international environmental NGO). They believe that Greenpeace's advocacy has frightened off investors and impeded community development. During the same protest, they also asked the local government to invite investment projects into their adat territory. The community believes that investment in their territory will improve their standard of living [33].

The cases noted above have shown how the adat community has made several adjustments in response to the euro-western style state governance and its development projects. To be able to secure their claims, the adat community has been urged to openly collaborate with some parties and reject alliances with others. In such situations, adat identity tends to be presented to meet the criteria demanded in the state's recognition politics, and international standards. Adat, hence, is associated with a distinctive ethnic group's demands for exclusive rights and authority.

This adjustment has then been followed by the "officializing strategy," conferring official status on adat elites as well as recognizing the authority of those elites to rule adat territory and community members ([34], pp. 295–318). This strategy is employed to turn adat elites into state officials (as members of the adat council in district government), or to make their unofficial adat power recognized by the state. As in the reconstruction of Nagari, West Sumatra, and Negeri and Maluku, some of the adat elites, retired migrants, and local intellectuals are seeking adat status as official power holders in the local administration [35–37].

This situation has undermined the villagers' confidence in their leaders, weakened customary institutions, created factions, and fractured kin relations [18]. Consequently, this revival could uproot the adat community from their traditions and substantive values. The technocratic response and approach of the adat resurgence has disrupted community solidarity, which is supposed to be a useful support system for both individuals and the community.

Adat Revivalism: Hidden Stressors on Adat Community Mental Health

The adat lifestyle has long been considered a traditional and harmonious way of life. In this sense, traditional practices are preserved, while ceremonies and symbols are promoted as an aspect of national identity and a tourism commodity. Up to now, adat has also been expressed as a new power in a cultural and political context. Adat elites and institutions were reborn and filled the positions of power provided by the Indonesia democratization process ([35], p. 2). They are expanding from the community level up to the provincial level, and even the national level. Many adat communities are involved in the political and legal struggles for state's recognition. Adat has also transformed as a political narrative to justify native tenure rights and, thus, to exclude migrants or vulnerable adat members from collective tenure allocation. This situation has led to prolonged conflicts with government and other development actors and causes friction within the adat community.

Illusion of Recognition and Individual Mental Health Issues

It cannot be denied that adat revivalism in this post-authoritarian context has changed the way the community exercises their beliefs, values, and norms. These changes emerged due to their need to re-articulate their adat identity and Indigeneity to fit the requirements of the present-day power structure and to continue to demonstrate their significance as a distinctive socio-cultural group. At this point, institutions and beliefs are being reshaped to support adat transformation and to enable them to occupy a more salient political and cultural space.

This recognition, which has become the focus of Indigenous movements since the Reform era, has been transformed into an illusion [38]. It has diverted the energy of many adat communities into seeking recognition, which requires a prolonged political and legal struggle. Silove et al. [39] show that long-running political violence and instability, a lack of justice, and ongoing socio-economic deprivations have resulted in maladaptive effects, such as explosive anger, residual anger among survivors, and social frustration. Tania Li [18] observed how the anger of impoverished villagers in plantation projects in Maluku has been aimed at their fellow villagers, especially those who were involved in signing away land that did not belong to them.

The internal fracturing of the adat community was described by Rukka Sombolinggi, Secretary General of AMAN, in the fifth Congress of AMAN in Tanjung Gusta, North Sumatra, 2017. She highlighted:

> From now on, what is really happening, the future challenge of the (adat) community movement is that we seem likely to be fighting with our own shadows. Why? Because many of the adat community will be diverted elsewhere. There are a lot of our friends, already recruited by companies. Already crossed. They will be our opponents. They are our shadows. [40].[10]

Being occupied with the struggle for recognition and internal fractures, the adat community tends to consider issues of mental well-being as "domestic" matters that are less urgent to resolve. This paradigm has led adat institutions to pay less attention to ensuring mental well-being in the community. Moreover, individual

---

[10] The original speech was delivered in Bahasa Indonesian: "*Mulai saat ini, yang sedang terjadi sebenarnya, tantangan gerakan masyarakat kedepan adalah kita akan seperti berkelahi dengan bayang-bayang sendiri. Kenapa? Karena banyak dari masyarakat adat yang akan dibelokkan kemana-mana. Sudah mulai banyak teman-teman kita, yang sudah direkrut oleh perusahaan. Sudah menyeberang. Merekalah yang akan menjadi lawan kita. Mereka adalah bayang-bayang kita.*"

well-being is seen as more likely to be located in the domestic sphere of the family, where adat authorities have less interest. Thus, collectiveness is being exercised only in the political struggle for state recognition, and it is rarely demonstrated in terms of achieving individual mental well-being.

This tendency can be found in several communities of Nagari in West Sumatra and Desa Pakraman in Bali, where field research has been conducted. Both are village-based adat communities that have gained recognition from local government and are respected because of their influence in local politics. According to some interviews with adat functionaries in both regions, they have a strong desire to be politically outstanding and to promote the adat as a cultural power. The protection of communal rights, group solidarity, and interaction with the financiers were discussed eloquently. However, when questions were asked about the role of adat institutions in caring for people with disabilities in their area, questions about the separation between *urusan pribadi* (personal affairs) and *urusan adat* (community affairs) were often raised. This separation implies that adat are less likely to consider mental health issues as their "public business."

Some of the adat leaders we interviewed claim that decisions about caring for people with disabilities (including mental health issues) are the family's domain. They believe that such issues are a part of a family's authority, which adat institutions should respect. This is interesting, since the same sources also mentioned *kebersamaan* (collectiveness) and *ikatan berkelompok* (in-group feeling) to differentiate the adat community from other communities in a general sense. The non-adat community is widely assumed to be a group that separates private and public matters explicitly. This group is considered individualist.

The adat authorities will become involved if there is a potential threat to the community or when a family openly declares their inability to care for one of their members. However, for the sake of harmony, the family response to these preferences is to remove the person with mental health issues (PMHI)[11] from wider sociocultural interactions in the community. The shame and the potential damage to social order become the main reasons for isolating PMHI from their community roots. Furthermore, this decision is followed by the *dispensasi* (dispensation or exemption) granted by the adat authorities to absolve them and their family from adat responsibilities.

Using the *dispensasi*, the Desa Pakraman in Bali chose to "free" PMHI from community meetings, ceremonies, and other adat activities. Although it has not been stated explicitly, the regular decision-making forums (*sangkep* or *rapat adat*) attended by adult males usually do not provide opportunities for women and PMHI to be involved. Thus, PMHI participation in social and cultural processes is only minimally accommodated. The adat provide "voluntary-based options," which

[11] To consider and to accommodate a dynamic perspective on mental health which evolved in adat community, we tend to use "person with mental health issue" (PMHI) rather than "person with psychosocial disability." The first term can cover more variation and symptoms of mental health issues, for example, intellectual disability, mental and behavioral disorders, as well as psychosocial disability.

either engage PMHI in adat activities or prevent them from disrupting social harmony in the community.

Therefore, the strong emphasis on the recognition of adat identity has confined the notion of community well-being to access to natural resources, food security, group identity, and the construction of Indigeneity. As a consequence, individual mental health issues have ultimately been confined to the family, as their responsibility alone. The priority given to the strategic areas stated above has led to a reduction in the community's awareness of psychosocial and well-being issues to the lowest possible level.

Creating Harmony in the Adat Community

In addition to the public–private distinction resulting from the prioritization of identity recognition, the approach to mental health issues in the adat community has also been influenced by notions of "collectiveness" and "harmony" in the group. These concepts maintain solidarity and sense of group order on the one hand, but they are prioritizing the interests of the community above those of the individual.

As a consequence, the distinctive presence of the individual is not expected to emerge in the public sphere. In Toraja, as Ibu Romba Sombolinggi (the Head of AMAN Toraja) mentioned, this dangerous situation became the starting point for determining the treatment of people with mental health issues. She stated that:[12]

> For a person with a mental illness, if he or she is considered dangerous, the community would usually build a hut for them or, most of the time, send them to the mental hospital. This action is taken to prevent the person with mental illness endangering other members of the community. Conversely, if they are not considered dangerous, the community will accept them as a common member. If there is any ceremony conducted by members of the community, and the person with mental illness comes to visit or just passes by, they will be invited to eat and also be given some food and meat for dinner. Healthy people will not get that kind of treatment.

Interestingly, this isolation does not just impact PMHI alone. Their family is often, albeit unintentionally, also isolated. This arises due to the assumption that mental health problems in a family are a collective fault. Some adat communities believe that the parents' or ancestors' karma can ripen in the next generation. The adat community in Bali, with their belief in *Karma Phala* (any conduct brings its consequence) and reincarnation, often associate disability with sins from a previous life that must be atoned for in the present.

---

[12] In Bahasa Indonesian: "*Untuk yang cacat mental atau gila biasanya dia dikirim ke rumah sakit jiwa atau dia dibikinkan pondok-pondok, kalau dia berbahaya ya. Biasanya sih diusahakan untuk dikirim ke rumah sakit jiwa, jangan sampai membayahakan orang lain. Kalau dia tidak membahayakan kemudian dia jalan di luar kalau ada orang makan ya biasanya dikasih makan. Dia tidak dibiarkan begitu saja. Di upacara adat juga begitu. Karena ini orang sedang punya banyak makanan kan. Kalau mau pulang juga dibungkuskan makanan, dikasih daging juga. Kalau orang sehat kan tidak mungkin dibungkuskan untuk makan malam.*"

This exclusion also derives from patriarchal constructions in the adat community. Since men are expected to bear public obligations, women—mothers, grandmothers, and sisters—have to stay at home to ensure the family is cared for. Women often spend time caring for PMHI as well as running the household business. This situation has prevented many from being fully active in the community. Consequently, women have become the most frequently excluded parties in the community's activities and decision-making.

Opportunities Arising from Development Projects and Adat Revivalism

Aside from the challenges which arose due to development projects and adat transformation during the post-Reform era, some opportunities also arose, thanks to common practices and local knowledge in the adat community. These strengths have included adat beliefs and values, which comprise the socio-cultural capital of the adat community, including a kin-based caring system and adat revivalism, which could be utilized by the community to attain better mental well-being for their members.

Adat Beliefs and Values as Cultural Capital

The findings of the Royal Commission on Aboriginal People (1999) as quoted in ([41], p. 333) argues that hundreds of years of colonization have not diminished Indigenous People's perceptions of their aboriginal identity. This persistent cultural perception has instead strengthened their "aboriginal" identity and will continue to do so in the future. According to Berry, colonialization and globalization have failed to homogenize culture and identity into a single concept. Although this does not mean that culture and identity are static concepts, this persistence provides evidence that the Indigenous community has adequate cultural capital to preserve their identity in the middle of a vortex of external influences.

In the Māori context, Durie [42] interestingly shows that there are six primary capacities that encourage the *whānau* (extended family) to achieve well-being: the capacity to care, the capacity for guardianship, the capacity to empower, the capacity for long-term planning, the capacity to endorse Māori culture, knowledge, and values, and the capacity for consensus. These capacities involve a wide range of life skills and actors that shape the *whānau* identity. These capacities focus not only on the community's choice of action and how individuals have responded to such action, but also how the community express their way of life and collective identity to the external actors. The challenge, then, remains how to position well-being and mental health issues as a collective experience, rather than as an individual matter such as physical health or the absence of disease [43].

In several findings in West Sumatra and Bali, the interaction between individuals and cultural space has played a significant role in promoting mental health issues in terms of shared values. Some space remains available for the participation of PMHIs and their families in community activities. The position of the adat authorities becomes crucial to determine the extent to which PMHIs can be involved, and what kind of community work can be offered to them. Opportunities are possible if the family is open to abandoning isolation-based caring and placing the PMHI back in the community.

Some people with disabilities in Bali are actively involved in the socio-cultural process of ceremony preparation. Some of them are also members of the *sekaa gong* (traditional musical group) which is responsible for the music performance in community rituals and ceremonies. In Bengkala village, there is a prominent *janger kolok* (traditional dance performed by a group of deaf dancers) that uses visual beats instead of audio to direct the deaf dancers. *Kolok,* in this village, has become an aspect of villagers' shared identity. Their sign language (which differs from universal sign language) is used in social interactions and in the local school. It is accepted as a second language in the community, as both deaf community members and non-deaf members are able to communicate in this language.

In Toraja, North Sulawesi, such involvement has also been quite common. Disability has not been considered as evidence of an imbalanced situation. As the Adat Leader of Sangalla stated:

> In Sangalla, a person with disabilities, a person with mental illness and an invalid are usually treated as (we treat) the "senior" members. Instead of being regarded as a curse, the condition of the person with mental illness is usually understood by the community. For the person who is unable to walk, he or she can get involved in an adat ceremony by working on things that can be done by just sitting. These people have received more privileges, those especially for people with mental or physical disabilities.[13]

The collectiveness and harmony which are central to adat values are surviving colonialism and globalization. As long as adat values are used to construct a shared identity, these values may encourage community awareness of individual and collective well-being. Mental health issues could then be framed as *urusan adat* (public affairs) instead of *urusan pribadi* (private affairs). This also demonstrates the capacity of the adat community to broaden its resurgence and strengthen solidarity due to what Durie [42] stated as a "positive identity."

---

[13] In Bahasa Indonesian: *"Kalau di Sangalla orang cacat, orang gila, orang invalid biasanya diberikan perlakukan yang lebih senior. Mereka tidak dianggap kutukan. Misalnya orang gila biasanya dimaklumi saja. Kalau orang yang cacat tidak bisa jalan misalnya ya dia bisa membantu dikasih duduk untuk mengerjakan sesuatu dalam upacara adat. Justru lebih banyak mendapat perlakuan yang diistimewakan utamanya cacat mental dan fisik."*

Kin-Based Caring System

Besides the territorial ties, adat communities in Indonesia are usually genealogically bound as kin groups. Most of them are predominantly patrilineal, except most of the community in Java Island (bilateral) and most of the community in West Sumatra (matrilineal). As practiced in many regions, kinship influences the right to control access to resources and income-generating opportunities [44], in addition to shaping patron-client and religious relations [45].

Although these three kinship systems are related to different parental lines, the male members of the family still predominantly lead decision-making processes. This advantage is often followed by responsibilities for caring for kin descendants. Most people in the Nagari (adat village) in West Sumatra are tied into the principle of *anak dipangku, kemenakan dibimbing*,[14] which means that *Mamak* (the uncle from the mother's line) has a responsibility to look after and foster, not only his own children, but also his nephews (the children of his sisters). This principle applies to the whole continuum of life, including birth, education, financial issues, and even choosing a life partner. In kin groups with strong kinship ties, *Mamak* is also actively involved in caring, fostering, and treating the children with psychosocial problems.

In the patrilineal community in Bali, sons and daughters are considered part of their father's kin. The boy will continue his father's lineage (*Purusa*-Bali), while the girl will move away from her father's kin and join her husband's family when she gets married (*Pradhana*-Bali). An unmarried woman will be the responsibility of her father and brother's family. This responsibility emerges because men hold a central position in the family decision-making system. It also comes as the consequence of male control over the kin's inheritance as well.

In the bilateral societies in most of Java, sons and daughters are members of both the father's and mother's families. The responsibility for caring and raising children is the responsibility of both kin until the children are *mentas* (mature). This term refers to a phase when the responsibility of kin drastically diminishes, after the child is married and able to take responsibility for themselves. Both sons and daughter have rights over the kin's inheritance.

These three kinship systems show that the extended family provides the structured social capital of the kin-based caring system. In this framework, none of the kinship systems provides room for individual isolation. Decisions on health, education, and marriage, as well as resource allocation, are made as kin decisions and not merely by members of the nuclear family.

Thus, the support system for achieving mental well-being in the adat community has been traditionally provided by the kinship system. Dube [44] stated:

> Kinship needs to be seen as providing the organizing principles for group placement and social identity, inheritance and resource distribution, socialization, post-marital residence and women's relationship to space, the formation of basic kin groups, marriage and conjugal relations, authority and power, and rights over children. The very notion of entitlement

---

[14] This proverb literally means that "child is on lap, while nephew is guided."

> to various kinds of resources including food, health and nutrition, and the obligations and responsibilities of members of the group in the business of living, can be understood by keeping in view the fact that it is the kinship system which provides the language for all these and gives them legitimacy.

For many Indigenous communities, ties in lineage-based kinship are more of a determinant than biological kinship. As Alvard [46] has proven in studies of traditional whale-hunting groups in Lamalera, East Nusa Tenggara, it is mutually beneficial for hunters when they are associated with others who are expected to share ideas about what constitutes normative behavior. This derives from what Griffin & West [47] identified as altruistic behavior, which influences the degree of cooperation.

As long as the altruistic behavior works as intended, the kin-based caring system is a possible gain. In this sense, the initiative and responsibility to ensure individual mental well-being do not exclusively belong to the nuclear family alone. As already shown in several regions, the adat community or the kinship group are responsible for the care and support of individuals within their group. It is institutionally embedded with other social mechanism including resources management and wealth distribution. The community-based caring system could also end the seclusion practiced through family-based caring systems.

Adat Revivalism: A Catalyst for Negotiating Better Mental Well-being

Within the present-day post-reform context, adat revivalism has focused on the struggle for recognition, political identity, and natural resource contestation. Nevertheless, the revival of the adat also offers opportunities for greater mental well-being. With this awakening, many adat communities are no longer as isolated as they used to be. They are able to connect their interests and power with state or non-state actors to service their basic needs in the economic as well as political spheres.

Given the fact that the adat are embedded in a larger political structure [48], the adat community actually has the power to promote mental health discourse in a wider context. The capacity of adat leaders and decision-makers has become much more developed during the Reform era. Better access to education, funding, and communication infrastructure, as well as support from the government, NGOs, or international initiatives, has enabled them to become involved in development programs and policy-making processes.

Although this involvement has led to the rise of adat elites and local aristocracies [49, 50], the revival of adat also encourages the youth in the community to be critically aware of their community's needs and dynamics. Better education, access to government and bureaucracy, interaction with NGOs and international initiatives will help them to develop critical thinking to buffer the dominance of the old elite.

The problem is, rather than responding to depression, trauma, and grief, unemployment, or a loss of cultural integrity, youth are more interested in heroic mobilizations and political confrontation. In the newly established Central Sumba District, for instance, the youth seem very keen to use violence and enforce the social exclusion of their political opponents ([50], p. 103).

Adat socio-cultural capital is more widely positioned as a symbol of resistance rather than exercised in common practices. Thus, the sense of shared identity is more aligned to identity politics than it is used to achieve well-being and social cohesion. With its improved capacities, and access to networks, adat revivalism should reconsider its orientation and begin to focus on allocating resources to build resilience, an empowered identity, and community solidarity.

Conclusion

During the democratization and decentralization of the Reform era, Indigenous communities (*Masyarakat Adat*) in Indonesia gained the momentum to reclaim their freedom to practice their traditions and authority over their territory. At the same time, injustices perpetrated by the government and related development projects have continued and are continuing. The pressures exerted by these projects are interconnected to the internal dynamics of the adat community. The most notable is the paradigm shift from "in-group feeling" to "common-struggle feeling," which the adat people call upon to make claims to ancestral land and natural resources.

The adat revivalism in the present-day post-authoritarian context is featured by the rise of political and legal power of adat communities. Notions of state recognition, legal status, and certainty of rights have dominated the community vision of what constitutes important interactions and well-being. The contemporary adat movement tends to prioritize the community quest to formal recognition and fulfillment of adat rights by the state. At the same time, mental health issues are relegated to the domestic sphere.

Nevertheless, several opportunities to address the mental well-being of community members have arisen due to the conditions mentioned above. Some adat communities have shown how the concept of collectiveness and disability can be articulated as a collective experience. For instance, the social inclusion of a person with mental health issues (PMHI) is accepted in Bengkala, Bali, and Sangalla, Toraja. In addition, the role of kinship systems in supporting mental well-being remains crucial. Kinship group is one of the power axes of the adat community that is able to influence domestic and public decisions within extended families. The kin-based caring system could offer a socio-cultural identity to all PMHIs and encourage them to be involved in public spaces.

The opportunities that are emerging as a result of adat political resurgence remain wide open. Adat communities engaged in state and NGO networks have become aware of the significance of their position as a local power. This self-appreciation could be further established if networks were able to direct support not only to the land-related resistance movement, but also to building confidence and internal solidarity. Better access to decision-making processes and development support would offer promising social capital to improve education, employment opportunities, and meet the other basic needs of the adat community.

Glossary

Adat Literally means custom. However, it is often associated with culture, tradition, and normative ordering in the community.

Adat revivalism The rise of adat, mostly in local politics and in the relationship of Indonesia indigenous people and the state.

Anak dipangku, kemenakan dibimbing Proverb from West Sumatera which means "child is on lap, while nephew is guided". It gives obligation to a male to look after his own children as well as his nephew.

Desa Pakraman Adat (customary) village in Bali.

Janger Kolok Traditional dance performed by a group of deaf dancers in Bengkala Village, Bali.

Mamak The uncle from mother's line in West Sumatera

Masyarakat Adat The Adat Community. This community base their life on their ancestral origins in a particular territory, that possess sovereignty over their land and natural resources, whose socio-cultural life is ordered by adat law, and whose adat institutions manage the continuity of their community (definition stated in first AMAN's Congress in 1999)

Mentas Javanese terminology to refer a mature status. This status is usually gained after the children conduct a marriage or when he or she is able to take responsibility for him/herself.

Nagari Adat (customary) village in West Sumatera

Negeri Adat (customary) village in Maluku

Pasung The practice to shackle or to lock up person with mental health issue in confined spaces

Tri Hita Karana Three causes of happiness (Balinese value on harmony)

References

1. Hansen KB, Jepsen K, Jacquelin PL. The indigenous world 2017; 2017. https://www.iwgia.org/images/documents/indigenous-world/indigenous-world-2017.pdf
2. Na'im A, Syaputra H. Kewarganegaraan, Suku Bangsa, Agama, dan Bahasa Sehari-hari Penduduk Indonesia: Hasil Sensus Penduduk Tahun 2010. Jakarta-Indonesia: Badan Pusat Statistik; 2011.
3. Erb M. Adat revivalism in western Flores: culture, religion and land. In: Davidson J, Henley D, editors. The revival of tradition in Indonesian politics: The deployment of adat from colonialism to indigenism. 1st ed. New York: Routledge; 2007. p. 295–318.

4. Research and Development Agency for Health. Riset Kesehatan Dasar; 2013. http://www.depkes.go.id/resources/download/general/Hasil%20Riskesdas%202013.pdf
5. Utami DS. Indonesia free from pasung. In: Presented at the 3rd global mental health summit. Bangkok: Thailand; 2013, August.
6. Human Rights Watch. Living in hell: abuses against people with psychosocial disabilities in Indonesia; 2016. http://www.hrw.org
7. Feith H. Repressive-developmentalist regimes in Asia. Alternatives Global Local Political. 1982;7(4):491–506. https://doi.org/10.1177/030437548200700406.
8. Henley D, Davidson JS. In the name of adat: regional perspectives on reform, tradition, and democracy in Indonesia. Mod Asian Stud. 2008;42(04) https://doi.org/10.1017/S0026749X07003083.
9. Tyson AD. Decentralization and adat revivalism in Indonesia: the politics of becoming indigenous. 1st ed. New York: Routledge; 2010. https://doi.org/10.4324/9780203849903.
10. Cohen A. The mental health of indigenous peoples: an international overview. World Health Organization; 1999.
11. Montiel CJ, Noor NM, editors. Peace psychology in Asia. 1st ed. New York: Springer; 2009.
12. Qurtuby SA. Peacebuilding in Indonesia: Christian–Muslim alliances in Ambon Island. Islam and Christian–Muslim Relations. 2013;24(3):349–67. https://doi.org/10.1080/09596410.2013.785091.
13. Bräuchler B. Reconciling Indonesia, grassroots agency for peace. 1st ed. London and New York: Routledge; 2009.
14. Cobo JRM. The study of the problem of discrimination against indigenous populations. Retrieved from United Nations Document E/CN.4/Sub.2/1986/7; 1986.
15. Martinez MA. Study on treaties, agreements and other constructive arrangements between states and indigenous populations; 1997, July. http://hrlibrary.umn.edu/demo/TreatiesStatesIndigenousPopulations_Martinez.pdf
16. Hodgson DL. Introduction: comparative perspectives on the indigenous rights movement in Africa and the Americas. Am Anthropol. 2002;104(4):1037–49. https://doi.org/10.1525/aa.2002.104.4.1037.
17. Henley D, Davidson J. Introduction: radical conservatism—the protean politics of adat. In: Davidson J, Henley D, editors. The revival of tradition in Indonesian politics: the deployment of adat from colonialism to indigenism. 1st ed. New York: Routledge; 2007. p. 1–49.
18. Li TM. After the land grab: infrastructural violence and the "Mafia System" in Indonesia's oil palm plantation zones. Geoforum. 2017; https://doi.org/10.1016/j.geoforum.2017.10.012.
19. von Benda-Beckmann F, von Benda-Beckmann K. Transforming traditions: myths and stereotypes about traditional law in a globalizing world. In: Presented at the EASA conference "experiencing diversity and mutuality". Ljubljana: Slovenia; 2008, August 26.
20. Arizona, Y., Malik, M., & Ishimora, I. L. (2017). Pengakuan Hukum terhadap Masyarakat Adat: Tren Produk Hukum Daerah dan Nasional pasca Putusan MK 35/ PUU-X/2012. Epistema Institute.
21. Bedner A, Huis SV. The return of the native in Indonesian law: indigenous communities in Indonesian legislation. Bijdragen Tot de Taal-, Land-En Volkenkunde. 2008;164(2/3):165–93.
22. Vel JAC, Bedner AW. Decentralisation and village governance in Indonesia: the return to the "Nagari" and the 2014 village law. J Legal Pluralism and Unofficial Law. 2015;47(3):493–507. https://doi.org/10.1080/07329113.2015.1109379.
23. Komnas HAM. Annual Report 2012; 2013. https://www.komnasham.go.id/index.php/laporan/2017/03/21/22/laporan-tahunan-komnas-ham-tahun-2012.html
24. Tim Nasional Inkuiri Komnas HAM. Inkuiri Nasional Komisi Nasional Hak Asasi Manusia: Hak Masyarakat Hukum Adat Atas Wilayahnya di Kawasan Hutan (1st ed.); 2016. https://www.komnasham.go.id/files/20160530-inkuiri-nasional-komisi-nasional-%24N60YN.pdf
25. The Jakarta Post. Govt to revive food estate project in Papua; 2015, April 16. The Jakarta Post website: http://www.thejakartapost.com/news/2015/04/16/govt-revive-food-estate-project-papua.html. Accessed 12 Sep 2018

26. Coordinating Ministry for Economic Affairs. Acceleration and expansion of Indonesia economic development 2011–2025; 2011. https://www.bappenas.go.id/index.php/download_file/view/11061/3437/
27. Nolan B. Destroying local livelihoods with Mifee; 2013, Jan 20. Available from Jakarta Globe website: http://jakartaglobe.id/archive/destroying-local-livelihoods-with-mifee/. Accessed 12 Sep 2018
28. Dewan Ketahanan Pangan (Indonesia), & World Food Programme. (2009). Peta ketahanan dan kerentanan pangan Indonesia, 2009 (a food security and vulnerability atlas of Indonesia, 2009). Jakarta, Indonesia: Dewan Ketahanan Pangan, Departemen Pertanian: World Food Programme.
29. Center for Agricultural Data and Information System Statistic of food consumption 2017; 2017. http://epublikasi.setjen.pertanian.go.id/download/file/388-statistik-konsumsi-pangan-2017
30. Jamaludin J. Kelaparan, 11 Orang Rimba Meninggal di Jambi; 2015, March 2. Tempo website: https://nasional.tempo.co/read/646497/kelaparan-11-orang-rimba-meninggal-di-jambi. Accessed 12 Sep 2018
31. Rafliana I, Arif A. Refleksi kritis atas ‘ketangguhan masyarakat’ akibat relokasi pasca bencana: Studi kasus mentawai, Indonesia. Prosiding PIT ke-5 Riset Kebencanaan IABI, 5, 14; 2018. https://seminar.unand.ac.id/index.php/iabi/pit5iabi2018/paper/viewFile/399/73
32. Lund C, Breen A, Flisher AJ, Kakuma R, Corrigall J, Joska JA, et al. Poverty and common mental disorders in low and middle income countries: a systematic review. Soc Sci Med. 2010;71(3):517–28. https://doi.org/10.1016/j.socscimed.2010.04.027.
33. Purba JR. Masyarakat Adat Papua Sebut Greenpeace Lakukan Intervensi Berlebihan; 2018, March 25. https://regional.kompas.com/read/2018/03/25/20020001/masyarakat-adat-papua-sebut-greenpeace-lakukan-intervensi-berlebihan. Accessed 13 Sep 2018
34. Acciaioli G. From customary law to indigenous sovereignty: Reconceptualizing masyarakat adat in contemporary Indonesia. In: Davidson J, Henley D, editors. The revival of tradition in Indonesian politics: The deployment of adat from colonialism to indigenism. 1st ed. New York: Routledge; 2007. p. 295–318.
35. Bräuchler B. The revival dilemma: reflections on human rights, self-determination and legal pluralism in eastern Indonesia. J Legal Pluralism Unofficial Law. 2010;42(62):1–42. https://doi.org/10.1080/07329113.2010.10756648.
36. Schulte Nordholt H, Van Klinken G. Renegotiating boundaries: local politics in post-Suharto Indonesia. Leiden: Brill; 2007a.
37. Schulte Nordholt H, van Klinken GA, editors. Renegotiating boundaries: local politics in post-Suharto Indonesia. Leiden: KITLV Press; 2007b.
38. von Benda-Beckmann F, von Benda-Beckmann K. Multiple embeddedness and systemic implications: struggles over natural resources in Minangkabau since the Reformasi. Asian J Soc Sci. 2010;38(2):172–86.
39. Silove D, Brooks R, Bateman Steel CR, Steel Z, Hewage K, Rodger J, Soosay I. Explosive anger as a response to human rights violations in post-conflict Timor-Leste. Soc Sci Med. 2009;69(5):670–7. https://doi.org/10.1016/j.socscimed.2009.06.030.
40. Damai A. Sang jendral masyarakat adat nusantara itu bernama rukka; 2017. https://www.youtube.com/watch?v=bVa1K1TCXGk. Accessed 2 Jan 2020
41. Berry JW. Globalisation and acculturation. Int J Intercult Relat. 2008;32(4):328–36. https://doi.org/10.1016/j.ijintrel.2008.04.001.
42. Durie M. Measuring Māori Wellbeing. Guest Lecture Series. Presented at the Wellington, New Zealand. Wellington, New Zealand: New Zealand Treasury; 2006.
43. King M, Smith A, Gracey M. Indigenous health part 2: the underlying causes of the health gap. Lancet. 2009;374(9683):76–85. https://doi.org/10.1016/S0140-6736(09)60827-8.
44. Dube L. Kinship and gender in south and southeast Asia: patterns and contrasts. New Delhi: Centre for Women’s Development Studies; 1996.
45. Faust K, Schweizer T, White DR. Kinship, networks, and exchange. Soc Forces. 1999;78(2):826. https://doi.org/10.2307/3005591.

46. Alvard MS. Kinship, lineage, and an evolutionary perspective on cooperative hunting groups in Indonesia. Hum Nat. 2003;14(2):129–63. https://doi.org/10.1007/s12110-003-1001-5.
47. Griffin AS, West SA. Kin selection: fact and fiction. Trends Ecol Evol. 2002;17(1):15–21. https://doi.org/10.1016/S0169-5347(01)02355-2.
48. von Benda-Beckmann F, von Benda-Beckmann K. Ambivalent identities; decentralization and Minangkabau political communities. In: Schulte Nordholt H, Van Klinken G, editors. Renegotiating boundaries: local politics in post-Suharto Indonesia. Leiden: Brill; 2007. p. 417–42.
49. Bakti AF. Family rule in Wajo, South Sulawesi. In: Schulte Nordholt H, Van Klinken G, editors. Renegotiating boundaries: local politics in post-Suharto Indonesia. Leiden: Brill; 2007. p. 373–86.
50. Vel JAC. Campaigning for a new district in West Sumba. In: Schulte Nordholt H, Van Klinken G, editors. Renegotiating boundaries: local politics in post-Suharto Indonesia. Leiden: Brill; 2007. p. 91–120.

Tody Sasmitha Jiwa Utama is a lecturer in Faculty of Law and researcher in Djojodigoeno Adat Law Center, Universitas Gadjah Mada (UGM), Indonesia. He was also a research fellow in several civil society organizations and research institutions such as HUMA, SAPDA, Epistema Institute, and PSKP UGM. Currently, he is the Editor in Chief of *Journal of Mimbar Hukum* and the Head of Research and Publication Unit in the Faculty of Law UGM. Tody is interested in socio-legal issues, particularly regarding the law and vulnerable groups, legal pluralism, and adat (customary) law. In recent years, he has participated in research related to women, disability and adat; the recognition of native tenure; and post-reform reconstruction of adat. He recently published "Impediments to Establishing Adat Villages: A Socio-Legal Examination of the Indonesian Village Law," in the *Asia Pacific Journal of Anthropology*. Some of his publications are available at https://ugm.academia.edu/todysasmitha.

Isnenningtyas Yulianti is a Researcher on Human Rights, Social and Political Issues. From 2006 to 2020, she worked at Komnas HAM. Now, she works for Social Ministry at Center for Research and Development of Social Welfare Services (Balai Besar Penelitian dan Pengembangan Pelayanan Kesejahteraan Sosial or B2P3KS) Yogyakarta. She earned her Master of Human Rights and Democracy from the Faculty of Politics and Government Studies, UGM. She has worked in economic, social and cultural rights issues, focusing mostly on persons with disabilities, women, indigenous peoples, and the Right to Food. She has also completed various studies, such as drafting the Draft of Persons with Disabilities and preparing a CRPD initiative report for Komnas HAM. She recently published an article "Unravelling Disability Participation in Indigenous Peoples" in the Journal of Southeast Asian Human December (2019), and "Komnas HAM and the Land Rights of Indigenous Peoples: National Inquiry as a New Mechanism for the Settlement of Disputes", Palgrave Macmillan (2020).

Nurul Saadah Andriani is the Director of SAPDA Foundation (Center of Advocacy for Women, Disability, and Children). She obtained her Master of Constitutional Law from UGM. Her research and advocacy centers on the rights of women and persons with disabilities, and especially on the violence faced by both vulnerable groups. Nurul has actively participated in the bill-making process of the Person with Disabilities and Government Regulation. Her book *Menguak Kekerasan terhadap Perempuan Disabilitas* (Revealing the Violence against Women with Disabilities) was published by SAPDA in 2012. Her most recent publication is *Penanganan Penyandang Disabilitas Berhadapan dengan Hukum di Lingkungan Pengadilan* (Court Case Handling of People with Disabilities), published by MaPPI and SAPDA in 2019.

Happiness, Underdevelopment, and Mental Health in an Andean Indigenous Community

Jorge Yamamoto, María Victoria Arevalo, and Sebastian Wendorff

An Unhappy Psychopathological Developed World

During the 1990s, original research on global happiness that included measures of subjective perceptions of well-being showed a paradoxical pattern: the countries of the self-described "First World" tended to be unhappier than the countries of moderate and moderate-to-low incomes [1–3]. This appears to contrast with the classic "happiness" indexes which, instead of using measures of subjective perceptions of well-being, use prosperity indicators such GDP, access to health services, education, and unemployment insurance [4, 5]. Thus, it should not be assumed that wealthy countries are happy countries. Furthermore, mental health is related to this paradoxical pattern. For example, in 2003, suicide levels were higher in developed countries such as Japan, Finland, Austria, and Switzerland (36.5–50 per 100,000) and lower in developing countries such as Peru, Guatemala, Dominican Republic, and Honduras (0–1 per 100,000) [6]. Statistics from 2015 indicate that Peru and Mexico have 5.0–9.9 per 100,000 suicidal rate compared to greater than 15 per 100,000 (the highest in the cited report) in the United States, Canada, Sweden, and

J. Yamamoto (✉)
Department of Psychology, Pontificia Universidad Católica del Peru (PUCP), San Miguel, Peru
e-mail: jyamamo@pucp.pe

M. V. Arevalo
Department of Psychology, Pontificia Universidad Católica del Peru (PUCP)/Peruvian Institute of Cognitive Behavioral Therapy, San Miguel, Peru
e-mail: mvarevalop@pucp.pe

S. Wendorff
Wellbeing, Culture and Development Research Group, Pontificia Universidad Católica del Peru (PUCP), San Miguel, Peru
e-mail: swendorff@pucp.pe

D. Danto, M. Zangeneh (eds.), *Indigenous Knowledge and Mental Health*,
https://doi.org/10.1007/978-3-030-71346-1_8

France [7]. Rates of depression and anxiety show a similar trend. In the Americas, the prevalence of depressive and anxiety disorders in terms of percentage of population are lower in Peru and Mexico than in the United States [8].

Our research group has been studying the happiness in what have been called "Third World" countries, with a special focus on communities of Indigenous People. We found elevated levels of well-being, particularly in communities of Indigenous People living in environments and lifestyles similar to those of their ancestors [9]. As supported by what Buss [10] states, an important part of Western unhappiness lies in the differences between the industrialized environment and ancestral lifestyles. Our interpretation is that this happened because the human brain and its mechanisms evolved to produce neurotransmitters of happiness in that ancestral environment. The urban way of life, particularly in economically developed countries, distances itself from these mechanisms, and thereby fails to activate these happiness neurotransmitter processes and "release happiness." For example, in Western cities natural landscapes that once displayed sources of food, shelter, and clean water are being replaced by landscapes full of glass and cement, with only small spots of green areas. Moreover, the intense interpersonal relationships within small groups of families and neighbours that used to generate networks of support, cooperation, and shared leisure time are being altered by the presence of a massive and anonymous social environment, characterized by extreme individualism and harsh competition.

How to Avoid the Contagion of Unhappiness and Psychopathology: An Emic Methodological Approach

The differences between Indigenous and urban levels of happiness are directly related to the differences in their conceptions, or emic understandings, of development. Frequently, Western scholars, practitioners, and "international development experts" assume a universal and unique model of development, which is closely related to the factors behind Western unhappiness, such as material goals and autonomy, as opposed to Indigenous interdependence and social security. They assume a sort of a contemporary version of the Ten Commandments in the agnosticized world. Therefore, Indigenous conceptions of development in non-Westernized groups should be a topic of research, not a practice of agnostic Western evangelism; this is not to extrapolate or impose the Western ideas of development but to investigate the different conceptions of development beyond Western thought.

In order to understand the singularity of Indigenous communities, as well as their values, and conceptions of development and happiness (which tend to be different and even opposed to those of academic researchers), an alternative methodology to the one commonly applied in psychology is needed [11]. One kind of typical cross-cultural research in psychology can be characterized by swift arrival of the field researchers who, after applying copious tests, return to the comfort of their hotel.

Using an ethnographic approach, living for some weeks in the communities, will provide the context for sensible interpretations. A non-emic approach is based on standardized tests, without the background information to make sensible interpretations. A lack of ethnographical support will not permit a researcher to discover if their conclusions are real or imaginary. The data could work as projective stimuli, which, with the help of Cronbach and collaborators, turn out to be statistically reliable. This is the established ethic approach: to start with researcher's hypothesis to be tested through some variations of the described methods. In contrast, the emic perspective grounds on the ideas and feelings of the population under research, using different methods to systematize them in a more transparent way.

The method proposed by our research group has three main steps. The first step is to conduct an ethnographic study of the group under research based on the coexistence with the community and the exploration of their geographical area, urbanism, local history, daily routines, and other similar aspects. This phase, which is surprisingly uncommon in the methodology of cross-cultural psychology studies, introduces the researchers to the unique behavioural patterns of communities of Indigenous People, which tend to pass unnoticed when only statistical significance levels, statistical power indexes, and the sizes of effects are analyzed. Without this phase, results would be incomprehensible, or worse, interpretations of these would be made based on the frustrations and happy memories of the researchers. Also, this ethnographic phase allows the Indigenous People to feel more comfortable with the presence of the researchers, as, having been victims of a systematic and long history of colonization, genocide, and exploitation, they tend to be particularly suspicious of non-community others. This trust must not be underestimated, as it can take months or even years for some Indigenous groups to express their ideas and emotions in an open manner. Otherwise, rapid data recollection can lead to the construction of an articulated, high-impact, high-cash, science-fiction story.

Once the local geography, cultural anamnesis, and the community's daily routines have been fully understood, the second phase of the proposed method, which consists of structured interviews with open-ended answers, must be carried out. To avoid the risk that unstructured interviews could easily end up covering topics of investigator's subjective interests (which are not necessarily important topics for the study participants), it is important to previously define key research variables, and to create neutral questions that allow respondents to answer using their own words, ideas, and feelings about the research variable. Although this step may sound simple, achieving a neutral question may take weeks of trial and error. The answers are then analyzed using the content analysis method, which allows the reduction of the open conversations into several categories that synthesize the main ideas that each participant openly expressed for each variable. This approach presents a complete list of the study subjects' collected answers that are related to the variables of interest within the sample. These categories will enable the construction of items to create a psychometric test with close-ended questions that fits the culture of the study.

Finally, the third phase consists of applying the test to a sufficient number of subjects to carry out statistic and mathematical analyses. Even though the third stage of the investigation is quantitative, the results are contrasted or triangulated with the previous qualitative phases. This, therefore, is an integration of qualitative and quantitative data.

Up to this point, we have addressed three principal topics: the paradox between happiness and industrialized development, how the human brain releases happiness whenever ancestral challenges are faced and, the need for an emic qualitative-quantitative methodology. What is the role of psychopathology in this scenario?

Over the past few decades, clinical psychology has started to broaden its traditional illness-based focus to include the study of well-being in a positive psychology approach. Psychopathology can be better understood in the context of general well-being, and this is particularly important in the understanding of Indigenous mental health. Environment, culture, and cultural shock can ignite unique processes that are not related to the understanding and standardized practices of psychopathology of economical developed countries. Hence, a study on happiness and development, with an exploratory link to psychopathology in an Andean Indigenous community, could provide the basis for interpretations of the connection between well-being, Indigenous studies, and psychopathology.

Andean Indigenous Happiness, Mental Health, and Development

In small Indigenous Andean traditional communities, a series of elements that are positively related to mental health can be found. To begin with, nuclear families provide high levels of support to their members, as do a cohesive extended family and strong support networks with friends. Psychological investigations have reported that these elements constitute factors that protect general health [12]. Second, these communities are usually located in natural and clean environments, where the landscapes have the beauty of natural reserves. Numerous studies support the fact that these environments have positive effects on well-being, improve mood and cognitive recovery after stress [13], increase cognitive performance [14], and improve emotional regulation [15]. Third, daily stressors of developed countries, such as financial debts, an anonymous, massive and hyper-hierarchized society, traffic, and gadgets, which serve as long-term sources of unhappiness, are absent. All these elements strengthen the hypothesis of the existence of a correlation between high levels of well-being and mental health.

There is no reliable national epidemiological study to support the hypothesis of positive mental health in Andean communities of Indigenous People. Available data provided by the Peruvian National Institute of Mental Health [16, 17] can differentiate between the urban capital of Peru and rural highlands. As seen in Table 1, there are no important differences between the psychopathology rates of the Peruvian rural highlands and those of urban Lima. The rates of the rural highlands are higher

Table 1 Epidemiological Data of Mental Health in urban and rural Peru

Psychopathology variables	Rural highlands	Metropolitan Lima and Callao
Percentage of the population that frequently experiences negative affects	10–28.8%	10–20%
Lifetime prevalence of psychiatric disorders	28.1%	26.1%
Most frequent psychiatric disorders and lifetime prevalence of each	Posttraumatic stress disorder (12.0%) Generalized anxiety disorder (5.0%)	Posttraumatic stress disorder (5.1%) Generalized anxiety disorder (3.0%)
Lifetime prevalence of suicidal ideation	7%	8.9%
Life prevalence of suicide attempts	0.6%	2.8%
Percentage of the population that, after having attempted suicide at least once, still thought it could be a viable solution to problems	33.3%	3.6%
Most frequent folkloric syndromes[a] and life prevalence of each	Susto (29.2%) Chucaque (23.9%)	Susto (8.9%) Chucaque (8.4%)

[a]Particular syndromes that exist only in native communities

in some areas, as we can see in the number of people who think that suicide could be a way to solve problems. Nonetheless, the number of respondents who attempted to commit suicide at least once was higher in Lima's urban zones. These paradoxical statistics are consistent with the little or absent differences between populations classified into urban and rural categories. In addition, previous studies carried out by our research group have shown that diverse factors may contribute to the low validity of some epidemiological diagnostics.

For instance, some questions may be valid for urban abstract mental processing but might be not appropriate for Indigenous People's different understanding. Moreover, cultural characteristics, such as the communication with ancestral spirits, may be confused with valid indicators of psychopathology in urban societies, which results in unreal mental health indexes. Furthermore, some indicators even show an opposing pattern. In 2007, a 7.9 Richter scale earthquake occurred in Peru. As part of a psychological support group, we found indicators of posttraumatic stress disorder (PTSD). The protocols of the Pan American Health Association considered that social isolation was a PTSD indicator and, hence, it was included as an item in their diagnostic test. However, we found that the PTSD from the earthquake was related to the opposite behaviour, in that Indigenous People didn't want to be alone after the trauma [18]. Finally, to date, no epidemiological data concerning the mental health of communities of Indigenous People has been found.

In this context, qualitative work should be the first step in the investigation of psychopathology in communities of Indigenous People.

Subjective Life Satisfaction

Subjective life satisfaction [19] is a crucial element in the understanding of the well-being of a community because it analyzes the principal goals that a particular group considers important in the pursuit of happiness. These goals are obtained using interviews with open-ended questions to ensure that the answers are not prompted by the researchers. Once a list of goals has been obtained, a psychometric test with close-ended questions is created to analyze the level of expectation for each of the goals. This approach allows researchers to identify the preference for some goals over others, as well as their variation in time.

For example, it can be found that in Andean cultures, family-oriented goals are more important than goals regarding material possessions. Equally, having children is not an important goal in groups of people that have not reached the culturally appropriate life-stage for marriage. Although these variations are obvious, traditional well-being measures do not record them accurately.

Once the necessary goals to achieve happiness and the level of expectation for each have been identified, the perception of achievement of each goal is found using quantitative methods. This establishes the difference between the expectation and the perceived achievement of each goal. For instance, a person who does not have the goal of having children and who does not have children should not consider himself unsatisfied by this fact. Given that he doesn't want children and he doesn't have them, he remains in a state of balance rather than unsatisfied. A person whose goals consist of moderate material aspirations and believes that he possesses that level of material goods will also be in balance and will not feel unsatisfied in that aspect. Likewise, if someone does not own a smartphone but does not want it or is not even aware of its existence, then that person cannot be unhappy about that circumstance.

Hence, this method helps to set what individual cultures propose as crucial aspects of happiness as the starting points of the investigation and enables the comparison of perceptions of achievement with levels of expectation. The subjective well-being component of this study will be measured using this method.

The description of what a culture considers important to be happy isn't the same thing as happiness. In other words, the identified goals or needs must be analyzed according to their effects on well-being. For example, a culture that considers daily drug usage a fundamental need will require a study that deepens the understanding of the implicit psychological processes underlying that behaviour. If indicators of hedonic adaptation, allostatic load, or personal and family disruptions are found, it would be obvious that this cultural need doesn't result in subjective well-being. Another example could be the materialistic goals, which are widely present in the United States culture and have systematically been negatively related to subjective well-being [20].

Subjective Development Satisfaction

The second study variable is development. As previously noted, contemporary Western culture assumes an axiomatic and supposedly universal model of development, based on economic progress and social security, although these also positively correlate with suicide rates and unhappiness. International organizations are the main actors of these tendencies. For instance, the United Nations proposes a "Decalogue," or a series of ideals to which all countries must aspire in order to be developed—and happy. However, these ideals do not match those that our research team has identified in happy communities of Indigenous People. In some cases, we have even found opposing conceptions of development compared to the "universal development" goals.

Alternatively, the study reported in this chapter shows the subjective development satisfaction index [21] of communities of Indigenous People, for which an emic approach begins by asking local settlers about the conceptions of development that they use. Once this information is collected, the next phase is a quantitative phase, with close-ended questions carried out to identify levels of expectation for each conception of development and their respective perceptions of achievement. The result is a contrast between the expectations and the perceptions of achievements, like the one discussed in the conception of subjective life satisfaction, but this time focused on the development of the community (hence, the name "subjective development satisfaction"). In this chapter, we describe this process.

An Exploration of Mental Health

During the ethnographic phase of our study, some villagers and community authorities asked the researchers if they could provide psychological support for some community members reporting psychological difficulties. It is important to clarify that there are no mental health services in the community. This requirement was atypical among the many studies in Andean and Amazonian communities conducted by our research group. It was an interesting opportunity for a qualitative exploration, beyond epidemiological studies, about mental health in Andean communities of Indigenous People. One of the most renowned psychotherapists of Lima conducted the diagnostic interviews and intervention therapy (considering the limitations implied by the location of this remote community). It is evident that this approach does not have quantitative validity, and more qualitative studies are required. However, these findings can be considered preliminary evidence, and can be discussed in the context of well-being and development in Andean communities of Indigenous People.

The small traditional communities of the Andes are cultural groups that have inherited the ancestral pre-Columbian legacy of the Andes. As it usually happens in different cultures around the world, this legacy has undergone a complex adaptation process. Here, the process has taken place since these communities have had to interact with other pre-Columbian cultures, with the culture of the European invaders and genocides, and with the multiple migrations of the Peruvian republican period. Thus, the small traditional communities of the Andes maintain patterns of social organization, worldview, and cultural practices rooted in the ancient culture but they also inherit a complex syncretism. Regarding this syncretism, the word "Indigenous" cannot be used as easily in the Peruvian Andes as it can be used in the Amazon or in North America. In the Andean context, this word has turned into an offensive one, as people consider it a term to describe a subjugated and archaic group or a person possessing many negative characteristics. In fact, the word is generally used as a form of insult both by non-Indigenous people and among Indigenous People. Therefore, if one asks someone if they consider themselves Indigenous or not, the person may feel offended and the answers they give would lack validity. However, this does not imply that persons cannot be considered Indigenous in an academic and political sense. In this chapter, we use the word "Indigenous" solely as an academic term. However, the culturally correct term is "Andean community" and the culturally sensitive academic term is "small Andean traditional community." The purpose of this chapter is to describe subjective life satisfaction, subjective development satisfaction, and the general mental health patterns in the small Andean traditional community of Purhuaracra.

The Small Traditional Andean Community of Purhuaracra

To understand each community within its historic, geographical, and contextual reality, short ethnographic studies were carried out. A researcher was assigned to the place of interest, where interviews and observation of participants took place. Documents and existing studies of the site were also revised. The data collection was done in the year 2009.

The study was conducted in the community of Santa Rosa de Purhuaracra, known as Purhuaracra. This place belongs to the district of San Pedro de Cajas, located in the province of Tarma, which is at the south of the department of Junin. The community can be reached by a one-hour walk at a local pace (two and a half hours at an urban foreigner pace) from the district of San Pedro de Cajas through a mountain hike. Alternatively, there is access by way of an unpaved road that starts at the district of Palcamayo. In an automobile, the ride lasts about half an hour, and the cost of a car ride can be of US$ 6.50. Also, people can take a van ride for $ 0.60 U.S.); however, the van will not depart while it still has vacant seats. The majority of people in Purhuaracra do not own cars or other similar means of transportation.

The community of Purhuaracra is built into a mountainside. The Negrohuanusha, Antipayarguna, Putayoc, Viscamachey, and Mochihuagana springs are large, flowing streams of the Purhuaracra River, which crosses the slope.

The community of Santa Rosa of Purhuaracra produces tubers, grains, and vegetables. Among the principal tubers produced are potatoes, oca, ullucus, and mashuwa; among the grains, barley, wheat, and quinoa; and among the vegetables, onions, celery, lettuce, spinach, carrots, beets, turnips, and green peas. The crops are harvested either for consumption or for sale.

Within the community, houses usually have two floors and are made from adobe. The local school has a nursery, and a classroom constructed of bricks and cement has recently been built. The local Catholic Church is being rebuilt out of bricks and cement as well. A communal building has recently been put into use as a medical centre. The main square is an empty space located in the middle of the community. There is also a football field in an empty area on the outskirts of the community.

As to the basic services available in this place, most houses have electricity and get their water from the springs, but they have no sewage system. There is public lighting in the main street. Health services are provided by a nurse who visits the community three times per week. Most inhabitants own cellular phones and there is a communal satellite phone. Local children receive the benefits of the "Glass of Milk" programme, which is a social programme created by the national government that offers infants and seniors of poor communities a daily food ration. The extent of the programme does not cover the whole community and the rations provided are more of a complement than a supplement of daily food requirements.

It is important to mention that, unlike in some countries, where governments may provide some economic support to Indigenous families, Peruvian people must survive and progress on their own. Housing spaces are built by community labour. Whenever a family wishes to build a home, they will prepare adobe blocks and collect wood and other building materials for months. Then, they will summon a *Minka*, which is a communal gathering in which people build the house of a community member in 1 or 2 days. The person who was helped will then return the favour whenever a neighbour has a similar need. The *Minka* is not some form of forceful reciprocal labour; such events are organized as huge parties where nice meals are provided and all participants share a festive sense of humour. These end up being fun, memorable days for the locals. Also, the *Minka* usually includes several ancestral Andean rituals that can include sacrificing animals in exchange for a blessing for the new house.

Although the Peruvian government does finance public lighting and sewage, it involves a slow and complex requisition process, only to be placed in a waiting list of hundreds of communities. As mentioned, although the government does not provide funding for the daily expenses of local people, there are some programmes like the "Glass of Milk." However, these are not permanent, and they depend on the decisions of the political office-holders, who usually want them to serve the objectives of their next electoral campaign rather than to generate sustainable change in the community.

According to the results of the 1998 census, which was the most recent one that included this community, there are 61 families and a total of 191 inhabitants, of which 93 are men and 98 women. Of these, 71 are under age 18. The present study reports that Purhuaracra has about 90 housing units, of which five are abandoned. The main language spoken is Spanish. Although most of the population is Catholic, the Evangelic church is also present.

The community of Purhuaracra was founded more than 90 years ago. The first inhabitants were shepherds who first knew the area because they took their cattle to graze in nearby fields, and then decided to set up a community and started building Andean agricultural terraces, called *andenes*. About 40 years later, the Cave of Antipa Yarguna was discovered, which is in present times a main tourist attraction in the area. The construction of the unpaved road, about 20 years ago, enabled people to sell local products in big cities, such as Tarma in the highlands, and Lima in the coast. The road boosted the economy of the region and therefore led to a diversification of crops that had initially consisted only of tubers.

The community had only a municipal agency, with a lieutenant governor. There is also an organization of irrigators, and all active farmers who own agricultural lands are required to join, to promote and secure the equitable distribution of irrigation water among its users. Another important entity is the community organization that represents the people that reside in the area. It seeks to promote the development of the community and defends their interests and rights. The president of the community, who is the head of the community organization, holds the most influential position. Given the absence of state authorities (there are no police departments or law courts, for example), the community organization, which has been ruling communities for centuries, are the primary agents of central administration. Its functions include administrating local justice systems, resolving conflicts, and organizing communal labour for the maintenance and construction of roads, irrigation ditches, and other buildings for public use. In general, Purhuaracra is a small state with informal autonomy, where the absence of the Peruvian government promotes communal organization. Thorough centuries of trial and error, it appears to be very functional.

The community's nursery school has a permanent teacher and there are approximately 15 enrolled children. The primary school, "IE 30845," has two multi-level classrooms: one for students in grades one to three and another one for students in grades four to six. There is also a principal. In total, the school has approximately 45 students. Young people who wish to receive secondary education must go to San Pedro de Cajas district, or move to the capital city, Lima. As it was mentioned before, the community receives weekly visits from a nurse whose medical treatments are palliative and rely primarily on medical herbs. In cases of emergency or more serious illnesses, patients are transferred to the Palcamayo medical centre or the Tarma hospital. The usual diseases found in this community are parasite infestations, malnutrition (mainly in children), and acute respiratory infections. All the characteristics mentioned here describe a relatively typical small traditional Andean community.

Subjective Life Satisfaction, Subjective Development Satisfaction, and Mental Health: Method

Structured interviews with open-ended answers were administered once the ethnographic report was completed. These results were then processed by way of a content analysis technique, in which interviews answers are summarized in categories. These categories were then converted into the items of a psychometric battery that was applied in a third round of fieldwork.

Participants

A quota sampling was conducted based on the location and distribution of the community households. The community was divided into four big zones, each being proportional to the number of families. A total of 30 interviews were conducted for the qualitative phase and 60 psychometric tests for the quantitative phase. Given the difficulties most of the population had in reading, the items were read out loud to the participants and the answers they gave were marked by the field researchers.

Measure

An in-depth interview following the emic well-being components protocol (*Entrevista de Componentes de Bienestar,* or ECB: Yamamoto [001]) was used, applying the modules of goals and Indigenous conceptions of development. Results from the content analysis of the in-depth interviews guided the creation of the items of a psychometric test. The test contained two scales: subjective life satisfaction and subjective development satisfaction. Both measured the importance of each goal (life and development) and their corresponding perceptions of achievement. These tests were created following a previously used methodology [21, 002].

Analytical Technique

For the qualitative phase, a heuristic content analysis technique was used to analyze the in-depth interviews. In this technique, the answers are grouped into minimal categories that express the essence of the ideas given by the interviewees. This allows the formation of a complete list of categories for each variable of analysis, and it represents the total number of answers given by the sample regarding a specific variable. Based on that list of categories, a psychometric battery was created.

The subjective life satisfaction coefficient utilizes two variables from the quantitative scale: the goals and the perception of achievement of those goals. A statistical contrast test, in this case, the Wilcoxon signed-rank test, is used to determine if there is a statistically significant difference between the importance of a goal and its satisfaction. If there is no difference, it is labelled as state of equilibrium; if the difference indicates that the importance of a goal is greater than the perception of achievement of said goal, it is labelled as subjective life dissatisfaction; if the difference indicates that the perception of achievement of a goal is greater than the importance of said goal, it is labelled as subjective life satisfaction. In the case of subjective development satisfaction, the same procedures and evaluation criteria apply, except that the compared variables are the goals of community development and the perception of achievement of community development goals.

An Equilibrated Subjective Life Satisfaction with Subjective Development Dissatisfaction in Purhuaracra

The statistical contrasts reveal a generalized equilibrium in the personal goals of Purhuaracra community villagers. As seen in Table 2, Satisfaction is observed particularly with the people's own children, as well as with having a peaceful and quiet life, living in harmony with the neighbours, and having a good relationship with God. It is important to note that the scientific literature of happiness points out that these elements are key in promoting subjective well-being.

Regarding development, as seen in Table 3, a general subjective dissatisfaction is observed. The main development goals are the official recognition of San Pedro de Cajas, support from the government and financial entities, support for livestock farming, and the installation of a sewage system. Although these goals represent indicators of development, the scientific literature suggests that they are not key to the promotion of happiness. In this chapter, we discuss how having a balanced subjective life satisfaction and a general dissatisfaction with development can be interpreted.

Indications of Low Psychopathology in Purhuaracra

As noted, at the request of community members and authorities, a renowned psychotherapist was recruited to provide free psychological assistance for those who considered it necessary. A total of 12 individuals attended the services, which is an important number of people considering the community's population size.

The most frequent problem consisted in mothers having to deal with their children's disobedience (five cases). This was related to four cases of physical aggression and yelling as means of punishment. There also was the case of a father who

Table 2 Subjective life satisfaction in Purhuaracra

	Mean		Wilcoxon test	
	Goal	Achievement	Asymp. sig. (2-tailed)	Significance level
Health	2.53	2.50	0.739	EQ
Daily meals	2.48	2.45	0.758	EQ
Education for one's children	2.42	2.15	0.027	EQ[a]
Having a good relationship with God and/or with the church	2.42	2.65	0.004	SAT[b]
Improvement of the community	2.37	2.17	0.060	EQ
Having a job that allows buying food and supplying needs	2.37	2.23	0.170	EQ
Having a room or house to live on	2.33	2.03	0.021	EQ[a]
To live in a clean and nice place	2.33	2.25	0.409	EQ
Good relations with the family	2.30	2.75	0.000	SAT[b]
Having a job so a salary can be earned	2.28	1.32	0.000	IN[b]
Shop, buying, and selling	2.27	2.02	0.026	EQ[a]
Owning things for the house such as pots and furniture	2.27	2.12	0.116	EQ
To progress [improve]	2.27	2.18	0.419	EQ
To be part of the community	2.27	2.45	0.079	EQ
To have a good behaviour	2.27	2.45	0.028	EQ[a]
Peace and quietness, as well as the absence of violence or crime	2.27	2.78	0.000	SAT[b]
Electricity, water, or sewerage	2.25	2.15	0.260	EQ
Public transport	2.25	1.97	0.019	EQ[a]
To be a professional	2.22	1.08	0.000	IN[b]
Clothes	2.20	2.18	0.847	EQ
Marriage	2.20	2.32	0.364	EQ
Education for oneself	2.20	2.43	0.027	EQ[a]
To get along with neighbours	2.20	2.55	0.000	SAT[b]
A phone or another form of communication	2.18	1.92	0.033	EQ[a]
Teaching others what one knows	2.18	2.30	0.178	EQ
Friendship	2.17	2.50	0.000	SAT[b]
To have leisure spaces like sport complexes	2.15	1.77	0.002	IN[b]
Organized participation between neighbours	2.15	2.18	0.724	EQ
To own a means of transportation	2.13	1.12	0.000	IN[b]
Electronic devices such as a television, blender	2.07	1.70	0.003	IN[b]
Children	2.07	2.47	0.003	SAT[b]
Partner	2.05	2.33	0.025	EQ[a]
To be an authority, have power	1.90	1.08	0.000	IN[b]

(continued)

Table 2 (continued)

	Mean		Wilcoxon test	
	Goal	Achievement	Asymp. sig. (2-tailed)	Significance level
Assisting parties [attending festivities]	1.47	1.88	0.000	SAT[b]
Organize and fund the annual community celebration	1.40	1.95	0.000	SAT[b]

EQ is equilibrium; SAT is Satisfaction; IN is dissatisfaction
[a]Dissatisfaction or satisfaction found at a 0.05 level of significance
[b]Dissatisfaction or satisfaction found at a 0.01 level of significance

Table 3 Subjective development satisfaction in Purhuaracra

	Mean		Wilcoxon test	
	Goal	Achievement	Asymp. sig. (2-tailed)	Significance level
Official recognition by San Pedro de Cajas	2.60	1.15	0.00	IN[a]
Health post	2.48	1.78	0.00	EQ
Improving the highway	2.48	1.92	0.00	IN[a]
Support from government and financial entities	2.47	1.27	0.00	IN[a]
Water for irrigation	2.47	2.20	0.023	EQ[b]
Sewage	2.42	1.00	0.00	IN[a]
Support for livestock farming	2.42	1.08	0.00	IN[a]
Improvement in education	2.40	1.97	0.00	EQ
Technical improvements in agriculture	2.38	1.35	0.00	IN[a]
Communal place	2.35	1.48	0.00	EQ
Improve the council building	2.35	1.57	0.00	EQ
Better community authorities	2.33	2.33	1.00	IN[a]
Television signal	2.27	1.02	0.00	IN[a]
Refurbishment of the Catholic Church	2.22	2.07	0.165	IN[a]
Internet	2.08	1.00	0.00	IN[a]

EQ is equilibrium; SAT is Satisfaction; IN is dissatisfaction
[a]Dissatisfaction or satisfaction found at a 0.01 level of significance
[b]Dissatisfaction or satisfaction found at a 0.05 level of significance

did not provide economic support to his family and, another case with someone who had difficulty in making decisions.

Three women were identified as experiencing anxiety associated with threatening conditions. The main situations that triggered these anxieties were having their children living away from home. Anxiety was also related to economic difficulties in raising and educating children (one case), the infidelity of the husband (one case), not knowing how to teach children how to do their homework (one case), menopause symptoms (one case) and the irrational core belief that "one is worth nothing if things are not done in the way one wants them to be done" (one case). Finally, social anxiety disorders were also identified (in two cases).

Strategies for intervention were picked according to the needs of each person. For instance, to aid in promoting the obedience of children, mothers were trained how to give orders without yelling or being physically aggressive to the child. Assertive training and modelling was used too. The same strategies were applied to train the mothers in expressing physical affection and appreciation of their children, as in congratulating them for their obedience or for achieving academic success.

Training in communication skills was given to people who presented relationship problems with their spouses. They were taught how to reach agreement and how to express concerns. Regarding the cases of social anxiety, the interventions consisted in helping the individuals understand that they had social skills, but because they anticipated failure, they did not use them. Also, they were taught the technique of reality testing, which consists in showing the individual that it is better to rely on evidence-based facts rather than in the anticipated threats they create, which are usually based on several assumptions that are not necessarily true.

Psychoeducational techniques were applied in all the cases, which allowed the individuals to understand the variables of their problems, recognize that their problems had viable solutions, and hence, ease their anxiety.

The final comments of the individuals included them feeling calmer because they had a better understanding of their situation and feeling grateful for the help received. A workshop for mothers to improve their abilities in establishing discipline and obedience in their kids was requested and it was carried out in a subsequent session.

The identified problems do not indicate the presence of severe psychopathology in the community; moreover, these are typical difficulties of a family's daily life. If this is the case in other, similar communities, a mental healthcare programme could include preventive practices such as a "parent's school," in which mothers and fathers are trained in how to teach their children to obey. This can be done by explaining to them the negative effects of physical punishment and of verbally reprimanding the child, as well as showing them more efficient and healthy alternatives. Another recommendation for prevention and intervention can be oriented to help improve communication between couples. All these techniques could be summed up as problem-solving strategies for a variety of difficult situations that may occur. The intervention can address issues concerning primary or even secondary prevention, with a special emphasis on the latter.

In conclusion, there were no indications of severe and generalized psychopathology related to life conditions of the community. The problems found were those that usually occur in human coexistence. Only in one case of social anxiety disorder was psychotherapy considered. Relaxation techniques and other cognitive techniques could be taught to this individual to help them cope. Local healthcare providers could also be trained in these, as at present time they do not know how to use them.

Discussion: Unhappiness, Overdevelopment, and Psychopathology

Results suggest complex interactions between a state of happiness based on a balanced subjective life satisfaction and low levels of subjective satisfaction with development. On an exploratory level, the combination of these could be related to low levels of psychopathology.

The community of Indigenous People of Purhuaracra is surrounded by a clean and beautiful natural landscape; it remains isolated from media influences and the use of electronic devices is minimal. The enormous amount of time that urban people usually spend on gadgets and media is replaced by interactions with friends and family. Although this might seem inconceivable for some, it can actually be really fun, relaxing, and debt-free. Hence, spending quality time with family and friends is a crucial aspect of daily life in traditional Andean communities, whereas it is a bit less frequent in Andean towns and cities.

The intense interactions with family and friends, which usually bring together a whole community due to their small size, are sources of a neurotransmitter named oxytocin [22, 23]. The production of this has been associated with lasting feelings of well-being [24] and only a few side effects have been identified. Hence, it could be argued that small, traditional Andean communities are oxytocinergic societies. This means, in psychological terms, that the abundance of positive affect that can be found in them could be related to the extended and closely knit interpersonal relationships between community members. These could generate the feeling of living in a community of Indigenous People with effective support networks.

The oxytocinergic Indigenous society could be the opposite of what occurs in what could be called dopaminergic societies, such as Western occidental ones, whose psychological correlates could be described as peaks of intense affects followed by emotional downfalls. This may be due to the scarce interpersonal relationships combined by an intense consumerism and exciting experiences, activities known to produce dopamine shots in the brain. These behaviours are also characterized by having high peaks of intense emotions followed by periods of acute negative affect. If this peak-and-fall emotional pattern is intense and prolonged, it may generate co-lateral effects such as habituation and allostasis, meaning that, in time, increased doses of the dopamine-boosting stimuli will be needed to feel the same effects as before.

Daily routines in Purhuaracra consist basically of a limited number of chores that require intense physical labour, such as irrigating the lands, sowing them, caring for the crops, harvesting them, taking care of the cattle, and attending the responsibilities people may have in the community. In these places, there is no such thing as going to the gym to do a "healthy" cardio and weight-lifting workout. Yet, in a natural way, these people have a magnificent daily session of what Western cultures recently call "functional training." A difficult hike for a skilled mountaineer can be the route from home to work for an Andean. Thus, a routine consisting of simple chores and intense physical activity will also result in high levels of well-being, as well as in physical and mental health [27–29].

In Andean communities, people wake up at dawn to go to their plots of land and attend to irrigation rotation and look after other maintenance and agricultural tasks as needed. They may also graze their cattle or participate in a community activities such as maintaining access roads and water canals. Children are not absorbed in gadgets; they usually have defined household chores, such as bringing water from the springs or firewood for the kitchens. Although this may qualify as "child labour" in some Western cultures and may seem inhumane for some (in fact, it is forbidden by the International Labor Organization), from an alternative perspective, one could consider that a true inhumane and terrifying act would be to give children addictive electronic devices of rectangular shape that would deprive them of interactions with their family members that also satisfy a range of vital needs. This "labour" is also an important educational source of values and provides a sense of integration relating work, fun, and family. Moreover, the ethnographic observations that were carried out in this study showed that kids perceived these chores as fun games. This can also be observed in a more general level, because Andean and Amazonian daily life consists of ongoing jokes, laughter and *buena onda*—positive vibes there is no need for buying toys or free leisure time, as these seem to be free in the Andean daily routine. In addition, children do have plenty of playing time with friends, using the woods, the ravines, and the fauna as toys.

The life goals that were ranked higher on average in Purhuaracra were consistent with this scenario. These were health, daily meals, education for one's children, having a good relationship with God, and the development of the village community. These are also strongly related to the needs of the human species in ancestral contexts, which is where the human brain wired its last important mutation before becoming a "modern" *Homo sapiens*. In those times, the primary necessities were the satisfaction of basic survival needs, the continuity and improvement of lineage via sons and nephews, and the protection that God's blessing provided. All of these could be the indicators that a tribe was progressing.

Four of the most relatively important life goals of the people of Purhuaracra are at balance, meaning that there is not a statistically significant difference between the expectation levels and perception of achievement of these. The goal of "having a good relationship with God" is satisfied, which means that the perception of achievement is greater than the level of expectation. Considering all goals, a state of equilibrium can be observed, rather than one of subjective life satisfaction. In previous studies, a state of equilibrium instead of a subjective life satisfaction was more positively related to subjective well-being in Andean communities. This may occur because a state of satisfaction may implicate a society model based on achievement and continuous progress, which, however, could be more susceptible to stress and hedonic adaptation. In other words, as demands become greater in time, stress, the possibilities of frustration, and the physiological and psychological resources needed to constantly achieve new goals will also increase. Facing constant challenges may favour hedonic adaptation, as the constant exposure to pleasant stimuli may produce a decline in the pleasant effects these generate [28]. In contrast, a state of equilibrium represented by a traditional life with a controlled increase of goals and challenges may offer a different scenario. However, the tendency to slow changing traditions may also be related to a limited development. Once again, there arise suggestions of a complex paradox between subjective well-being and development.

Subjective satisfaction with development was found to be low—that is, generally unsatisfied—in Purhuaracra. The development goals are specific to the actual context of the community, which suggests that, as soon as Purhuaracra is politically recognized (political recognition is one of the more important development goals), another development goal would appear. The fact that development goals are closely related to specific contexts has been found in other studies about emic conceptions of development.

The most important goals regarding development were political recognition of the community's autonomy, as mentioned; a health post; improvement of the highway; more support from government and financial entities; and water for irrigation. Of these, the availability of health posts as well as water for irrigation are crucial elements for the community's development. As noted regarding life goals, being healthy was the most important goal for subjective life satisfaction, and having a health post would, at the community level, be fundamental for its achievement. This suggests that Purhuaracra's development goals are related to the context of their own situation, such as geography and needs, but also have issues related to core elements for survival and development.

A health post is the satisfied development need. Paradoxically, it does not have minimal medical equipment or a doctor. This demonstrates the importance of understanding subjective satisfaction as a contrast between expectations and achievements. Even though there is no 24-hour service, or a proper medical doctor, there is satisfaction. Nonetheless, the satisfaction may decline, and when it does, the search for more frequent service will start. Once this is obtained, the satisfaction could be experienced again. Eventually, it will decline and a more ambitious goal, such as having a licenced doctor present a few days a week, will surge. As in a circle, in the context of little development regarding health services, the road to progress may generate a positive hedonic impact, just as when rewards are given after each completed task in a video game. Yet, if we imagine a game in which all levels and rewards are obtained at once, the result would probably be quite boring. As this analogy shows, it is possible that, in a society in which social security systems are flawless and have nothing to improve, people could feel a hedonic void. Therefore, a strong state with the capacity to avidly and rapidly fulfil the basic needs of its population might generate a subjective satisfaction with development, yet its positive emotional impact will never be as high as the one generated by a weak state, where improvements tend to be difficultly obtained through tough negotiations and petitions brought about by the community's collective organization.

The pleasure produced by this ongoing improvement, which is a mechanism hardwired into the brain, may be a positive force for survival and getting ahead. However, when an equilibrated development is achieved, and resources are widely available, a rush to achieve things that are not related to the hardwired brain may arise. As a consequence, achieving these other goals will not result in the production of neurotransmitters of happiness. If these goals are oriented toward a competitive social dynamic instead of a cooperative life that promotes interdependence, close family bonds, and interactions with friends, then one of the most important boosters of happiness neurotransmitters will be inhibited. This further illustrates the paradox between (over)development and happiness.

Water for irrigation was another important development goal that appeared to be in balance. Given that Purhuaracra is an agricultural community, water is essential for their survival and development, and a crucial component of a good place to live. Official political recognition of the community, improvement of the highway, and support from government and financial entities are perceived by the community as goals that have not been satisfied. This dissatisfaction could be interpreted either as a frustration or a challenge. Given that the human brain has evolved in a context where extreme survival challenges were present, living in an environment in which everything is already "solved" (high levels of security and few survival-challenging goals left to achieve) may cause a sub-activation of challenge-pleasure neurotransmitters. This can be related to having no new vital tasks to deal with, or having vital tasks substituted by masturbatory-evolutionary chores as video games, sports, and compulsive consumption. As result, this absence of challenges could contribute to short-term hedonic peaks but long-term reduced levels of subjective well-being, more depressive episodes, and greater risk of psychopathology.

The hypothesis of the "zoo well-being syndrome" [9] proposed that urban societies with high levels of security could generate low levels of well-being and depression. Human beings have just not evolved enjoying the security provided by nature; rather, their ancestral story has been filled with great difficulties and challenges that favoured the development of a powerful hedonic system that allowed the species to adapt to these. Neuroscience investigations bring evidence of the existence of a related happy virtuous cycle. It activates itself whenever survival challenges are faced and immediately, the stress circuits are initiated. This is followed by increased levels of cortisol, which is a biomarker of stress. Cortisol then generates the production of oxytocin, which is felt as a motivation to seek for support in close relationships. When a person perceives that the support is being reciprocated, then the levels of cortisol are reduced and opioids are produced [29, 30]. Hence, when survival problems are being faced, although the presence of stressors may be high, subjective and physiological stresses are reduced. Moreover, a state of happiness emerges, resulting from the increased levels of opioids.

In contrast, if an Indigenous society had all its survival challenges solved at once by some sort of Scandinavian social security system, what was a step-by-step "real life video game" could turn into a deactivation of the challenge—collective agency—achievement—pleasure mechanism, which could promote depression and be related to psychopathological outputs. Therefore, a strong and rich state, oriented by the ideals of modern development and social security, could promote an environment that causes important reductions in levels of well-being, and potentially increases the rates of psychopathology. In contrast, an absent state with limited resources, could promote among communities of Indigenous People the development of a sense of belonging to the earth and the belief that certain situations can be changed, step by step. These steps can, in turn, be challenges that promote cooperation and, when fulfiled, could lead to a video-game-like pleasure of achievement—in other words, happiness, slow-aged development, and mental health.

The hypothesis of the "zoo well-being syndrome" proposes an explanation of unhappiness levels in the self-proclaimed "First World." This hypothesis can be extended to some of the so-called communities of Indigenous People in overdeveloped countries, magnificent ancient cultures incarcerated in prisons that go by the name of reserves.

It is important to note that these reflections are speculative, and more and epidemiological studies (with culturally sensitive measures) are needed. We are not suggesting by any means that Andean Indigenous communities should not receive more support from the state, nor do we believe that support that is being given to Indigenous groups in countries with strong governments should be reduced. We are strongly suggesting that the modern conceptions of happiness and development and their effects on mental health needs to be a topic of research and discussion. We are also suggesting that in contrast to the modern conceptions of well-being and development, the deep evolutionary roots of human nature should be considered as a foundation for happiness, development, and mental health. We also propose, based on the case presented in this chapter, that mental health prevention and intervention in Indigenous cultures should be revisited by giving proper consideration to the Indigenous culture and context, and not based on the policy-makers' culture, prejudices, and unhappiness.

Finally, we believe that we have to learn from Indigenous societies, instead of providing them with a model of unhappy development. The processes of cultural devastation imposed on United States and Canadian Indigenous groups are not only a matter of human rights; they are also a matter of lack of intelligence and sensitivity.

Acknowledgements The study reported in this chapter was supported by a grant from Pontificia Universidad Catolica's Dirección de Gestión de la Investigación. The authors are grateful to Jesus Aparicio, Cinthya Diaz, Cintia Arbulú, and Gonzalo Pons, research assistants for the study, and to Mariana Yompian for the assistance in writing this chapter. We are particularly grateful to Ramiro Castro, community leader of the Andean Indigenous Village of Huagapo, our main supporter and friend of our research group. We are also deeply grateful to the community leaders of Purhuaracra, Luciano Favian and Freddy Sánchez, for their logistical support, advice, and kindness.

References

1. Abdallah S, Michaelson J, Shah S, Stoll L, Marks N. Happy planet index: 2012 report. A global index of sustainable well-being. London: New Economics Foundation; 2012.
2. Abdallah S, Thompson S, Michaelson J, Marks N, Steuer N. The (un)happy planet index 2.0. London: New Economics Foundation; 2009.
3. Marks N, Abdallah S, Simms A, Thompson S. The unhappy planet index. London: New Economics Foundation; 2006.

4. Helliwell J, Layard R, Sachs J. World happiness report 2017. New York: Sustainable Development Solutions Network; 2017.
5. OECD. How's life? 2013: measuring Well-being. Paris: OECD Publishing; 2013. https://doi.org/10.1787/9789264201392-en.
6. WHO. Suicide rates; 2003. htttp://www.who.int/mental_health/prevention/suicide/suiciderates/en/
7. WHO. Sucide rates; 2015. http://gamapserver.who.int/gho/interactive_charts/mental_health/suicide_rates/atlas.html. Accessed 4 Feb 2018.
8. WHO. Depression and other common mental disorders: Global Health estimates. Geneva: World Health Organization; 2017.
9. Yamamoto J. The social psychology of Latin American happiness. In: Rojas M, editor. Handbook of happiness research in Latin America. Dordrecht: Springer; 2016. p. 31–49. https://doi.org/10.1007/978-94-017-7203-7_3.
10. Buss D. The evolution of happiness. Am Psychol. 2000;55(1):15–23.
11. Yamamoto J. Universal needs, cultural goals and development in context. towards a science of development. In: Rojas M, editor. The measurement of progress and well-being. Proposals from Latin America. Ciudad de Mexico: Foro Consultivo Científico y Tecnológico, AC; 2011. p. 93–102.
12. Reblin M, Uchino BN. Social and emotional support and its implication for health. Curr Opin Psychiatry. 2008;21(2):201.
13. Van den Berg AE, Jorgensen A, Wilson ER. Evaluating restoration in urban green spaces: does setting type make a difference? Landsc Urban Plan. 2014;127:173–81.
14. Berman MG, Jonides J, Kaplan S. The cognitive benefits of interacting with nature. Psychol Sci. 2008;19(12):1207–12.
15. Johnsen SÅK, Rydstedt LW. Active use of the natural environment for emotion regulation. Eur J Psychol. 2013;9(4):798–819.
16. Instituto Nacional de Salud Mental "Honorio Delgado—Hideyo Noguchi". Estudio Epidemiológico de Salud Mental en Lima y Callao—Replicación 2012. Lima: Instituto Nacional de Salud Mental "Honorio Delgado—Hideyo Noguchi"; 2013.
17. Instituto Nacional de Salud Mental "Honorio Delgado—Hideyo Noguchi". Estudio Epidemiológico de Salud Mental en la Sierra Rural 2008. Lima: Instituto Nacional de Salud Mental "Honorio Delgado—Hideyo Noguchi"; 2009.
18. Yamamoto J, Arévalo MV, Wendorff S. Diagnóstico e intervención psico-social en el terremoto de Pisco e Ica del 2007. Lima; 2008.
19. Yamamoto J, Feijoo AR, Lazarte A. Subjective wellbeing: an alternative approach. In: Copestake J, editor. Wellbeing and development in Peru. Local and universal views confronted. New York: Palgrave McMillian; 2008. p. 61–101.
20. Kasser T. Materialistic values and goals. Annu Rev Psychol. 2016;67(1):489–514. https://doi.org/10.1146/annurev-psych-122414-033344.
21. Yamamoto J, Meza R. Concepciones nativas de desarrollo y bienestar. Análisis intercultural de conflictos. Iquitos: Consorcio Focal Bosques—Instituto de Investigación de la Amazonía Peruana; 2004.
22. Yamamoto, J. El protocolo de entrevista a profundidad de componentes de bienestar. Pontificia universidad católica del Perú. Documento inédito. 2004.
23. Yamamoto J, Feijoo AR. La escala psicométrica de bienestar WQP. Pontificia universidad católica del Perú. 2005.
24. Donaldson ZR, Young LJ. Oxytocin, vasopressin, and the neurogenetics of sociality. Science (New York, N.Y.). 2008;322(5903):900–4. https://doi.org/10.1126/science.1158668.
25. Grewen KM, Girdler SS, Amico J, Light KC. Effects of partner support on resting oxytocin, cortisol, norepinephrine, and blood pressure before and after warm partner contact. Psychosom Med. 2005;67(4):531–8. https://doi.org/10.1097/01.psy.0000170341.88395.47.
26. Ishak WW, Kahloon M, Fakhry H. Oxytocin role in enhancing Well-being: a literature review. J Affect Disord. 2011;130(1–2):1–9. https://doi.org/10.1016/j.jad.2010.06.001.

27. Penedo FJ, Dahn JR. Exercise and Well-being: a review of mental and physical health benefits associated with physical activity. Curr Opin Psychiatry. 2005;18(2):189–93.
28. Rosenbaum, S., Tiedemann, A., & Ward, P. B. (2014). Meta-analysis physical activity interventions for people with mental illness: a systematic review and meta-analysis. J Clin Psychiatry, 75(0), 1–11.
29. Warburton DE, Nicol CW, Bredin SS. Health benefits of physical activity: the evidence. Can Med Assoc J. 2006;174(6):801–9.
30. Frederick S, Loewenstein G. 16 Hedonic adaptation. In: Kahneman D, Diener E, Schwarz N, editors. Well-being. The foundations of hedonic psychology. New York: Russell Sage; 1999. p. 302–29.
31. Heinrichs M, Baumgartner T, Kirschbaum C, Ehlert U. Social support and oxytocin interact to suppress cortisol and subjective responses to psychosocial stress. Biol Psychiatry. 2003;54(12):1389–98. https://doi.org/10.1016/s0006-3223(03)00465-7.
32. Taylor S, Gonzaga G. Affiliative responses to stress: a social neuroscience model. In: Harmon-Jones E, Winkielman P, editors. Social Neuroscience. Integrating biological and psychological explanations of social behavior. New York: The Guilford Press; 2007. p. 454–73.
33. UN General Assembly. Transforming our world : the 2030 agenda for sustainable development. United Nations; 2015.

Jorge Yamamoto is a Professor in the Psychology Department of Pontificia Universidad Catolica del Peru. He is also Founder of B y P Bienestar y Productividad Consultancy Group. Among other works, Yamamoto is author of *La Gran Estafa de la Felicidad* (2019); "The Social Psychology of Latin American Happiness," in M. Rojas (Ed.), *Handbook of Happiness Research in Latin America* (2016); "Necesidades universales, su concreción cultural y el desarrollo en su contexto: hacia una ciencia del desarrollo," in M. Rojas (Ed.), *La medición del progreso y del bienestar: Propuestas desde América Latina* (2011); "Un regard alternatif sur la subjectivité: le bien être des communautés andines," *Connexions* (2008); with A. R. Feijoo and A. Lazarte, "Subjective Wellbeing: An Alternative Approach," in J. Copestake (Ed.), *Wellbeing and Development in Peru: Local and Universal Views Confronted* (2008); and with R. Meza, *Concepciones nativas de desarrollo y bienestar: Análisis intercultural de conflictos* (2004).

María Victoria Arévalo is a Professor in the Psychology Department of Pontificia Universidad Catolica del Perú. She is Director of Studies at Instituto Peruano de Terapia Conductual Cognitiva. She is also a recipient of the National Psychology Award, 1994, awarded by the Peruvian Psychological Association. Arévalo's relevant publications include "Stress and extreme poverty in Peruvian women," *World Psychiatry* (2007).

Sebastián Wendorff is a Researcher on Well-being with the Culture and Development Research Group, Pontificia Universidad Católica del Perú. He has a Master's degree in research and intervention in social psychology at the Universitat Autónoma de Barcelona. He works as a social psychologist with research in stress, attitudes, subjective well-being, and close relationships. He is also a Presidente de la República Postgrado Internacional Scholarship winner. Wendorff's relevant publications include *Diagnostic of Habitability of Emergency Temporary Housing in Peru*, IEEE first Sustainable Cities Latin America Conference, with D. Rondinel, A. Acevedo, D. Albadra and N. Paszkiewicz (2019).

The Jewish People and Indigenous Resilience

Havatzelet Yahel

Like many Indigenous groups around the world, the Jewish people have suffered throughout history from various prohibitions and restrictions, forced assimilation and migration, bullying and deportations [1]. In different places, they have been treated as inferior to others and have been sent to live in ghettos. Their history is permeated with pogroms and killings and, in the mid-twentieth century, the Holocaust—a merciless, systematic genocide, in which 6 million Jews were murdered [2]. Many others were starved, tortured, and suffered from physical and mental trauma.

However, when we look at the Jewish people during the past decades, we witness an outstanding case study of resilience. We see a story of exceptional recovery from the ashes of the Holocaust, via a remarkable process of collective healing and growth. The Jewish people became a unique instance of a group of people who returned to their ancient homeland in order to revive their communal life and renew their biblical language, traditional calendar, and religious rituals. In 1948, the Jewish people gained independence and re-established a Jewish state.

In this chapter, I examine the Jewish people's resilience within the framework of Indigenous resilience studies. To that end, I look for examples of Jewish resilience practices that are similar to those described in the Indigenous literature. I do not claim, however, to provide a comprehensive analysis of all Jewish resilience and healing methods, and I certainly do not pretend to declare that I have found the key or keys to their relative success.

H. Yahel (✉)
Ben-Gurion Institute for the Study of Israel & Zionism, Ben-Gurion University of the Negev, Midreshet Ben-Gurion, Israel
e-mail: yahelh@bgu.ac.il

D. Danto, M. Zangeneh (eds.), *Indigenous Knowledge and Mental Health*,
https://doi.org/10.1007/978-3-030-71346-1_9

Not much has been written about the Jews in the context of the broader Indigenous international phenomenon. This chapter is the first discussion of Jewish resilience as part of the broader Indigenous framework that I know of.

First, I provide an overview of the development of the Indigenous discourse in the international arena. Next, I briefly introduce the literature on the resilience of Indigenous People. Following that introduction, I review the long history of the Jewish people and their resilience, first only in general terms, and then examining some of the means and methods of resilience they have used to ensure their historical and cultural continuity. Finally, before my concluding remarks, I shed light on three prominent figures whose writings can help in the understanding of the Jewish way of thinking and means and methods of resilience.

Indigenous Discourse in the International Arena

The use of the term "Indigenous" to describe groups of people, in its current political meaning, developed mainly in the nineteenth and the twentieth centuries. It gained momentum in recent decades with the assistance of the international platform given to Indigenous People's movements. These include, among others, working groups, regional and international forums, media coverage, experts and advisers, and generous funding. In 2007, the United Nation (UN), by a very large majority, adopted the Declaration on the Rights of Indigenous Peoples (DRIP). The DRIP is designed, first and foremost, to safeguard the survival and success of the Indigenous way of life, its cultures, and its traditions.

It seems that in the twenty-first century, the Indigenous discourse is more appealing than ever, and gradually, an increasing number of groups wish to be included.

The member states in the UN could not reach agreement about which groups should be defined as "Indigenous People." Therefore, the DRIP does not include a definition. This creates confusion, vagueness, and uncertainty in the use of the term. Without a clear definition, the protection and the limited resources that the international community has dedicated to Indigenous Peoples could reach groups that have minimal similarities with each other. While there are countries where the bare existence of an Indigenous People was recognized long ago, as with the North American Indians, there are many places where indigeneity is debated, and where questions arise as to the validity of such claims regarding particular groups. One of these places is the State of Israel, where competing groups claim the same territory based on historical ties. Many scholars have offered definitions [3–7]. One of the first and most used definitions was given by José Martinez Cobo [8]:

> Indigenous communities, peoples and nations are those which, having a historical continuity with *pre-invasion and pre-colonial societies* that developed on their territories, consider themselves *distinct* from other sectors of the societies now prevailing in those territories, or parts of them. They form at present *non-dominant sectors* of society and are determined to preserve, develop and transmit to future generations their ancestral territories, and their

> ethnic identity, as the basis of their *continued existence as peoples*, in accordance with their *own cultural patterns, social institutions and legal systems* [emphasis added] ([8], p. 29).

Yahel, Kark, and Franzman [7] offered a list of parameters commonly used when describing Indigenous communities: They are original inhabitants who have lived on the land from time immemorial, before imperialist newcomers arrived; they had pre-colonial sovereignty; they have experienced oppression by a foreign culture and legal regime; they have a unique common relationship, of a spiritual nature, with the land on which they lived or have lived; they are distinct, nondominant populations, with separate customary, cultural, economic, social, and political institutions; and they identify themselves and are recognized by others as Indigenous. Siegfried Wiessner, former Chair of the International Law Association (ILA) Committee on the Rights of Indigenous Peoples, wrote:

> Indigenous communities are still best conceived of as peoples *traditionally regarded, and self defined, as descendants of the original inhabitants of lands with which they share a strong, often spiritual bond.* These peoples are, and desire to be, culturally, socially and/or economically distinct from the dominant groups in society, at the hands of which they have suffered, in past or present, a pervasive pattern of subjugation, marginalization, dispossession, exclusion and discrimination. [emphasis added] [103]

Wiessner stressed that while the first sentence of his definition expresses indispensable elements to the characterization of a people as Indigenous, the second sentence includes features and experiences of the ideal type of an Indigenous community which may be lacking in individual cases. Following Weissner's definition in describing the history of the Jewish people means elaborating on elements of origin, self-perception, spiritual connection to land, and international recognition.

Resilience and Mental Healing of Indigenous People

Many studies have dealt with the difficulties faced by Indigenous People and the special ways they have developed in order to cope with them. This book focuses on means and methods of resilience that have been developed by Indigenous Peoples in various parts of the world, and hence, in this chapter, I am also focused on this aspect.

Numerous studies have indicated that there are places in the world, such as North America, where Indigenous Peoples suffer from extraordinary challenges, including higher rates of mental health problems. Several scholars have pointed to the social origin of the problems and have therefore argued for the promotion of social and political solutions. The mental health issues that Indigenous Peoples suffer from include higher rates of suicides, addictions, such as alcoholism and drugs, violence, intergenerational trauma, depression, and pervasive demoralization [9–14]. Kirmayer, Simpson, and Cargo [10] emphasized the need of people studying the situation to go beyond the individuals while looking for healing. They looked at the

Indigenous identity as a unique resource for mental health ([10], p. 21). In a later study, Kirmayer et al. [15] raised their concern that "exclusive attention to individual mental health problems may deflect attention from the larger social structural problems …" ([15], p. 27).

Scholars have suggested ways and practices that can help in the recovery processes. Kirmayer et al. [10] stressed three major aspects of resilience: "[k]nowledge of living on the land, community connectedness, and historical consciousness" ([10], p. 21). In an earlier study, Kirmayer, Brass, and Tait [9] pointed to the role of community institutions, and mainly the importance of group's control over them. They also stressed the place of cultural continuity ([9], p. 614). The role of cultural continuity is also emphasized in Chandler and Lalonde's studies [16, 17].

Marsh et al. [12] found that strengthening cultural identity, community integration, and political empowerment improved mental health, and they called for blending Indigenous and Western healing methods [12]. The significance of the land in the healing process is emphasized in the study by Matthew and colleagues ([18], pp. I–XV). Additionally, Brady [19] raised concerns that using cultural and spiritual ways of healing (culture as treatment) is ineffective to deal with addictions, unless they succeed also in creating a platform that disvalues such activities.

In 2009, Chandler and Lalonde [17] offered variables of "cultural continuity" that are correlated, according to them, with fewer suicides. These include traditional lands; self-government; community control over services of education, police, fire, and health; cultural facilities; participation of women in local governance (a measure that is important within the historically matrilineal First Nations in Canada); and provision of child and family services within the community (pp. 238–9).

Poonwassie and Charter [20] suggested empowering approaches to heal Indigenous communities. They argued that traditional Indigenous cultures have a broad worldview that includes the perception of "the wheel of life" and specific cultural imperatives. These influence their beliefs and actions and therefore must be learned and respected in order to support the healing process. Arguing that each nation should identify its own Healers and healing process, they have elaborated on several healing approaches that are important for the empowering process: storytelling, teaching, and sharing circles, participation in ceremonies, and the use of role modeling ([20], pp. 65–69). In addition, they point to the importance of collaborations and supporters from outside, such as governments that "understand and accept that Aboriginal people have practiced viable healing methods based on their worldview throughout their history …" ([20], p. 70).

Kirmayer et al. [21] have indicated several strategies which have been implemented by different Indigenous communities and have helped their resilience. Their list included narratives of historical identity and continuity, and the revitalization of culture, language, and tradition. They gave examples of the Mohawk people who found pride in their resistance ability, the Métis, who are proud of being self-reliant and resourceful, and the Inuit, whose concept of resilience has resonated with the concept of hope—"Faced with adversity, people talk of hope and wait for it to reveal itself" (p. 88).

Later in this chapter, I look at examples of the approaches that have been implemented by the Jewish people in their resilience and healing process.

The Jewish People—Historical Landmarks

The history of the Jews and their emergence onto the world stage are popular and highly debated research topics. Various scholars hold different approaches to the earliest date one can point to "Judaism" or "Jewish people." Some scholars argue that either Jewishness is merely a religion or, otherwise, a relatively new invented phenomenon of the late nineteenth century [22]. However, these views remain in the margins and does not hold true for the prevailing Jewish perception as well as academic circles [23].

The Jewish people, also called People of Israel (A'm Israel), were originally an Iron Age Semitic-speaking population that developed a distinct monotheistic religion. Jewish ethnicity and religion are strongly interrelated. Judaism, although it has changed greatly over the years, is the traditional faith of the Jewish people. They have a canonical collection of texts, most notably, the Hebrew Bible [Tanakh]. Parallel to the Tanakh is the oral history [Oral Torah], which includes traditions and discussions of Jewish Sages (Chazal).

According to the Jewish faith, the relations between the Jewish people and Eretz Israel (the Land of Israel) are spiritual and were the result of divine promise. The promise is described in the book of Genesis (15:18–21) and states that God made a convent with Abraham, the founding father of the Jewish people, and promised that his descendants would inherit a land from the Red Sea to the Mediterranean Sea, and from the desert to the Euphrates River (as in Exodus 23:31).[1] God confirmed the promise to Abraham's son Isaac, and then to Isaac's son Jacob (Genesis 26:3). This promise is embedded in the term "Promised Land." The biblical story continues that Jacob, who was awarded the name Israel (Genesis 32:29),[2] was invited to Egypt by Pharaoh, the king of ancient Egypt. He immigrated with 10 of his sons, and joined their long-lost brother, Joseph (Genesis 46:5). This is the period known as the patriarchal age, around the seventeenth century BCE.[3] During their time in Egypt, a new king enslaved the group (Exodus 1:13), from now on called Sons of Israel (Bnei Israel), Israelites, or People of Israel in the Bible (Exodus 1:9). According to the book of Exodus, Moses was chosen by God to lead their exodus from Egypt to Eretz Israel (Exodus 3:9–17). On their way through the desert, the Twelve Tribes of Israelites, descendants of the 10 sons of Jacob and the two sons of Joseph, received

---

[1] The borders are mentioned several times. See for example: *Exodus* 23:31.

[2] See also Knohl [24].

[3] See theories about the Patriarchal Age in Finkelstein and Silberman [25].

the Ten Commandments (Exodus 20:2–14, Deuteronomy 10:4). Moses' successor Joshua led the Israelites to conquer Canaan.

The promise, the journey, the exile, and the return to the land are central motives in the Jewish historical narrative [26]. In Eretz Israel, the Israelites were sovereign under a sequence of biblical judges and kings. King David made Jerusalem, also called Zion, his capital (II Samuel 5:6–10; First Chronicles 11:4–19; [25]).[4] Solomon, David's son, built the First Temple in Jerusalem. After his death, the monarchy split into two: the Kingdom of Israel in the north of Eretz Israel and the Kingdom of Judea (Yehudah) in the south [27, 93]. During the eighth century BCE, the Kingdom of Israel was conquered and its people were exiled by the Assyrians (II Kings 17:6; I Chronicles 5:26; Jerusalem Talmud, Sanhedrin, 10:6).[5] The fate of the Assyrian's exiles is unknown (Babylonian Talmud, Sanhedrin, 84:1; Yevamot, 17:2).[6] Modern Jews are considered to be the descendants of the people of the Kingdom of Judea, who were themselves later exiled by the Babylonians during the sixth century BCE (Jeremiah 52:12ff; II Kings 25:8). A considerable segment of the population was deported,[7] and this had traumatic and unforgettable effects on Jewish life and Jewish thought. The period of exile developed and shaped the Jewish collective identity and religion, as the Sages were focused on continuity on the one hand, and change in accord with the new conditions on the other, mainly reshaping traditions and rituals that were connected to Eretz Israel and the Temple [31].

According to biblical sources, Cyrus, king of Persia, ended the Babylonian captivity after 70 years [32–34].[8] This event is called the Return to Zion (Shivat Zion) in Jewish tradition, and from then on, the word Zion has also referred to Eretz Israel in general, even though the return was only to some areas, mainly Judea. The returnees rebuilt the Second Temple in the same place as the first in Jerusalem (Ezra 2; Babylonian Talmud, Megila, 17:2; Jerusalem Talmud, Brachot 2:4) (see Fig. 1 Jewish praying in the Western Wall in Jerusalem).

Eretz Israel was under the control of various non-Jewish rulers over the course of approximately four centuries. The Maccabean revolt took place against the

[4] Scholars debate over the extent and existence of the United Kingdom during David and Solomon periods. See Finkelstein and Silberman [25].

[5] Tiglath-Pileser III of Assyria in 733 BCE, and the final destruction of the kingdom by Sargon II in 722 BCE. Descriptions of the event can be found in many sources such as *II Book of Kings*, 17:6; I *Books of Chronicles*, 5:26; *The Jerusalem Talmud*, Sanhedrin, 10:6.

[6] References to them are found in Talmudic sources such as the *Babylonian Talmud*, Sanhedrin,84:1; *Babylonian Talmud*, Yevamot, 17:2. Some scholars such as Parfitt Tudor argue that the ten tribes are a myth [28]. Over the years, several hypotheses have been raised regarding the affiliation of groups as descendants of the 10 tribes, but no clear evidence has been found [29, 30].

[7] In 597 BCE and again in 586 BCE by the Neo-Babylonian Empire under the rule of Nebuchadnezzar II

[8] The exact time of the return is disputed. Details on the exile periods are in the Books of Ezra (1:1–4) and Nehemiah; however, scholars regard them as tendentious ([34]; Free Vos Howard 1992; [32]).

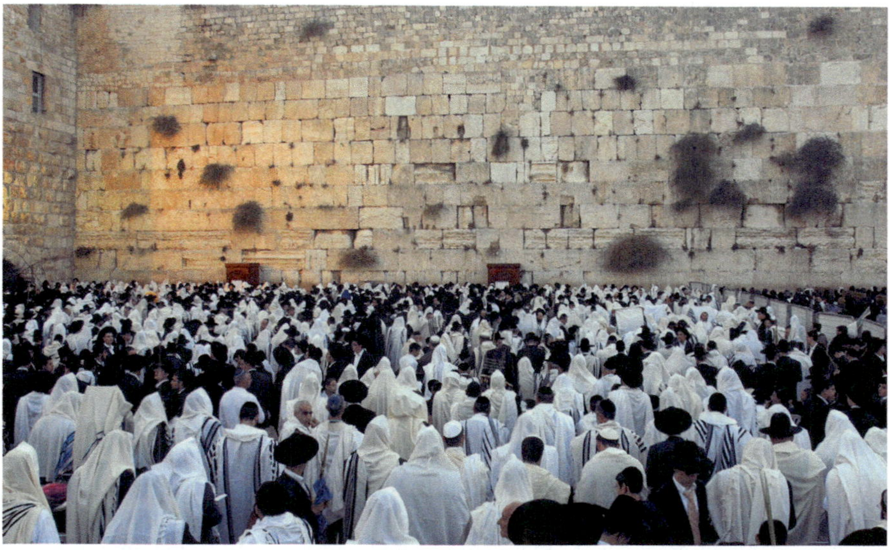

Fig. 1 Worshippers praying at the western wall in Jerusalem during the "Succot" holiday. Photo: Mark Neyman. 17 October 2008. Source: National Photo Collection, Israel Government Press Office

Hellenistic regime which converted Jerusalem into a Greek polis (II Maccabim 4; [35]). After several years of battle, the Seleucid Empire agreed to a political compromise and granted the Jewish Hasmonean leadership religious autonomy in Judea [36, 37].[9] In the following years, religious autonomy was gradually extended to political independence [99–101]. In 140 BCE, under the reign of Shimon, the Seleucids abolished the collection of taxes, while in 129 BCE, Judea was freed from Seleucid rule [38]. The Hasmonean dynasty expanded their conquests to the north and to the east [39, 40, 92]. Jewish culture and traditions were instituted in Judea, Edom, Transjordan, and the Golan, where the Jews were the majority population [41].[10]

The independent Jewish Hasmonean kingdom was ended by the conquest of Pompey in 63 BCE, and it was turned it into a Roman protectorate. This loss of independence lasted until the establishment of the State of Israel, more than 1800 years later.

The Romans ruled, with some minor hiatuses, for the next seven centuries. During their rule and as an outcome of a Jewish revolt, the Second Temple was

[9] Hanukka, a Jewish holiday is celebrated as a reminder of the Maccabees' victory and the rededication of the Temple. The story of Hanukkah is preserved in the First and Second books of Maccabees [36, 37].

[10] There were massive conversions in the annexed territories, such as the Edomites [41].

destroyed [42], a large part of the Jewish population were massacred and enslaved, lands were confiscated [43], and the Jewish community in Eretz Israel was almost exterminated [44].

The Jewish community in exile established alternative religious centers; the strongest developed in Babylon. With no Temple, the Jewish political and religious leadership that remained had to face the problematic reality and make adjustments. The Sanhedrin [Jewish court] played a central role in the new circumstances. The Sages collected and recorded the Oral Torah, developed the Yeshivot (Jewish rabbinic academies), and structured the Jewish way of life in the Diaspora. The belief that life in the Diaspora was temporary, while constantly being reminded of Eretz Israel, helped in preserving the unity and continuity of the people [45]. Meanwhile, following the Muslim conquest of Eretz Israel in the seventh century, there was increased movement of Arab immigrants. Over the next nine centuries, various foreign Muslim and non-Muslim occupiers controlled the region [46].

In the Diaspora, under Christendom and Islam, Jewish communities maintained their institutions and central Yeshivot in Babylon and Eretz Israel. Occasionally, Jewish communities suffered from the tyranny of the regimes and the hostility of local residents in areas where they were hosted and lived. With the emergence of nation-states, Jews had to make political compromises. They were asked to give up their uniqueness and to assimilate into the host nation-state in order to become an equal or merely tolerated religious or ethnic minority. But the new era of Enlightenment did not favor the Jews. In many places, a modern form of anti-Semitism emerged. As Jews became disillusioned with their dream of integration as equals in the general society, and as they were excluded from emancipation, some Jewish groups believed that the long-standing territorial connection to Zion could provide the solution for the collective future of the Jewish people [47]. The Zionist movement gathered momentum while promoting the idea that the only solution was the revival of Jewish culture and Hebrew language, the ingathering of the exiles in Zion, and the establishment of independent Jewish sovereignty. To that end, the Zionist movement established cultural, educational, and economic bodies, and acted externally in order to get international recognition for the inherent right of the Jewish nation to return to its historical and spiritual homeland. The Balfour Declaration, issued by the British government in 1917, and the terms of the British Mandate for Palestine in 1922 are two important expressions of Zionist success in gaining such external recognition [89].

However, in the following years, while Jews and Arabs argued about the future of the Jewish people in the Eretz Israel, the cruelest and most terrible plot in the modern era against the Jewish people was put into effect—the Holocaust. A systematic annihilation of the Jewish people was carried out by Nazi Germany, resulting in the murder of an estimated 6 million Jews [48–50]. The Holocaust trauma affected not only Jewish survivors, but also their second and third generations and further expanding circles [51].

Finally, in 1947 the UN General Assembly voted in favor of the partition of Palestine into two separate states [52]. This decision was the ultimate expression of the international community in recognizing the right of the Jewish people for sovereignty and to revive their communal life in their ancient homeland. The State of Israel's Declaration of Independence anchored the basic beliefs and aspirations of the Jewish people, while regarding Eretz Israel as the birthplace of the Jewish nation, where their spiritual, religious, and political identity was shaped (Ministry of Foreign Affairs; [53, 96]).

The Jewish people had regained sovereignty in the land of their ancestors. Since then, 70 years have passed and the lives of the Jewish people in Israel are tremendously different, in many physical and mental aspects, from the lives of the majority of their ancestors. The Israel of today, although far from perfect, and suffering from security challenges, social gaps, the conflict between Arabs and Jews, and other major concerns, is a developed country and a vibrant democracy, with a rich cultural and spiritual life. It is an Organization for Economic Co-operation and Development member, ranking 22 out of 189 in the UN Human Development Index of 2019 [54].[11] Furthermore, in an index that measures people's happiness by countries, the World Happiness Report (WHR), published by the UN Sustainable Development Solutions Network, ranked Israel 11 out of 156 countries [55]. The rate of suicides in Israel is one of the lowest in the Western world [56].[12] Israel has recently become known as the "start-up nation," famous for its having more start-up companies than large, peaceful, and stable nations [57].

Jewish Sources of Resilience

From the abovementioned general literature on indigeneity, we may draw up a list of the main Indigenous sources of strength. That list includes historical continuity and cultural identity; storytelling, teaching, and sharing; knowledge of living on traditional lands; community connections; self-governance institutions and control over services; and language, pride, resourcefulness, and hope. Having reviewed some of the more significant chapters of Jewish history, I turn now to the people's means and methods of resilience and some of the ways in which they used them, keeping in mind that others exist.

Jewish historical continuity, cultural identity, and storytelling of collective memory: During the years of existential difficulties, Jewish people used a variety of tools

[11] This index focuses on the richness of human lives while integrating three basic dimensions of human development: life expectancy at birth; mean years of schooling and expected years of schooling which reflect the ability to acquire knowledge; and gross national income per capita which reflects the ability to achieve a decent standard of living [54].

[12] Preceded only by Greece and Cyprus [56].

and mechanisms to ensure their historical and cultural continuity. They retain the Jewish canonical book, the Bible, which provided the shared historical narrative of the Jewish people. The oral traditions of the Halakha developed and framed Jewish cultural identity. The Halakha was transmitted orally for hundreds of years until it was put into writing. It contains the central body of Jewish religious laws, and it shaped Jewish daily life for generations. The Halakha laws played a major role in preserving the separateness of the Jewish people. The Halakha books include interpretation of biblical texts. Alongside the Halakha, the compendium of Haggada (legends, lore) also developed as part of Jewish cultural heritage [58]. The Haggada includes Jewish folklore and anecdotes, as well as moral and practical advice [59, 60]. Jewish cultural continuity was also strengthened by a focus on constant learning, debating, and analyzing Jewish texts. These shaped and developed Jewish philosophy and ways of thinking. The collection of literature, along with placing learning at the center of life, played an important role in making Jewish knowledge accessible to the members of the communities and thus preserving it.

The act of transmitting Jewish collective memory is prominent in Jewish daily life. Some historical events are included in daily prayers. All chapters of the Torah (the first five books of the Tanakh) are read in an annual cycle. Each week one chapter is read, taught, and explained in the synagogues. Furthermore, traditional rituals of history telling are included on special days. The most popular is the Seder, a ceremony during Passover dinner, when families traditionally gather and spend the evening telling the younger generation the story of the Jewish Exodus from Egypt (see Fig. 2 a family celebrating the Seder).

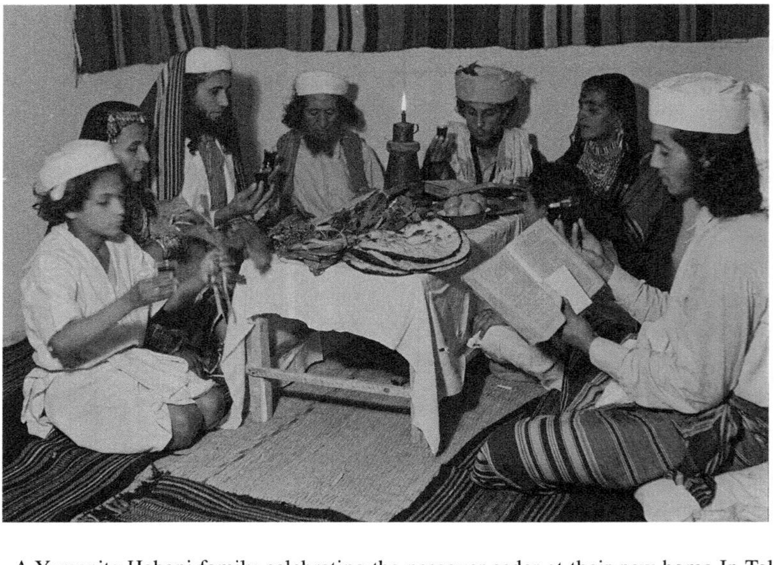

Fig. 2 A Yemenite Habani family celebrating the passover seder at their new home In Tel Aviv. Photo: Kluger Zoltan. 1 April 1946. Source: National Photo Collection, Israel Government Press Office

Resourcefulness and *pride:* Many biblical stories emphasize the resourcefulness and the ability of the people who survived, when acting against all those who tried to vanquish them. The story of David's victory over Goliath, the giant Philistine, is perhaps the most well-known (I Samuel, 17–18). Resourcefulness is also the essence of several Jewish celebrations. The celebration of Purim, another Jewish holiday, is an example in which the Jews commemorate the resourcefulness of Queen Esther and her uncle, Mordechai, who rescued the Jewish people from an attempt by Haman, the Persian king's deputy, to kill them all (Book of Esther). The Passover Seder is one example of the ability of the Jews to escape from a strong army. The Jewish holiday of Hanukah commemorates the rededication of the Second Temple in Jerusalem at the time of the Maccabean Revolt against the Seleucid Empire. The importance of the need to refer to successes was understood by the Zionist movement; while calling for the Jewish Return to Zion, they found symbols of courage and resourcefulness in the stories of the Maccabees as well as in other stories of victories and ancient achievements [61, 62, 90].

Community: There many examples acknowledging the vital function of community for public resilience and survival. When the Second Temple was destroyed, the Jewish Sages commanded the building of synagogues as places for communal Jewish gathering and praying. The Hebrew term for synagogues is Beit-Knesset, which means a house of gathering. The obligation to pray together in synagogues put the community in the center of Jewish life, and enabled those who were illiterate to hear a prayer from a public emissary. In other words, the public was obliged to gather and create a framework of spiritual support (Babylonian Talmud, Berachot, 8:1).[13] Furthermore, to ensure that people would gather together, a quorum of 10 Jewish adult men (Minyan) is required for certain religious rituals (Bablonian Talmud, Berachot, 21:2). The Torah also contains many provisions designed to protect and support the weak by creating welfare bodies. Society bears responsibility for each of its members, especially the less fortunate ones, and the strength of society rests on the way it protects its weakest members (Deuteronomy 24:10–22, 14:28–29; Leviticus 22:20–23; [63]). Many of the Commandments are connected to helping the poor and needy, while promoting ideas of social justice (Deuteronomy 15:11; Leviticus 23:22).[14]

Language: Common language is also a source of strength for the Jewish people. During many decades in the Diaspora, Hebrew was taught as a holy language and was used for the reading of the Torah. It was common for Jewish children at an early age to memorize biblical texts in Hebrew by heart and to gain skills in Hebrew writing and reading. Retaining the knowledge of Hebrew alongside their local language in the Diaspora enabled Jews around the world to stay connected. When the State of Israel was established, Hebrew became its spoken and official language.

[13] The ones who do not join are called "bad neighbours." *Babylonian Talmud*, Berachot 8:1.

[14] *Deuteronomy* 15:11: "For the poor will never cease out of the land; therefor I command you, you shall open wide your hand to your brother, to the needy and to the poor, in the land." *Leviticus* 23:22 commands not to harvest the corners of the field, or to pick the last fruit from the tree, to be left for the poor. Contribution of the tenth part of production to widows and the orphans.

Hope: The concept of hope is also a basic theme [64–66]. In the Jewish context, hope is highly connected to the memory of exile and freedom. The hope for a better future helped to maintain Jewish peoplehood during the long periods of exile. The exact character of Jewish hope, its precise role in Jewish life, and what exactly it meant during history became a focus for studies [67]. The term "hope" plays an important role in Jewish daily rituals, prayers, religious Jewish music *(Piyyut)*, songs, and literature. The best evidence for the centrality of hope for the Jewish people can be understood by the fact that the State of Israel adopted "HaTikva" (The Hope) as its national anthem. The words of the anthem reflect the spiritual, historical, and even existential connections between the Jewish people and Zion, and the hope of being free people in their own land.

Self-governance institutions: These were integral to the Jewish people's lives for thousands of years. One example is the establishment of a judicial system by Moses, either symbolic or not, as described in the book of Genesis. That institution more or less functioned for generations (Genesis 18; [68]), from the period of Moses' rule, through the days of the judges and kings, to the establishment of the Great Sanhedrin and the leadership of high priests, presidents, and Supreme Court judges. Even when the Jews were dispersed throughout the Diaspora, they maintained and financed self-governance institutions, such as appointed rabbis and self-help associations [69, 70].[15] This was done with or without outside approval. Furthermore, communities in the Diaspora maintained connections with each other and shared a web of knowledge and values and offered help when needed. When the Zionist movement emerged, it was able to make use of that web of communication to spread its ideas.

Traditional lands: The vital role that the land of Eretz Israel played in Jewish people's lives is manifested in their prayers, rituals, and customs. As Eliezer Schweid put it: "The Bible is more than simply the collection of ideas, concepts, and symbols that the Jewish people has drawn upon, directly or indirectly, in every generation; it is in itself the spiritual link between the people and its land" [45]. From the book of Genesis we learn of the covenant between God and Abraham relating to the Promised Land. The Bible continues with numerous events, physical and spiritual, that occurred in Eretz Israel. When the Temple was built, it became the central holy place for Jewish worship and pilgrimage. Even when the Temple was destroyed, while the majority of the people lived in the Diaspora, Jerusalem in particular and Eretz Israel in general did not lose their spiritual roles [71]. The need to return to ancestral land is strongly manifested in the Jewish texts and traditions. Examples can be found in Jewish prayers that abundantly quote from the Book of Psalms (Psalms 120–134). When praying, Jews constantly remind themselves of the temporary exile and pray for a return to their homeland. The phrase "Next year in Jerusalem!" *(LeShana Habaah BeYerushalayim)* marks the end of the Yom Kippur service in the synagogue as well as the end of the Passover Seder [72]. Prayers in the Diaspora are directed toward Eretz Israel (Tosefta, Berachot, 3:16 [102]).

[15] One example is the case of the Jewish communities in Italy [69, 70].

Moreover, the Hebrew calendar is based on the seasons of the year in Eretz Israel. Each of the central three Jewish festivals, Passover, Shavuot, and Sukkoth, are connected to a particular agricultural season (Deuteronomy, 16:1; Exodus 24:22, Deuteronomy 16:13). The specific ceremonies on these holidays and others are specifically related to the realities of life in Eretz Israel.

Influential Statements of Resilience from Jewish Leaders

Jewish sayings, phrases, and poetry can provide additional insights for understanding Jewish sources of resilience. To the best of my knowledge, these examples give a proper representation of the sources of strength that have evolved over the years, as well as the way the Jewish people view themselves, their tasks, and their connection to Eretz Israel. In this section, I present three examples of statements taken from different periods in Jewish history. These words greatly influenced subsequent generations. They have been cited on numerous occasions and are often included in public speeches and lectures. They are regularly taught in schools and have become an integral part of the Israeli curriculum. The first example is a Talmudic phrase quoting Hillel the Elder who lived approximately 2000 years ago; the second is a section of a poem by Yehuda Halevy, dating from about 1000 years ago, and the third are words written by Theodore Herzl 120 years ago.

"If I Am Not for Myself, Who Will Be for Me?"

The first example is perhaps the most famous saying of Hillel the Elder [91]. Hillel was a predominant Jewish leader and scholar who died in 10 CE [73].[16] He was the president of the Sanhedrin during the reign of Herod. The independent state ruled by the Hasmoneans came to an end with the victory of Pompey in 63 BCE, and Judea was forced to become a protectorate of Rome, which is remembered as a traumatic event. Herod, who came to power under the aegis of the Roman Empire, used terror to secure his throne. That included the execution of 21 members of the Sanhedrin. Although Herod renovated Temple Mount, the Jewish traditional way of life was challenged [74, 97, 98]. In that highly problematic and challenging context, Hillel the Elder tried to preserve the Jewish way of life [75]. As written in Tractate Avot [Sayings of our Fathers] in the Talmud, Hillel said:

> If I am not for myself, who will be for me?And when I am only for myself, what am I?And if not now, when? (Pirkey Avot 1:14)

The three rhetorical questions, when put together, create a powerful demand for self and relationship reflections, as well as a call for action [75]. "If I am not for myself,

[16] His exact age is uncertain. According to Jacob Neusner, he was born in 50 BC [73].

who will be for me? And when I am only for myself, what am I?" The first step is for people to find their own individual powers within themselves. But individual self-empowerment is not enough. The self becomes meaningful in a group and as part of a community. Therefore, the combination of the two questions leads to the understanding that when helping their companions, one is actually acting on their own behalf. The third question is actually a call against the tendency to postpone the things they must do. When all the three questions are put together, they create a call for individuals to act, to collaborate and act together to change the current situation now, and not wait for the future. Hillel's precept was seen by future generations as a call for action. In his studies, Marshal Ganz uses Hillel's three-question statement as a starting point for his analysis of social movements [76]. In sum, no one will help the Jewish people unless they help themselves. Therefore, they should create self-help institutions and take care of their community, and their actions must be "now"!

"My Heart is in the East"—The Longing for Zion

Judah Halevi was one of the greatest Jewish philosophers and poets of the Middle Ages, as well as being a physician. He was probably born in 1075 in Toledo. At that period, Spain was divided between Muslim Almoravids and Christian crusaders, and Halevi residences were divided between the two regions [77, 78].

His work was written in an era known as the "golden age" of Jewish culture in Spain. However, his poems express the understanding that although Jewish life seemed, at the time, relatively good in Spain, things were about to change for the worse [79–81]. And indeed Christian intolerance in Western Europe and elsewhere had led to a series of forcible conversions or expulsions. The final accord in Spain, the Alhambra Decree of 1492, culminated a sequence of restrictions and persecutions against non-Christians, including the Jews, and brought to an end the old and prosperous Jewish community in the Kingdoms of Castile and Aragon and its territories [82, 94].

In his poems, Halevi expressed deep longing for Zion, and the philosophical and religious view that Jewish fulfillment and redemption could only be achieved in Eretz Israel. He decided to leave Spain in order to realize his love for Zion and to travel and live there. It was then part of the Latin Kingdom of Jerusalem. It appears that he arrived in Jerusalem in 1141, but died soon after. The circumstances of his journey and his death are under scholarly debate [79–81].

One of his more studied poems describes his love and longing for Zion:

> My heart is in the East, and I am at the ends of the West;
> How can I taste what I eat and how could it be pleasing to me?
> How shall I render my vows and my bonds, while yet
> Zion lies beneath the fetter of Edom, and I am in the chains of Arabia?
> It would be easy for me to leave all the bounty of Spain—
> As it is precious for me to behold the dust of the desolate sanctuary.

In his emotional words, Halevi expresses his spiritual bonds to the place. For him, the ruins of the Temple are more precious than all the wealth of Spain. He gives the reader a feeling of his deep sorrow at being distant from the land and reflects that he can only fulfill himself in Zion. Halevi's beautiful poem belongs to the literary genre known as "Songs of Zion." He wrote a total of about 750 poems, of which 35 are Songs of Zion. This genre was followed through the years by many others [83, 84]. It describes the longing for Eretz Israel, sorrow for the destruction of the Temple, the exile of Jewish people, and the hope for redemption and revival of the "People in the Land."

"If You Will It, It Is No Dream"

The statement "If you will it, it is no dream" was written by Theodor Herzl in his utopian novel *Altneuland* (The Old New Land) published in 1902 [85, 95].[17] Herzl was born in 1860 in Budapest, Hungary, and died in 1904 in Austria. He was a doctor of law, a political activist, a playwright, an author, and a journalist.

The eighteenth and nineteenth centuries, the era of the Enlightenment in Europe, did not favor the Jews. In many places, modern forms of anti-Semitism emerged. The pogroms against Jews spread and caused a growing number of Jews to flee, mainly to the United States. As Jews became disillusioned with the dream of integration and emancipation, initiatives for a Jewish national solution began to appear. In that context, Herzl founded and led the Zionist movement (see Fig. 3 Herzl at the first Zionist Congress in Basil). Within a short time, he became the senior representative of the Jews throughout the world. He is regarded as the father of the State of Israel. The Zionist movement, with Herzl as its leader, was successful in community building and in Jewish self-empowerment. Its goals included the Return to Zion, the ingathering of the Jewish in exile, the revival of Jewish culture and the Hebrew language, and the establishment of an independent Jewish sovereignty. Such sovereignty will be achieved by the *Geulat HaKarka* (redemption of land), a biblical term for returning land to its lawful owners which was used by the Zionist movement as a call for collective purchase and settlement of the land in Zion [86].

Herzl led the first Zionist Congress in 1897. The conference declared that "Zionism aims at establishing a publicly and legally assured home in Palestine for the Jewish people." For that mission, several institutions were created including the Zionist General Council, a public bank as the financial instrument, and the Jewish National Fund to purchase land in Eretz Israel for Jewish settlement.

Altneuland was published 5 years after the first Jewish Congress. In the novel, Herzl presents his vision for a Jewish state in the Land of Israel. His empowering statement refers to the ability of Jews around the world to revive Jewish communal life in their homeland. Herzl argues that such a vision is not a dream or a fairy tale;

[17] *Wenn ihr wollt, ist es kein Märchen.*

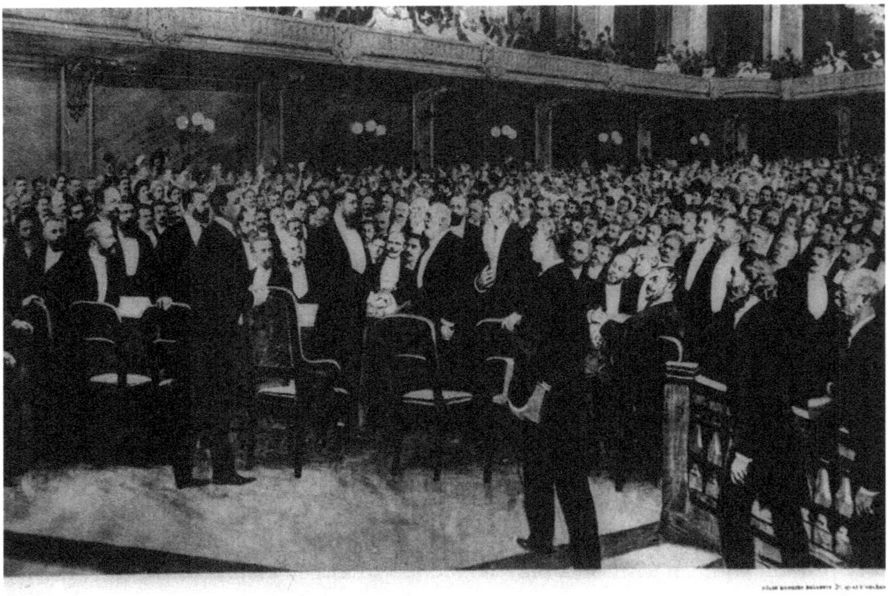

Fig. 3 Theodor Herzl at the first Zionist congress in Basel. 25 August 1897. Source: National Photo Collection, Israel Government Press Office

it can become reality and will materialize if people choose to put words into actions. The power is in people's hands. Herzl's vision helped the Zionist movement to persuade many mainly Jewish youth from all over the world to join the Zionist movement and to return to Zion. All those who followed the Zionist call and return to Zion, along with other Jews who left on time before the German Nazis took over Europe, survived the Holocaust. Herzl's statement of empowerment is regularly taught and discussed in schools and youth movements [87].

Looking Forward

An analysis of the Indigenous resilience theory provided me with new tools to look at the Jewish people's challenges and accomplishments. To that end, I surveyed resilience knowledge and then used it in examining the Jewish people, beginning with a brief description of the history of the Jewish people. I have looked at parameters such as traditions, rituals, community institutions, language and learning, connection to the land, and the role of hope. I have also provided some specific examples. My findings are that the case of the Jewish people is an overwhelming example of good implementation of the use of Indigenous resilience methods.

In his book *Imagine Zion*, Ilan Troen wrote about the Zionist pioneers who, after 2000 years in exile, were able to return to their ancestral lands, ingather their people, revive their language, gain recognition, and create the basis for a Jewish sovereign state: "[The] 'ingathering of the exiles,' whether one believes it is the fulfillment of a Divine promise or a necessary pragmatic response of Jews to persecution in the lands where they sojourned, has signified an unprecedented opportunity and challenge" [88].

In this chapter, I have discussed the resilience of the Jewish people by examining them within the framework of an Indigenous People, shedding light on some of their sources of resilience while examining the historical context. However, mine is not meant to be an exhaustive discussion on the matter, but rather an opening for future research. I hope that the case study of the Jewish people in the context of Indigenous resilience will continue.

References

1. Ostrer H. Legacy: a genetic history of the Jewish people. Oxford: Oxford University Press; 2012.
2. American Jewish Committee. "The Jewish population of the world." In American-Jewish year book. Jewish Virtual Library; 2016. http://www.jewishvirtuallibrary.org/jewish-population-of-the-world.
3. Anaya JS. Indigenous peoples in international law. New York: Oxford University Press; 2004.
4. Daes, E. A. (1996). "Working paper on the concept of "indigenous people"". U.N. ESCOR, commission on human rights, sub-commission on prevention of discrimination and protection of minorities. U.N. Doc E/CN4/Sub2/AC4/1996/2.
5. International Law Association Committee on the Rights of Indigenous Peoples. Final Report 75th ILA Biennial Meeting, Sofia. August 26–30; 2012.
6. Kingsbury B. Indigenous peoples in international law: a constructivist approach to the Asian controversy. Am J Int Law. 1998;92(3):414–57.
7. Yahel H, Kark R, Franzman SJ. Negev Bedouin and indigenous people: a comparative review. In: Chand R, Nel E, Pelc S, editors. Societies, globalization and marginalization: marginal regions in the 21st century. New York: Springer; 2017. p. 121–44.
8. Cobo JM. The problem of discrimination against indigenous populations. Report submitted to the United Nations—Indigenous Peoples; 1987.
9. Kirmayer LJ, Brass GM, Tait C. The mental health of aboriginal people: transformations of identity and community. Can J Psychiatry. 2000;45:607–16, 609.
10. Kirmayer LJ, Simpson C, Cargo M. Healing traditions: culture, community and mental health promotion with Canadian aboriginal peoples. Austr Psychiatry. 2003;11(Supplement):15–23.
11. LaFromboise TD. American Indian mental health policy. Am Psychol. 1988;43(5):388–97.
12. Marsh TN, Coholic D, Cote-Meek S, Najavits LM. Blending aboriginal and Western healing methods to treat intergenerational trauma with substance use disorder in aboriginal peoples who live in northeastern Ontario, Canada. Harm Reduct J. 2015;12(1):14.

13. Royal Commission on Aboriginal Peoples. Choosing life: special report on suicide among aboriginal people. Ottawa: Supply and Services; 1995.
14. Wexler LM, Gone JP. Culturally responsive suicide prevention in indigenous communities: Unexamined assumptions and new possibilities. Am J Public Health. 2012;102(5):800–6.
15. Kirmayer LJ, Tait CL, Simpson C. The mental health of Aboriginal peoples in Canada: Transformations of identity and community. In: Kirmayer LJ, Valaskakis GG, editors. Healing traditions: the mental health of aboriginal peoples in Canada. Vancouver: UBC Press; 2009. p. 3–33, p. 27.
16. Chandler MJ, Lalonde C. Cultural continuity as a hedge against suicide in Canada's first nations. Transcult Psychiatry. 1998;35(2):191–219.
17. Chandler MJ, Lalonde C. Cultural continuity as a moderator of suicide risk among Canada's first nations. In: Kirmayer LJ, Valaskakis G, editors. Healing traditions: the mental health of aboriginal peoples in Canada. Vancouver: UBC Press; 2009. p. 221–48.
18. Matthew W, McDonald M, Irlbacher-Fox S, Coulthard G. Learning from the land: Indigenous land-based pedagogy and decolonization. Decolonization Indigeneity Education Society. 2014;3(3):I–XV.
19. Brady M. Culture in treatment, culture as treatment: a critical appraisal of developments in addictions programs for indigenous North Americans and Australians. Soc Sci Med. 1995;41(11):1487–98.
20. Poonwassie A, Charter A. An aboriginal worldview of helping: empowering approaches. Can J Couns. 2001;35(1):63–73.
21. Kirmayer LJ, Dandeneau S, Marshall E, Phillips MK, Williamson K. Rethinking resilience from indigenous perspectives. Can J Psychiatr. 2011;56(2):84–91.
22. Sand S. Eich VeMatai Humtza HaAm HaYehudi? (When and how the Jewish nation was invented?). Tel Aviv: Resling (Hebrew); 2008.
23. Shapira A. The Jewish-people deniers. Israel J Israeli History. 2009;28(1):63–72.
24. Knohl I. Jacob-el in the Land of Esau and the roots of biblical religion Israel. Vetus Testamentum. 2017;67:481–4.
25. Finkelstein I, Silberman NA. The Bible unearthed: Archaeology's new vision of ancient Israel and the origin of its sacred texts. New York: The Free Press; 2001. p. 319–25.
26. Sacks J. Tikkun Olam: perfecting God's world. In: Breger MJ, editor. Public policy and social issues: Jewish sources and perspectives. Westport CN & London: Praeger; 2003. p. 35–48.
27. Finkelstein I. The sociopolitical organization of the central hill country in the second millennium B.C.E. In: Biran A, Aviram J, editors. Biblica archaeology today, 1990, Pre-congress symposium—population, production and power. Jerusalem; 1993. p. 119–31.
28. Tudor P. The lost tribes of Israel: the history of a myth. London: Phoenix; 2003.
29. Benite ZB. The ten lost tribes. New York: Oxford University Press; 2009.
30. Weil S. Beyond the Sambatyon: the myth of the ten lost tribes. Tel-Aviv: Beth Hatefutsoth, The Nahum Goldman Museum of the Jewish Diaspora; 1991.
31. Busteney O. The Judean exiles in Babylonia: survival strategies of an ethnic minority. In: Mor M, Pastor J, Ronen I, Ashkenazi Y, editors. For Uriel: studies in the history of Israel in antiquity. Jerusalem: The Zalman Shazar Center; 2005. p. 53–77.
32. Becking B. We all returned as one!: critical notes on the myth of the mass return. In: Lipschitz O, Oeming M, editors. Judah and the Judeans in the Persian period. Eisenbrauns: Winona Lake, IN; 2006.
33. Free JP, Vos HF. Archaeology and Bible history. Grand Rapids, MI: Zondervan; 1992.
34. Winkle RE. Jeremiah's seventy years for Babylon: a re-assessment. Part I: the scriptural data. Andrews Univ Seminary Stud. 1987;25(2):201–14. http://www.otgateway.com/articles/1987-2-04.pdf
35. Schalit A. The Hellenistic age: political history of Jewish Palestine from 332 B.C.E. to 67 B.C.E. London: W.H. Allen; 1976.

36. Popović M. The Jewish revolt against Rome: interdisciplinary perspectives. Leiden & Boston: Brill; 2011.
37. Rappaport U. Toldot Israel BeTkufat HaBayit HaSheni (the history of Israel during the Second Temple period). Tel-Aviv: Amihay (Hebrew); 1983.
38. De Lange N, editor. The illustrated history of the Jewish people. London: Aurum Press; 1997.
39. Schäfer P. The history of Jews in the Greco-Roman world: the Jews of Palestine from Alexander the great to the Arab conquest. London & New York: Routledge; 2003.
40. Schürer E, Vermes G, Millar F, Black M. The history of the Jewish people in the age of Jesus Christ. London: Bloomsbury; 2014.
41. Shatzman I. "Al Giyuram Shel HaEdomim" (On the conversion of the Edomites). In: Mor M, et al., editors. For Uriel; studies in the history of Israel in antiquity. Jerusalem: The Zalman Shazar Center (Hebrew); 2005. p. 213–41.
42. Goldwurm H. History of the Jewish people: the second Temple era. Brooklyn, NY: Mesorah Publications; 1982.
43. Flavius J. The Jewish war. Reprint. New York & London: Oxford University Press; 2017.
44. Yadin Y. Bar-Kokhba: the rediscovery of the legendary hero of the last Jewish revolt against Imperial Rome. London: Weidenfeld & Nicolson; 1978.
45. Schweid E. The land of Israel: national home or land of destiny. London & Toronto: Herzl Press Publications; 1985.
46. Gil M. A history of Palestine, 634–1099. Cambridge: Cambridge University. Press; 1997.
47. Goldstein Y. We were the first: a history of Hibat Zion, 1881–1918. Jerusalem: Bialik Institute; 2015.
48. Bauer Y. A history of the holocaust. New York: Franklin Watts; 2001.
49. Dawidowicz LS. The war against the Jews, 1933-1945. New York: Open Road Integrated Media; 2010.
50. Marrus MR. The darkest hour. In: de Lange N, editor. The illustrated history of the Jewish people. London: Aurum Press; 1997. p. 255–302.
51. Kellermann NPF. Holocaust trauma: psychological effects and treatment. New York & Bloomington: iUniverse Inc.; 2009.
52. UN General Assembly. A/RES/181(II) of 29 November 1947. https://unispal.un.org/DPA/DPR/unispal.nsf/0/7F0AF2BD897689B785256C330061D253.
53. Yahel H. Israel declaration of independence and the indigenous discourse. In: Elboim D, editor. Megilat Ha'atzmaum—Talmud Israeli. Rishon Lezion: Bina & Yediot (Hebrew); 2019. p. 80–1.
54. UN Development Program, Human Development Report 2019, New York. http://hdr.undp.org/en/content/2019-human-development-index-ranking
55. Helliwell J, Layard R, Sachs J. World Happiness Report 2018. New York: Sustainable Development Solutions Network; 2018. https://s3.amazonaws.com/happiness-report/2018/WHR_web.pdf
56. World Health Organization. World health statistics data; 2015. http://apps.who.int/gho/data/node.sdg.3-4-data?lang=en.
57. Senor D, Singer S. Start-up nation: the story of Israel's economic miracle. New York, NY: Twelve; 2011.
58. Bialik HN. Halacha and Aggadah. New York: Schocken; 1977.
59. Bialik HN, Ravnitzky YH. The book of legends: legends from the Talmud and Midrash. New York: Schocken; 1992.
60. Sebba-Elran T. From Sefer Ha'aggadah to the Jewish bookcase: dynamics of a cultural change. Jewish Studies Quarterly. 2013;20:272–95.
61. Azaryahu M, Kellerman A. Symbolic places of national history and revival: a study in Zionist mythical geography. Trans Inst Br Geogr. 1999;24(1):109–23.

62. Don-Yiḥya E. Hanukkah and the myth of the Maccabees in Zionist ideology and in Israeli society. Jew J Sociol. 1992;34(1):5–23.
63. Mandell S. The road to resilience: from chaos to celebration. London: The Toby Press; 2015.
64. Bloch E. The principle of hope. Cambridge, MA: MIT Press; 1986.
65. McDonald J, Stephenson AM. The resilience of hope. Amsterdam & New-York: Rodopi; 2010.
66. Rosmarin DH. Grateful to God or just plain grateful? A comparison of religious and general gratitude. J Posit Psychol. 2011;6(5):389–96.
67. Chalier C. Jewish hope versus revolutionary hope. In: Namli E, Svenungsson J, Vincent AM, editors. Jewish hope, utopia, and revolution. Amsterdam & New York: Rodopi; 2014. p. 23–32.
68. Carmichael CM. Joseph, Moses, and the institution of the Israelite judicature. In: Coleson JE, Matthews VH, editors. Go to the land I will show you. Winona Lake, IN: Eisenbrauns; 1996. p. 15–25.
69. Bonfil R. "HaKehila HaYehudit BeItaly BeTkufat HaRenaissance" (the Jewish Community in Italy during the renaissance). In: Grossman A, Kaplan Y, editors. Yemei HaBeinaim VeHaet HaHadasha HaMukdemet (the middle ages and the early modern period). Jerusalem, Zalman Shazar Center for Jewish History (Hebrew); 2004. p. 197–220.
70. Cooperman BD. Ethnicity and institution building among Jews in early modern Rome. Assoc Jewish Stud Rev. 2006;30(1):119–45.
71. Bar D. LeKadesh Aretz: HaMekomot Hakdoshim HaYehudim BeMedinat Israel (Holy places in the State of Israel). Jerusalem: Yad Ben-Zvi Press & Ben-Gurion Research Institute for the Study of Israel and Zionism, Ben-Gurion University of the Negev Press. (Hebrew); 2007.
72. Medoff R, Waxman CI. Historical dictionary of Zionism. NY & Abingdon: Routledge; 2012.
73. Neusner J. From politics to piety: the emergence of pharisaic Judaism. Oregon: Wipf & Stock; 2003.
74. Schalit A. King Herod: portrait of a ruler. Jerusalem: Bialik Institute; 1960.
75. Buxbaum Y. The life and teachings of Hillel. Lanham, Md: Rowman & Littlefield Publishers; 2008.
76. Ganz M. Why stories matter: the art and craft of social change. Sojourners; 2009. https://sojo.net/magazine/march-2009/why-stories-matter.
77. Gerber JS. My heart is in the East…. In: de Lange N, editor. The illustrated history of the Jewish people. London: Aurum Press; 1997. p. 141–98.
78. Weiss S. Biblical hermeneutics in the thought of R. Solovetchik: A preliminary appraisal of the influence of R. Yehuda Halevi. In: Kanarfogel E, Schwartz D, editors. Scholarly man of faith. Brooklyn, NY: Ktav Publishing House; 2018. p. 27–48. & Jerusalem: Urim Publications.
79. Kaplan GB. Review of: the compunctious poet: cultural ambiguity and Hebrew poetry in Muslim Spain. Hisp Rev. 1993;61(3):405–7.
80. Lobel D. Between mysticism and philosophy: Sufi language of religious experience in Judah HaLevi's Kuzari. Albany NY: SUNY Press; 2000.
81. Singor I, et al. Judah Ha-Levi. New York, Funk & Wagnalls Company: Jewish Encyclopedia; 1901–1906.
82. Roth N. Conversos, inquisition, and the expulsion of the Jews from Spain. Madison, WI: University of Wisconsin Press; 2002.
83. Doron A. Yehudah Haleṿi: Mivḥar Ma'amre Biḳoret Al Shirato (Yehuda Halevi: a selection of critical essays on his poetry). Tel Aviv: HaḲibuts HaMe'uḥad & Ḳeren Tel-Aviv LeSifrut VeLeOmanut (Hebrew); 1988.
84. Fleische E. Shirat HaKodesh Ha'Ivrit BeYemei HaBenayim (Hebrew liturgical poetry in the middle ages). Jerusalem (Hebrew): Magnes; 2007.
85. Herzl BZ. Altneuland. Leipzig: Hermann Seemann Nachfolger; 1902.
86. Kark R. Geulat HaKarka BeEretz Israel (Land Redemption in Eretz Israel). Jerusalem: Yad Ben-Zvi (Hebrew); 1990.

87. Cohen E. Herzl said … an exemplary community in Zionist thought. Jerusalem: Shalom Hartman Institute and Be'eri; 2012. https://shi-webfiles.s3.amazonaws.com/Beeri_2012_Herzl_TeachersGuide.pdf
88. Troen IS. Imagining Zion: dreams, designs, and realities in a century of Jewish settlement. New Haven: Yale University Press; 2011. p. xiii.
89. Balfour Declaration, Israeli Ministry of Foreign Affairs; n.d.. http://www.mfa.gov.il/mfa/foreignpolicy/peace/guide/pages/the%20balfour%20declaration.aspx.
90. Ben-Gurion D. "HaTafkid HaHalutzi BeKibutz Galuyot" (the pioneering role in the ingathering of the exiles). In: Ben-Gurion D, editor. Hazon and Derech (vision and way). Tel Aviv: Am Oved. (Hebrew); 1950. p. 20.
91. Eden Y. Individual and society: Teacher's guide. Jerusalem: Shalom Hartman Institute and Be'eri; 2012. http://meyda.education.gov.il/files/mazkirut_pedagogit/toshba/Madrih.yahid.final.pdf
92. Elior R. Zikaron and Shichecha: Sodan Shel Megilot Midbar Yehuda (memory and oblivion: the mystery of the Dead Sea scrolls). Jerusalem and Tel-Aviv: Hakibuts Hameuchad & Van Leer Institute (Hebrew); 2009.
93. Galil G. The chronology of the kings of Israel and Judah. Leiden: E. G. Brill; 1996.
94. Shirman H. HaShira HaIvrit BeSfarad VeBeProvance (Hebrew poetry in Spain and Provence) I Part 2. Jerusalem & Tel-Aviv: Mosad Bialik (Hebrew); 1961.
95. Herzl T. Old-New land. Translation Levensohn, L. New York: Bloch Publishing Co. & Herzl Press; 1941.
96. Israel Declaration of Independence. Israel Ministry of Foreign Affairs; n.d.. http://www.mfa.gov.il/mfa/foreignpolicy/peace/guide/pages/declaration%20of%20establishment%20of%20state%20of%20israel.aspx.
97. Knoblet J. Herod the Great. Lanham, Maryland: University Press of America; 2005.
98. Netzer E. The architecture of Herod, the great builder. Tübingen: Mohr Siebeck; 2006.
99. Rappaport U. Sefer Maccabim I (Book of Macabees. Translation, Introduction and interpretation). Jerusalem: Yad Yizhak Ben-Zvi. (Hebrew); 2004.
100. Tcherikover V. Gzerot Antiochus VeBa'ayoteihen (Antiochus edicts and their problems). Jerusalem: Eshkolot, Magnes; 1954.
101. Tcherikover V. Hellenistic civilization and the Jews. New York: Atheneum; 1975.
102. Tosefta, Berachot, 3:16. Based on Erfurt manuscript by Moses Samuel Zuckermandl. Jerusalem: Vaharman Books; 1963. Retrieved from http://www.hebrewbooks.org/20419
103. Wiessner S. Indigenous peoples: the battle over definition. The Legal Geography of Indigenous Communities: Negev Bedouins in Comparative Perspective. Research Workshop. Ben-Gurion University of the Negev, October 24–27; 2016.

Havatzelet Yahel is a senior faculty member at the Ben-Gurion Research Institute for the Study of Israel & Zionism, Ben-Gurion University of the Negev. She received her PhD from the Hebrew University of Jerusalem, MPA from the Harvard Kennedy School of Government after receiving the Israel Wexner fellowship for excellence in the public sector, and BA in Economy and in Law from Tel-Aviv University. Yahel was the Deputy to the Southern District Attorney (Civil Matters) at the Ministry of Justice in Israel.

Dr. Yahel's work is multidisciplinary and includes research on minorities and Indigenous communities, land rights and land settlements, historical geography, and legal history. Yahel is the author of numerous publications; recent works among them include "The Conflict over Land Ownership and Unauthorized Construction in the Negev," "Israel's Declaration of Independence and the Indigenous Discourse," and "Bedouin Settlement Proposals in Pre and Early Days of the State of Israel."

Part IV
Culture and Treatment

Alcohol Use and Resilience among the Indigenous Tuvinians of Siberia

Anastasia Peshkovskaya, Nikolay Bokhan, Anna Mandel, and Irina Badyrgy

Introduction

Siberia is home to 65 groups of Indigenous People, including Tuvinians, Buryats, Khakases, Khants, Yakuts, and Altaians. Tuvinians [1], Buryats [2, 3], Khakases [4], and the southern Altaians are Central-Asian Mongoloids. Despite differences in culture and anthropomorphological traits, these Indigenous People have lived together in the same territory for many years. There is no overt discrimination or ethnic prejudice among them. Moreover, there are many mixed families [5].

However, current world trends associated with migration, acculturation, and technological changes in society are having an impact both on Indigenous Peoples' social sphere and on their health [6–8]. The trend to depopulation of the Indigenous ethnic groups can be observed today with statistics on health. One of the main driving factors of this trend is the high level of alcohol abuse [9–12].

A. Peshkovskaya (✉)
Mental Health Research Institute, Tomsk National Research Medical Center of the Russian Academy of Sciences, Tomsk, Russia

Tomsk State University, Tomsk, Russia
e-mail: peshkovskaya@data.tsu.ru

N. Bokhan
Mental Health Research Institute, Tomsk National Research Medical Center of the Russian Academy of Sciences, Tomsk, Russia

Siberian State Medical University, Tomsk, Russia
e-mail: mental@tnimc.ru

A. Mandel
Mental Health Research Institute, Tomsk National Research Medical Center of the Russian Academy of Sciences, Tomsk, Russia

I. Badyrgy
Social Policy Committee, Kyzyl, Republic of Tyva, Russia

D. Danto, M. Zangeneh (eds.), *Indigenous Knowledge and Mental Health*,
https://doi.org/10.1007/978-3-030-71346-1_10

The problem of alcohol use and dependence among the Indigenous People of Siberia has gained considerable attention of researchers within the past three to four decades [13–20]. The Mental Health Research Institute (MHRI), Tomsk National Research Medical Center of the Russian Academy of Sciences is the largest research center in Russia for studying the mental health of Indigenous People. As a long-term member of the World Association of Cultural Psychiatry (WACP), and the International Association of Ethnopsychologists and Ethnopsychotherapists (IAEE), MHRI is now one of the centers for global cooperation between Russian and foreign scientists. MHRI develops and implements new medical and psychological technologies to the regions of Eastern and Western Siberia, as well as the Far East of Russia. A number of MHRI researchers, including the authors of this chapter, regularly participate in scientific expeditions (Fig. 1).

Over the past 5 years, the authors were actively involved in scientific expeditionary work in the Republic of Tyva, where they conducted clinical, genetic, and psychological studies on the Tuva Peoples' mental health and provided a series of medical and psychological consultations. The authors are also involved in dialog with the Tuvinian medical community and Tuva Republic Ministry of Health to develop an effective approach to protecting the mental health and resilience of the Indigenous People of Siberia and the Far East (Fig. 2).

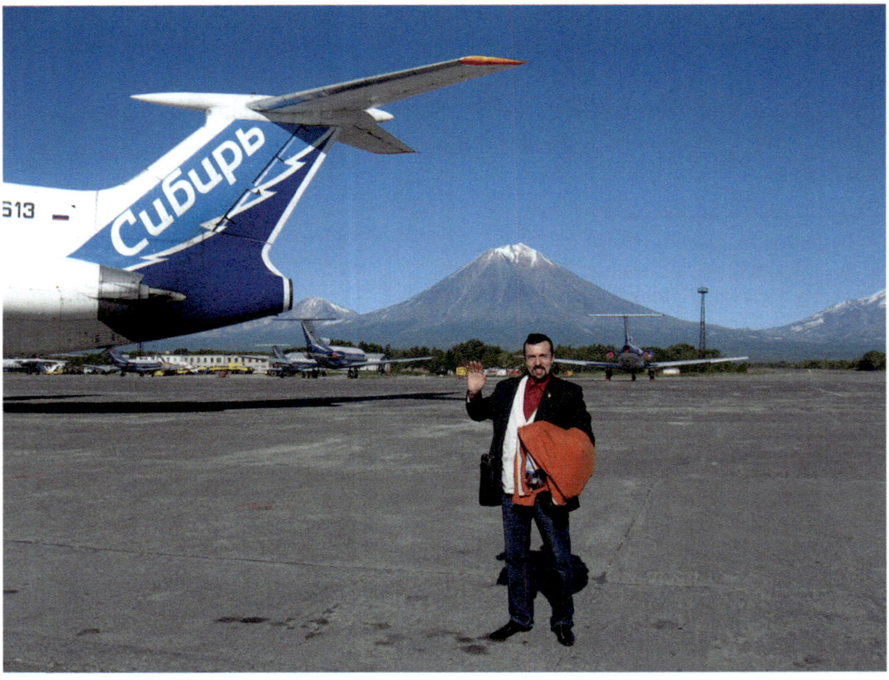

Fig. 1 Academician of the Russian Academy of Sciences, Director of Mental Health Research Institute, Professor Nikolay Bokhan in Kamchatka Region, Russia

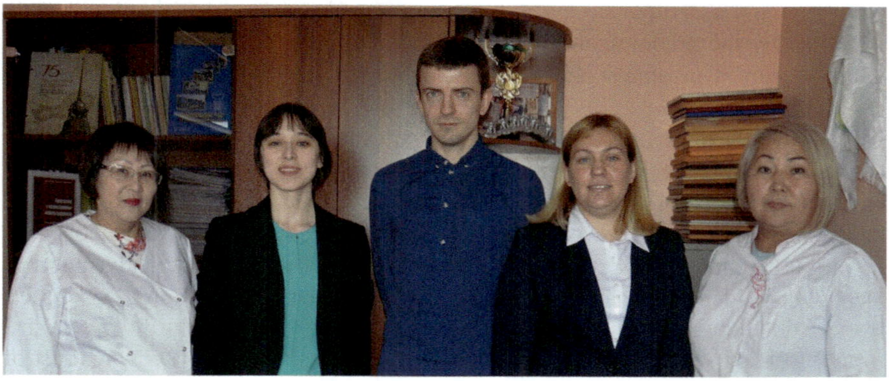

Fig. 2 Anastasia Peshkovskaya (second in the row, L-R) with Irina Badyrgy (first in the row, L-R) and colleagues during scientific expedition to the Republic of Tuva

We consider the mental health research among Indigenous ethnic groups extremely important for better understanding causes, risk factors, and the clinical picture of alcohol-use disorders in Indigenous People as well as for improving the efficiency of their therapy.

Alcohol-Related Challenges Among Tuvinians

Tuvinians are one of the numerous Indigenous Peoples of Siberia. Tuvinians live in the Republic of Tyva region of the Russian Federation. In 2016, 5354 patients with substance-use disorders (1.7% of the total number of the population of the Republic) were registered in the territory of the Republic of Tyva. Most of those registered (78.1%) were patients with alcohol dependence, alcoholic psychoses, and persons using alcohol with harmful consequences.

In 2016, 3929 patients with alcoholism were registered by the substance abuse service of the Republic of Tyva—equal to 124.48 per 10,000, or 1.2% of the population. In comparison with 2015, when 129.74 to 124.48 per 10,000 of the population were registered, the average prevalence of alcoholism, including alcoholic psychoses decreased by 4.1%. The number of persons reported with harmful alcohol use was 255 persons in 2016. The general incidence of harmful alcohol use was 4.97 per 10,000 of the population.

The clinical picture of alcoholism in Tuvinians had the following features: alcoholism co-occurred with psychotic disorders; alcoholic psychoses occurred in the form of abortive delirium with hallucinosis. In addition, Tuvinians had a high rate of alcoholism: in the majority of patients (44%), it was formed in 3–5 years of systematic alcohol use. Tuvinians had a lower tolerance for alcohol. Affective disorders, dysphoria, and depression were diagnosed as co-occurring pathology. Most Tuvinians had an impulsive variant of craving for alcohol, frequently manifested in paroxysm and accompanied by an acute anxiety. The clinical picture was heavily weighted by the predominance of a severe non-regressive variant of alcoholism, which occurred in almost 40% of Tuvinians, as well as very short remissions (44%) [21].

This data gave evidence of the extreme relevance of alcohol-related problems among Tuvinians. At the same time, the results of the published studies showed the essential influence of ethnicity on clinical and dynamic characteristics of alcohol dependence [22–24]. However, studies on the prevalence and features of alcoholism in various groups of the population of Tyva are few. The psychological aspects of alcohol dependence formation in Tuvinians are also not studied enough.

Tuvinians, the People of Tyva

Tuvinians are continental Mongoloids, one of the Indigenous Peoples of the Altai-Sayan uplands in the south of Siberia. About 95% of Tuvinians live in the territory of the Republic of Tyva, as a part of the Russian Federation. The Republic of Tuva is located in the central part of the Asian continent between the south of East Siberia and the north of the Republic of Mongolia (Fig. 3).

The population of the Republic of Tuva is 318,550 (2017); population density is 1.89 persons/km^2. The urban population makes up 54.03% (2017). Most of the population of the Republic are of Indigenous Tuvinians (80%), including Tuvinians Todzhints—an ethnic group with a lower population and one of the smaller tribes of the North. More than 16% of those living in the territory of the Republic are ethnically Russian.

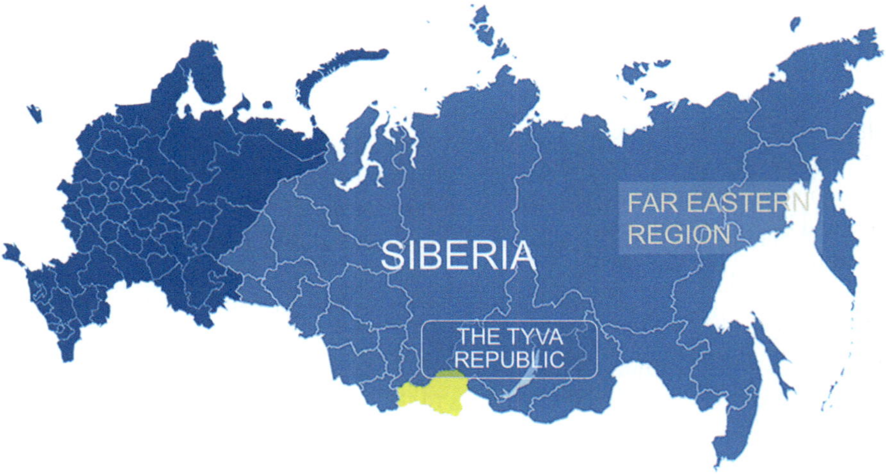

Fig. 3 Geographical location of the Republic of Tuva, Russia

According to their origins, the Tuvinian language is one of the Altai group of languages, which is a part of Turkic group of languages. Their traditional religion is Buddhism, maintaining elements of more ancient beliefs such as shamanism. Cattle breeding has been the primordial main occupation of Tuvinians. Most of those engaged in cattle breeding led a nomadic life. From boiled fermented milk they brewed an alcoholic drink known as *araga*. *Araga* was considered a sacred drink. The use of *araga* made a sacral sense, as the drink was used in various ceremonies. There was an ancient mystical taboo forbidding its use by women and children, and also by men aged 30 years and younger.

For centuries, the developed tradition of the use of a dairy *araga* created certain biochemical processes in the consumption of alcohol among Tuvinians which do not coincide with those in Caucasians. As a result, consumption of a culturally alien product (such as Western alcoholic drinks) has much more serious consequences for Tuvinians.

The Source of Strength and Resilience

Tuva is attractive in its rich historical and cultural heritage and its preserved ethnic culture. The culture of Tuvinians is surprisingly diverse and unique. Here, in Tuva, traditional occupations and beliefs have become the source of strength for life in the modern world. Many have come to Tuva only to fall into a completely different time, in another world and reality. It seems as if time and technology do not have power over life in some corners of the Tuva region. Visitors and travelers are surprised at how much the Tuvinian people have preserved their own traditions and their distinctive culture, which manifests itself in everything—hospitality, behavior, way of life, mentality, music and dance culture, art, and everyday life. We see horses, sheep, and cows grazing freely in the endless expanses of today's Tuva. Women and men of Tuva still cook traditional dairy products, ride horses, and practice throat singing.

Traditional Tuvinian houses, known as *yurts*, are widespread (Fig. 4).

A *yurt* is divided into two sides, the right for women and the left for men. Guests should go to the left (men's) side of the yurt. Friendly hosts pour fragrant green tea with milk, offer traditional food, consisting mainly of dairy products and meat, and ask you about your homeland and your life. Such hospitality comes from the depths of the centuries and is passed on from generation to generation.

Just as they did a 1000 years ago, the Tuvinians consecrate mountains, rivers, and *arzhaans* (curative springs), worship sacred places, build *ova* (heaps of stones), and ask for well-being for their relatives and friends.

Today, the national cultural traditions of the Tuvinian people fulfill the most important adaptive function for people in the modern world. Recognition at the state level of the importance of the national Tuvinian culture contributed to the active revival and scientific understanding of the Tuvan people's culture. Since the 1980s, traditional holidays such as Shagaa, the New Year's lunar calendar holiday have

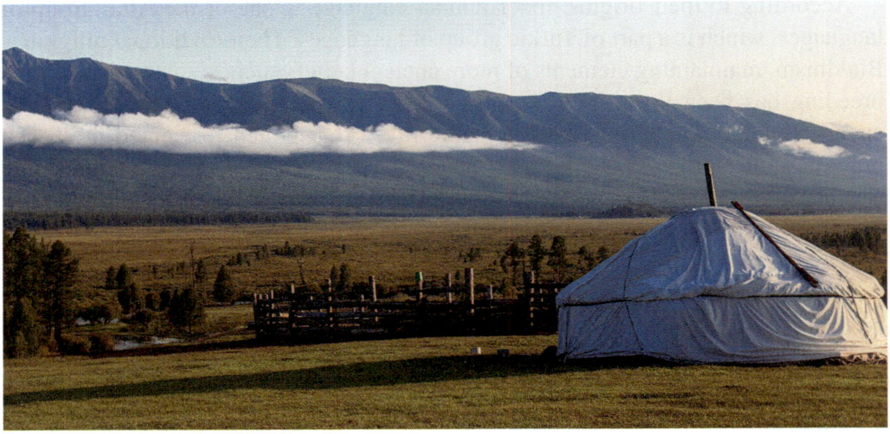

Fig. 4 Traditional Tuvinian house, a *yurt*. Photo by Valery Irgit

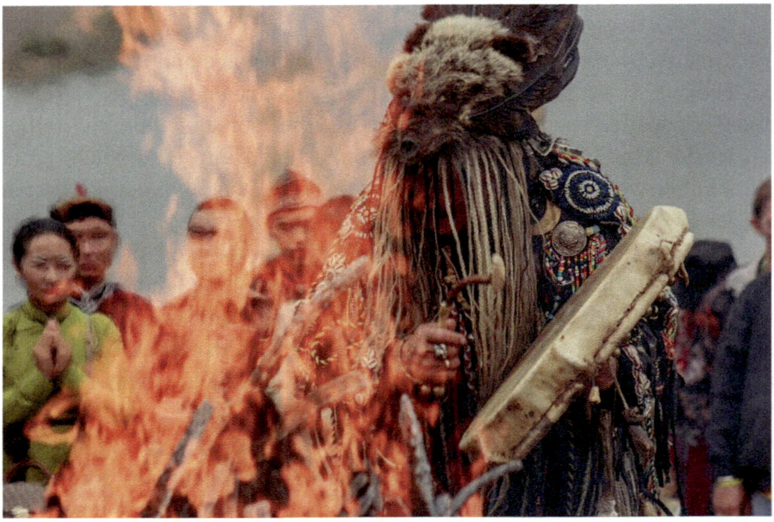

Fig. 5 The shamanistic rite at the festival Khomei in the Center of Asia. The place is Aldyn-Bulak, the Republic of Tuva, 2019. Photo by Valery Irgit

been revived. A number of cultural traditions are gaining political recognition and official status since 1990. Shagaa and Naadym, the holiday of the cattle breeders, have been declared state holidays of the Republic of Tuva since 1991 [25]. Today, a large number of festivals devoted to traditional arts and music are celebrated in Tyva (Fig. 5).

The foundation for the development of national culture is language. In 1991, the Tuvan language was given the status of the official language of the Republic of Tuva along with the Russian language. Today, the overwhelming majority of Tuvinians speak the Tuvinian language, a part of the Altaic language group [26].

There is an active process of new development of old traditions. In art, there are many traditional art masters. There is a transfer of knowledge, so new generations of masters are growing up. In the sphere of religion, various organizations of shamans and Buddhists exist. The role of clan communities is also still significant in Tuvinian society.

Clan Communities and Their Role in Health and Treatment

Tribal and clan communities are an important feature of Tuvinian culture. Traditionally, the clan is a group of people who have a common ancestor. Today, clan communities are a stable community of people connected by blood-related ties. Each clan community has a system of stable relationships between all community members [27].

Importantly, the clan community is the bearer of both spiritual and moral values and norms of behavior. Since ancient times, clan communities have closely followed a person's developmental process, their behavior, their self-awareness as a representative of a clan community, and their relationships with relatives, the surrounding society, and nature.

For example, according to the ancient rules of the clan communities, children from 3 to 15 years were partly involved in labor. Girls at the age of 5 could already milk goats. Boys could graze goats and lambs. At the age of 14, the boy should be able to pin a sheep and the girl to clean the insides of the slaughtered ram [28]. Traditionally, it was desirable for young people 16–29 years old to have a well-off family. People in middle age, from 30 to 55 years, were allowed to visit weddings, drink two drinks of alcohol, and offer blessings for others [28, 29]. In later adulthood, from 46 to 61 years of age, people should have gained a great life experience and a clear mind. In old age (from ages 61 to 81), people should have the strength to withstand the most difficult life challenges. And from the age of 81, they are the people who have created material and spiritual values for the present and future generation; they have the privilege of paying ritual tribute to the ancestors on the day of *Shagaa*, the lunar calendar's New Year's Day. Elderly people also are treated with respect as the bearers of wisdom. Clan members seek their advice and opinion on a wide range of life situations.

In ancient times, the rules of the clan communities regulated not only the daily routine of the clan but also offered behavioral models for clan members, including a model of alcohol-use behavior. Today, clan communities monitor the strengthening and transfer of Traditional Knowledge in families. Clan communities still act as a regulator of behavioral norms among community members. Thus, clan communities act as an informal system of protecting and educating children, caring for the elderly, and supporting sick community members. Every clan community has its sacred places. Community members meet from time to time to help each other and to hold charitable events related to the coming of the New Year, weddings, the birth of children, mourning, and so on.

The number of clan communities in Tuva is still large. For example, there are 19 clan communities today in the town of Chaata in the Ulug-Khem region of Tuva [30]. All 19 clan communities of Chaata have preserved a number of traditions, some of which are described below [31].

Adoption of orphaned relatives: Traditionally, representatives of the clan never give orphans to someone else's (unrelated) family and do not send them to orphanages and boarding schools.

Establishing a conscientious attitude to adopted children: Foster parents adhere to the democratic style of education, in which they give the child the right to be independent, without infringing on his or her rights and at the same time demanding the fulfillment of feasible duties. Trust, warm feelings, and reasonable care usually find a response in the child's soul, and explanations of the cause-effect relationships of a particular action allow children to form self-control and motivation.

Providing material assistance to low-income families and older people over 70 years of age: Assistance is provided on the eve of the traditional New Year's holiday with wishes of health and happiness. Heads of clans, town administrators, and school directors all participate in the organization of charity activities.

Shagaa, the New Year's holiday: Clan communities usually celebrate Shagaa together. The main idea is the veneration and praise of mothers—mothers, grandmothers, and great-grandmothers). There are numerous contests held, among them a contest to compile a family tree, a national clothes contest, and a Tuvinian songs contest. The culminating competition is the Huresh (traditional fighting) contest, in which all the fighters of the clan communities compete. Winners are awarded valuable prizes, for example, digital devices, gold and silver jewelry, horse gear, and agricultural equipment.

Veneration of ancestral lands and spiritual objects: Each clan community regularly pays homage to its ancestors and their ancestors' places of residence. The greatest attention on these special days is given to children. Children are told of the most important information: the history of their family and relatives. Issues of friendship and responsibility are discussed. Children observe how the ceremony of consecration of a spiritual object is conducted, and how to how to act with spiritual objects like special plants, symbols, stones, images on a stone, and so on.

Outdoor recreation: In this tradition, Tuvinians go to mountains, rivers, and other natural places to rest, to discover mental and physical recovery, and to communicate with clan members, or to spend some time alone.

Mutual assistance: Tuvinians have a constant tradition of expressing joy and empathy to clan members in special circumstances. These can be the birth of children, weddings, and anniversaries when clan members congratulate the family and make a significant contribution to their budget. Expressing condolences and rendering assistance is also a tradition of the Tuvinian people. During mourning, the suffering people are supported; responsibilities are shared among relatives. Everyone who comes into a family house brings food or money and performs rituals [31].

Significantly, clan communities also support their members who have problems with alcohol abuse. Clan members, especially the head of the clan, interact with the attending physician and participate in rehabilitation. Outdoor recreation and involvement in traditional occupations become important elements of the rehabilitation process. The rules developed by the clan community to regulate alcohol-use behavior and the support of the clan head are factors that help community members remain in remission. Moreover, the Council of Elders engages in the prevention of alcohol-use disorders and the promotion of a healthy lifestyle. Thus, the national culture is a source of strength and resilience for the Tuvinians. Traditions, closeness to nature, and support of the clan community have become a huge source of healing power for these people in the modern world.

Conclusion

Tuvinians are a good example of resilience due to the strong role of clan communities in supporting patients through treatment and in their involvement in the prevention of alcohol-use disorders and the promotion of a healthy lifestyle. Moreover, traditional Tuvinian occupations and beliefs have become a source of strength for life in the modern world. Nowadays, traditional origins of resilience and community support became extremely important to survive worldwide pandemic crisis [32, 33].

Placing our results in a global context, we should note that the problem of a high level of alcohol abuse among Indigenous ethnic groups is similar for countries around the globe [34–39]. We suggest that inadequate attention to the ethnic factor, which undoubtedly modifies the clinical picture of mental illness, often leads to errors in diagnosis, including the delineation of mental norms and pathology, incorrect therapeutic tactics, and incorrect planning of preventive measures. We stress that competence in ethnic and cultural specifics of mental health can determine new opportunities for heightening the efficiency of therapy, prevention, and rehabilitation of Indigenous People.

References

1. Bokhan N, Mandel A, Abolonin A, Peshkovskaya A, Nazarova I, Belokrylov I. Cognitive functioning in alcoholic patients and efficiency of their correction with use of individualized therapy. Eur Psychiatry. 2016;33(Suppl):S351. Abstracts of the 24th European Congress of Psychiatry. https://doi.org/10.1016/j.eurpsy.2016.01.993.
2. Dashieva BA, Kupriyanova IE. Factors influencing on mental health state of schoolchildren from Buryat rural population. World Cultural Psychiatry Res Rev. 2009;(Suppl S1):139–41.
3. Rakhmazova LD, Semke AV, Ochirova IB. Rasprostranennost' shizofrenii v Buryatii [prevalence of schizophrenia in Buryatiya]. Sibirskij vestnik psihiatrii i narkologii. 2012;3(72):18–20.
4. Taliyanova TI, Korobitsina TV. Osobennosti potrebleniya alkogolya bol'nymi—korennymi zhitelyami Respubliki Khakasii, stradayushchimi zavisimost'yu ot alkogolya [Peculiarities of

alcohol use in patients-natives of republic of Khakasia suffering from alcohol dependence]. Sibirskij vestnik psihiatrii i narkologii. 2011;3(66):85–8.
5. Sokolova Z. Peoples of West Siberia. Ethnographic review. Moscow: Nauka; 2000.
6. Pinedo M, Zemore S, Cherpitel C, Caetano R. Acculturation and alcohol use: the role of environmental contexts. In: Schwartz SJ, Unger J, editors. The Oxford handbook of acculturation and health. Oxford: Oxford University Press; 2017. https://doi.org/10.1093/oxfordhb/9780190215217.013.18.
7. Schwartz SJ, Unger JB, Zamboanga BL, Szapocznik J. Rethinking the concept of acculturation: implications for theory and research. Am Psychol. 2010;65:237.
8. Voevodin I, Peshkovskaya A, Galkin S, Belokrylov I. Social Adaptation and Mental Health of Foreign Students in Siberia. Sotsiologicheskie issledovaniya. 2020;(11):157–161. https://doi.org/10.31857/S013216250010306-9.
9. Jargin SV. Alcohol and alcoholism in Russia: insider's observations and review of literature. J Addiction Prevention. 2016;4(1):6.
10. Kozlov AI. Potreblenie alkogolja i svjazannye s alkogolem problemy u korennogo naselenija Severa Rossii [Alcohol consumption and alcohol related problems of the indigenous people of Russian north]. Narkologija. 2006;10:22–9.
11. Krasnov V, Bokhan N. Russian federation. In: Bhugra D, Tse S, Ng R, Takei N, editors. Routledge handbook of psychiatry in Asia. Abingdon: Routledge, Routledge Handbooks Online; 2015.
12. Maximova IV, Berezovskaya MA. Epidemiologicheskie issledovaniya alkogol'nykh rasstroystv v Krasnoyarskom Krae [Epidemiological studies of alcohol use disorders in Krasnoyarsk Krai]. Sibirskij vestnik psihiatrii i narkologii. 2017;1(94):76–80.
13. Bisaliev RV, Krechina EV, Khaninev NF. Jetnokul'tural'nye aspekty alkogol'noj zavisimosti [Ethnocultural aspects of alcohol addiction]. Nevrologicheskij vestnik. 2011;XLIII(1):68–75.
14. Bokhan NA, Mandel AI, Peshkovskaya AG, Badyrgy IO, Aslanbekova NV. Ethnoterritorial heterogeneity of alcohol dependence formation in the native population of Siberia. Zhurnal Nevrologii i Psihiatrii Imeni S.S. Korsakova. 2013;113(6):2013. Available at: https://www.scopus.com/inward/record.uri?eid=2-s2.0-84940309786&partnerID=40&md5=6dbbcf6b5c4f8c3a5cbe5c9e7a5d155c.
15. Dmitrieva TB, Polozhy BS. Etnokul'tural'naya psikhiatriya [Ethnocultural psychiatry]. Moscow: Meditsina; 2003.
16. Galkin SA, Peshkovskaya AG, Simutkin GG, Roshchina OV, Ivanova SA, Bokhan NA. Disorders of spatial working memory in affective disorders with mild current depression and their neurophysiological correlates. Zhurnal Nevrologii i Psihiatrii imeni S.S. Korsakova. 2019;119(10):56–61. https://doi.org/10.17116/jnevro201911910156.
17. Korolenko CP, Bochkareva NL. Osobennosti kliniki i techeniya ostrykh alkogol'nykh psikhozov na Kraynem severe [Features of clinical picture and course of acute alcoholic psychoses in the far north]. In: Osobennosti nekotorykh ekzogennykh intoksikatsiy v usloviyakh Severa [Features of some exogenous intoxications in the conditions of the north]. Novosibirsk, pp. 62–73; 1982.
18. Peshkovskaya AG. Do you draw with your patients? Cognitive deficiency diagnostics in alcohol-use disorder: a drawing as a neuropsychological method. Eur Neuropsychopharmacol. 2019;29(Supplement 6):S501–Sd502. https://doi.org/10.1016/j.euroneuro.2019.09.781.
19. Galkin SA, Peshkovskaya AG, Roshchina OV, Kisel NI, Ivanova SA, Bokhan NA. Features of brain activity in alcohol dependence in the task of inhibitory control. Bulletin of Siberian Medicine. 2020;19(4):38-45. https://doi.org/10.20538/1682-0363-2020-4-38-45.
20. Galkin SA, Peshkovskaya AG, Simutkin GG, Vasil'eva SN, Roshchina OV, Ivanova SA, Bokhan NA. Impairments to the functions of spatial working memory in mild depression and their neurophysiological correlates. Neurosci Behav Physiol. 2020;50(7):825–829. https://doi.org/10.1007/s11055-020-00973-4.
21. Koshkina EA, Kirzhanova VV, Babicheva LP, Mugantseva LA. The activity of drug addiction service of the Russian Federation: An assessment of statistical parameters and an analysis of results. Zhurnal Nevrologii i Psihiatrii imeni S.S. Korsakova, 2013;113(6–2):3–8.

22. Matveeva NP. Prevalence, risk factors and clinical dynamics of alcoholism and alcoholic psychoses among indigenous people of the Republic of Sakha (Yakutia) (ethnocultural, rehabilitation aspects). PhD thesis, Tomsk; 2010.
23. Polozhy BS, Kolotilin GF, Kudryavtsev YD. Klinicheskie osobennosti alkogol'noy zavisimosti u korennykh narodov Khabarovskogo kraya [Clinical features of alcohol dependence in indigenous people of Khabarovsk Krai]. Rossiyskiy psikhiatricheskiy zhurnal. 2001;3:24–7.
24. Mandel A, Peshkovskaya A, Bokhan T, Badyrgy I. Ethno-cultural context of clinical-psychological interrelationships in alcohol dependence. World Cultural Psychiatry Research Review (WCPRR), 2015;10(2),74–78.
25. Kuzhuget AK. Dukhovnaya kul'tura tuvintsev: struktura i transformatsiya [The spiritual culture of the Tuvinians: structure and transformation]. Kemerovo: KemGuki; 2006.
26. Suzukey VY. Muzykal'naya kul'tura Tuvy v XX veke [Musical culture of Tuva in the XX century]. Moscow: Kompozitor; 2007.
27. Sadokhin AP, Grushevitskaya TG. Etnologiya [Ethnology]. Moscow: Academy Publishing Center; 2000. p. 304.
28. Kenin-Lopsan MB. Traditsionnaya kul'tura tuvintsev [Traditional culture of the Tuva people]. Kyzyl: Nauka; 2006.
29. Kenin-Lopsan MB. Tyva Chonnun ydyktyg chanchyldary [Traditional ethics of Tuvinians]. Kyzyl: Tuvan Book Publishing House; 1994. p. 1994.
30. Sundai GD. Family community as a guarantor of childhood protection: history, current state and prospects. In: Proceedings of the republican scientific-practical conference dedicated to the 90th anniversary of M. B. Kenin-Lopsan, p. 11–15; 2015.
31. Dazhy-Davaa AO. Life traditions of the clan communities. In: Proceedings of the republican scientific-practical conference dedicated to the 90th anniversary of M. B. Kenin-Lopsan, p. 19–21; 2015.
32. Júnior JG, Moreira MM, Pinheiro WR, de Amorim LM, Lima C, da Silva C, Neto M (2020) The mental health of those whose rights have been taken away: An essay on the mental health of indigenous peoples in the face of the 2019 Coronavirus (2019-nCoV) outbreak. Psychiatry research, 289, 113094. https://doi.org/10.1016/j.psychres.2020.113094
33. Galkin SA, Peshkovskaya AG, Ivanova SA, Bokhan NA. Cognitive impairment in patients after COVID-19. Yakut Medical Journal. 2021;1(73):69-72. https://doi.org/10.25789/YMJ.2021.73.19.
34. Chartier K, Caetano R. Ethnicity and health disparities in alcohol research. Alcohol Res Health. 2010;33:152–60.
35. Herbert S, Stephens C. Alcohol use and older Māori in Aotearoa. J Ethn Subst Abus. 2015;14(3):251–9.
36. Hesselbrock MN, Hesselbrock VM, Segal B, Schuckit MA, Bucholz KK. Ethnicity and psychiatric co-morbidity among alcohol dependent persons who received inpatient treatment: African Americans, Alaska natives, Caucasians and Hispanics. Alcohol Clin Exp Res. 2003;27(8):1368–73.
37. Ramamoorthi R, Jayaraj R, Notaras L, Thomas M. Epidemiology, etiology, and motivation of alcohol misuse among Australian aboriginal and Torres Strait islanders of the northern territory: a descriptive review. J Ethn Subst Abus. 2015;14(1):1–11.
38. Skewes MC, Blume AW. Ethnic identity, drinking motives, and alcohol consequences among Alaska native and non-native college students. J Ethn Subst Abus. 2015;14(1):12–8.
39. Bokhan NA, Mandel AI, Gusamov RR. Mental and behavioral disorders in substance use among adolescents under conditions of the far north. Alaska Med. 2006;49:251–4.

Anastasia Peshkovskaya Researcher in the field of *clinical* psychology, member of the International Association of Ethnopsychologists and Ethnopsychotherapists (IAEE), Laureate of the Tomsk Region Award for Excellence in Science (2019). Her research program involves cross-cultural investigations with particular focus on clinical and neuropsychological aspects of alcohol-use disorder. Anastasia has a leading position in scientific expeditionary projects on the prevalence of mental disorders, its social and psychological determinants in the youth of remote Siberian regions, as well as in the Indigenous population of Russia. Anastasia is affiliated with Mental Health Research Institute, Tomsk National Research Medical Center, Russian Academy of Sciences, and National Research Tomsk State University.

Nikolay Bokhan Professor, Full Member of the Russian Academy of Sciences, President of the International Association of Ethnopsychologists and Ethnopsychotherapists (IAEE). His primary scientific interests are regional problems of addiction psychiatry, psychopharmacological and non-pharmacological therapeutic strategies for drug use disorders treatment. He also acts as a supervisor in research on transcultural problems of addiction in Mongolia and Russia. In 2004, Professor Bokhan was granted the title Honored Scientist of Russian Federation. Since 2013 he has served as the Director of Mental Health Research Institute, Tomsk National Research Medical Center of Russian Academy of Sciences. He is also affiliated with the Siberian State Medical University, Tomsk, Russia.

Anna Mandel Professor, Leading Researcher at the Addiction Department, Mental Health Research Institute, a member of the Scientific Council of Tomsk National Research Medical Center of Russian Academy of Sciences, Tomsk, Russia. Professor Mandel's research program focus on alcohol and drug use disorders, and its regional and ethnic aspects.

Irina Badyrgy Deputy Chair of the Tyva Republic Parliament, Chair of the Social Policy Committee Irina Badyrgy acts as a co-organizer of scientific expeditionary projects in the Republic of Tyva.

Reclaiming Our Identity Through Indigenous Cultural Generative Acts to Improve Mental Health of All Generations

Jordan P. Lewis

From 1762, when Russian ships first arrived at what is now known as Alaska, the purchase of Alaska by the United States in 1867, and statehood in 1959 [1], and as a result of colonization, including boarding schools, missionaries, and Western practices, Alaska Natives have lost their land, cultural values, and traditional spiritual practices. These losses have resulted in negative self-perception, diminished sense of pride, and the development of maladaptive behaviors (drinking, violence, depression, suicide) used to numb the pain of their lost identity [2]. These behaviors have a negative impact on younger Alaska Natives and change families and community relationships. Despite the history, a segment of Alaska Natives experiences "cultural motivations" to "become who they are meant to be" and age successfully by transmitting these motivations to others to ensure they age well and become who they wish and are meant to be. These cultural motivations, which are introduced to us as youth through the teachings of our Elders, remain present consciously or subconsciously throughout our lives living as Indigenous peoples. It is not until later in life, when we approach Eldership, that these lessons reemerge and become the foundation for our own lives as well as what we pass on to youth.

My impetus for this chapter stems from the groundbreaking work by the late Gerald Mohatt and his team at the Center for Alaska Native Health Research. This work is referred to as the People Awakening Study, which explored life-history narratives looking for factors that helped Alaska Native Elders to quit drinking, maintain their sobriety, and remain on their journey to recovery. It was found that what contributed to long-term recovery was filling expected roles as an Elder in their family and community, sharing their wisdom and experiences gathered over a lifetime, and being willing to pass on these stories of recovery, strength, and

J. P. Lewis (✉)
University of Minnesota Medical School, Duluth Campus, Memory Keepers Medical Discovery Team, Duluth, MN, USA
e-mail: jplewis@d.umn.edu

D. Danto, M. Zangeneh (eds.), *Indigenous Knowledge and Mental Health*,
https://doi.org/10.1007/978-3-030-71346-1_11

compassion for their cultural values, beliefs, traditions, and families. These acts fit within Erikson's notion of "generativity," where adults and older adults are concerned about future generations, sharing their knowledge and skills, and leaving a legacy that improves society.

In this chapter, grounded in generativity and Indigenous theories, I discuss the cultural motivations Alaska Native Elders used to replace unhealthy behaviors that lead to improved mental health, stronger sense of self, and "becoming who they were meant to be." When engaging in Indigenous cultural generative acts [3], Alaska Native Elders share experiences to encourage others to learn from their experiences and avoid similar challenges, discover their cultural motivations to live the life they imagined, and reclaim their identity as healthy Alaska Natives. This journey, of becoming who you are meant to be, to heal future generations, is depicted in Fig. 1.

Figure 1 outlines the journey for Indigenous Elders and how early life experiences, while difficult, are lessons on how to live life to the fullest, take those lessons to improve their daily life, and also pass those lessons along to others who may be struggling. I discuss this journey, starting with the adversities faced by many Indigenous peoples, with a focus on Elders, and how those adversities led to Elders reaching a turning point in life, and through motivations and supports, they reconnected to their cultural, familial, and community identity. Reclaiming their healthy Indigenous identity, and not keeping those lessons to themselves, has enabled them to achieve Eldership through Indigenous cultural generative acts.

A segment of the Alaska Native population has struggled, or currently struggles, with adversity throughout their lives, including substance misuse, trauma, racism, relocation, and other challenges that may continue to impact their lives, preventing them from achieving their idea of Eldership based on what they witnessed growing up among their Elders. Some of the struggles may also prevent them from engaging and teaching cultural values and practices, which we refer to as Indigenous cultural generative acts. These acts can include teaching younger people cultural practices, and, on a deeper level, the underlying values and worldview of their culture, as well as sharing their experiences with adversity and how they overcame those challenges. We can learn from those who share their lived experiences of recovery [4] because they have lived through the challenging times and gained personal insight and lessons they can pass down.

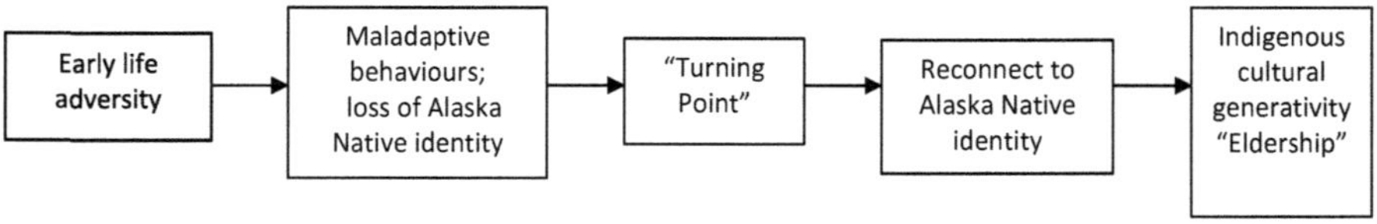

Fig. 1 Journey of "Becoming who I am meant to be" to heal the Seventh Generation through Indigenous cultural generativity

Need for a Paradigm Shift

Indigenous community research partners, including those working in partnership with Alaska Natives, advocate for a shift from a pathology-based to a strengths-based approach to serving Elders and communities, as well as developing programs and services to address mental health. Rather than focusing on problem behaviors and highlighting deficits, a strengths-based approach instead highlights individuals and subgroups that exemplify successful treatment outcomes or who have been protected from active mental health problems [5]. This approach has been similarly emphasized for more than two decades by Alaska Native and other Indigenous community leadership [6, 7]. A shift in focus to those who are successful contributes to our understanding of the protective factors from adverse mental health outcomes [8] and can guide Indigenous communities and providers in efforts to develop programs and services built upon individual, family, community, and spiritual and cultural strengths. In particular, it is important to highlight these cultural strengths that exist in Indigenous communities; these strengths include values based on family, clan, tribal affiliation, and spirituality, as well as engagement with and support from the community [5], and they also serve as cultural motivations for Elders to step into Eldership roles and mentor the Seventh Generations to live healthy and productive lives.

Turning Point

Alaska Natives, and other Indigenous peoples, have lost their land, cultural values, and spiritualty, resulting in negative self-perception, a diminished sense of pride, and the development of maladaptive behaviors (drinking, violence, depression, suicide) used to numb the pain of their stolen identity. These behaviors negatively impact younger Indigenous Peoples and change families and community relationships. Despite the history, a segment of these populations experiences a turning point in life to "become who they are meant to be" and they age successfully through the transmission of these experiences. Turning points vary for each person, but they have included the birth of a grandchild (and becoming a grandparent) or being asked by the community to fill the role of Elder, serve on Tribal Council, or work with youth; these roles are not compatible with poor health behaviors and choices.

When Elders, and others, after reaching their turning point, reconnect with their cultural values through engagement in personally and culturally meaningful roles and activities, they begin to heal and become who they are meant to be. In addition to the family, other sources of social support include friends and others in the wider community who provide opportunities to be engaged [9–12] in meaningful activities and events.

Paul Spicer [13] found that American Indians and Alaska Natives understood their role of teaching and helping others in their family and community, which supported their desire to overcome and avoid challenges they experienced in the past. Sondra Burman [4] found that, in addition to wanting to strengthen relationships with family and community members, a majority of American Indians and Alaska Natives want to be role models and share their experiences to ensure others do not face similar challenges. Spicer's [13] study explored recovery as a cultural process, involving the restoration of the cultural self, concluding that drinking is incompatible with a proper way of life for Indigenous people; through abstaining, people in recovery have been able to restore themselves to this proper Indigenous way of life and serve as role models for others. As we partner with Indigenous Elders and communities, this focus on strengths will build trust and open the dialog for them to share their journeys of recovery; we are asking them to share what they are doing right, what has enabled them to overcome adversity through reconnection to their culture, community, and family, and, when they feel ready, to share their experiences with others. This sharing is important because it enables Elders to share lessons learned, mentor others, as well as heal themselves through sharing.

Concept of Generativity and Its Role in Mental Health

A key element of a psychosocial development theory by Erik Erikson (1997) is the concept of generativity, which is defined as the urge to contribute to the well-being of other people, particularly the younger generations. John Kotre [14] defines generativity as the desire to invest one's substance in forms of life and work that will outlive the self. Although already identified as a topic associated with successful aging (in, for example, [15, 16]), generativity has not received much attention in the mental health or Indigenous literatures. Very little research, if any, has been conducted with Indigenous populations and their understanding of generativity and its role in well-being and mental health. Yet the concept can be applied to most Indigenous Elders with their desire to be involved with their family, teach, and engage in cultural practices, and pass on their knowledge and language to others to ensure they have the tools, stories, and wisdom to become healthy Indigenous peoples. Baltes and Baltes [17] discussed generativity and wisdom as important elements of a standardized definition of an ideal state of growing older. Achieving generativity, along with good health, should be considered strong indicators of successful aging [18] and mental well-being. George Vaillant [19] stated, "The mastery of generativity should be strongly correlated with successful adaptation to old age, for to keep it, you have to give it away" (p. 220), which is the same sentiment expressed by Indigenous Elders in their desire to pass on what they know to the younger generations. Through this sharing, Indigenous Elders grow stronger and healthier, and the stories they share grow; from sharing about overcoming adversity and what that has taught them in life and also being able to share stories of how life has changed after reconnecting with culture and becoming who they were meant to be.

In his later years, Erikson expanded the concept of generativity one step further to encompass caring for the wider community, social institutions, and the environment, which he labeled as "grand-generativity" [20]. This concept is thought to allow Elders to express care, to be engaged and valued by others, and to leave a legacy of themselves [21, 22], which directly applies to the cultural values practices of Indigenous Elders. According to Kotre [14], there are four types of generativity (biological, parental, technical, and cultural), and this study focuses specifically on cultural generativity, which is another form of grand-generativity. The importance of a wider concern with passing on social traditions, morals, and cultural values (as opposed to practical skills passed on through other forms of generativity) has been recognized with the concept of cultural generativity [14, 23, 24]. Expressions of cultural generativity are practiced and encouraged by the older adult's awareness and acceptance of being connected to their relatives and community members who have passed on and the younger generations (Seventh Generation) who will continue on and carry the legacy they learned as recipients of the cultural generative acts of their elders [25]. Kotre [14] states that generative cultures, communities, and individuals must be concerned not only with the physical (biological) survival of their children but also with their psychological and moral development, which is a major focus of why Indigenous Elders take on roles to pass on their knowledge and wisdom.

According to the literature, cultural generativity does not happen all at once; it is an ongoing process throughout one's life. To begin, you need a sense of belonging to a culture in order to feel responsible for passing it on [26]; the individual must experience a sense of belonging to that culture or feeling wanted and needed by their family and community (that is, meaningful engagement). Research has consistently demonstrated that self-reported generative concern shares a significant, positive relationship with measures of life satisfaction, self-esteem, happiness, and a sense of coherence [24, 27, 28]. Generativity is a complex stage of development that involves cultural demand, inner desire, concern, belief, commitment, action, and narration [29]. All of these actions focus on individual and community-based goals of caring for, and contributing to, the well-being and advancement of future generations. Indigenous Elders share their stories and experiences to serve as role models and teach others how to successfully navigate difficult life situations, but also how to live a healthy and productive life and serve as a role model in their family and community [30]. Hong Kong's older adults, aware of the gap between their knowledge and current social and technological developments, transmit moral and behavioral attitudes mostly by sharing stories of hardship in the old days and being a model of character, as a way of creating a more lasting influence [31] on the younger generations.

Indigenous Elders tend to be considered "keepers of the meaning," which is a term coined by psychoanalyst George Vaillant to define a person who is located between the seventh and eighth stages of Erikson's stages of development (between generativity and ego-integrity). These individuals are concerned with preserving a culture's traditions in order to preserve their way of living and being for future generations and to teach them how to live a life according to their cultural values. In a study by Ronald J. Manheimer [26], his subjects demonstrated a capacity to transform an experience of failure or personal agony into a morally instructive account that functions to redeem the past and throw light on the present and future. What makes the narratives of his subjects redemptive is the way a source of pain, anger, vulnerability, trauma, or humiliation becomes a vehicle leading to pleasure, satisfaction, strength, solace, and pride; what Kotre [14] himself calls the "transformation of defect" (p. 263). Through a lifetime of experiences, reflection, and teachings, Indigenous Elders were able to transform their past misfortunes, hardships, and personal challenges because they could place their personal experiences in a broader context, which enabled them to find common words for their struggles and provided a community with whom they could share their experiences (that is, family members, community members, others in recovery). Not only were they willing to share these experiences, but they grounded them in the cultural values and customs of their family and community and used them as vehicles to teach lessons and appropriate behaviors through storytelling.

According to Kotre [14], when a person practices cultural generativity, they share a story that draws from a system of symbolically encoded meanings (for example, language, tradition, concepts, cultural values, foods) to formulate and pass on a story that has psychological power and a moral message. These stories are not only recalled for the teller, reminding them of where they have been and how far they have come but also memorable and a lesson for the listener. From Kotre's [14] account, it seems that it is in the passage of story from teller to listener that "outliving the self" takes place. It is in the movement between one person who has shaped an account in the context of a sharable culture and the recipient, who understands how to receive this account, that the communal self is born, freed from the private self of inner reflection or even the social selves of family and community life [26].

While cultural generativity is a term discussed in the generativity literature, it is not often associated with Indigenous Elders or referred to as a way of preserving an Indigenous culture, passing down cultural values, or teaching lessons to the youth. I believe this chapter is unique highlighting how the act of passing down cultural values, life stories, and traditional practices provided these Indigenous Elders with an opportunity to reflect on their experiences and share lessons learned, which has a positive impact on their mental health and well-being. These acts also enable Elders to share stories that preserve their history, language, and cultural practices and values. A second unique aspect is that Indigenous Elders share all of this with others, not as a way to preserve their own legacy, but to ensure the health and well-being of their families and communities; they wish to leave the world better than they found it and ensure their families and communities have the tools, stories, and values to live a healthy and productive life through engagement in activities that are meaningful and enable them to be proud, despite previous challenges or adversity. Elders share their stories of adversity, not as a way to bring up the past and feel shame, but to take the experience as a lesson to learn from to ensure we avoid similar situations in the future and continue to do the best we can with what we have. As we think about mental health and overcoming challenges, such as addiction, these Elders reflect back on their last drink, when they were at their lowest, or what they lost connection to others, not to talk about how bad life was, but to highlight the dangers of mental health challenges, but also share how wonderful life is when sober and well. Elders remind us that our past does not define us, nor should we relive those memories as a punishment or be ashamed, but to reflect on those moments that defined us and put us on a new path of healing and recovery. Everything happens in life for a reason, and we need to reflect on those experiences to learn the lesson, apply it to our lives, and, when the timing is right, share our own journey on how we became who we were meant to be.

Generativity Mismatch and Poor Mental Health

One of the challenges facing Elders across the globe, but particularly Indigenous Elders, is the receptivity of younger generations to these stories and lessons shared by the Elders. Youth today are raised in a technological society, and many younger children have never lived without a cellphone, computer, or television in their home. Indigenous Elders grew up in a very different world, some without electricity, growing up in sod houses, and living completely off the resources of the land. Their stories of childhood are not the same as children's today, so we are beginning to see a gap between Elders and youth and common topics of interest. What Elders wish to share and pass down does not align with the interests of our Indigenous youth, and we need to continue working collaboratively with Indigenous Elders and communities to address the generative mismatch and technological gaps. Without common interests, where Elders feel heard and appreciated, they will disengage and discontinue their sharing, resulting in poorer mental health outcomes and disengagement, which can also lead to poor health.

Sharing Your Journey Heals Everyone

Indigenous Elders witnessed positive changes in their own lives once they changed their lifestyle and began their journey toward the Elder they are meant to be. These changes are motivated by cultural factors I have grouped under four thematic categories: family influence, role selection and socialization, cultural activities and community engagement, and spirituality. In the following discussion, I do not describe Elders' reasons for quitting drinking, but rather their motivations for their changing their drinking behaviors and sharing what has enabled them to heal and begin their journey of recovery and Eldership.

Growing up, we interact and spend time with Elders in our homes and communities, and they are sober, leaders in the community, and always happy to share. As we grow up and experience the world, some of us venture into unhealthy lifestyle choices or experience mental and physical health challenges. Elders become Elders in their families and communities, not by self-nomination, but because others notice their wisdom and experiences. As a result of this external recognition of their status as a respected Elder, they make choices to change behaviors and begin to live a clean and healthy life, so they can begin to live the life expected of them, a role they envisioned since they were children. Moreover, as Elders, they can pass on their traditional knowledge, teach how the Native ways of living used to be, and work with the community to ensure a healthy and productive future grounded in these cultural ways, including a strong sense of community. These Elders wish to pass on their traditional culture and the values that played an important role in their own lives, as well as share how spirituality played a critical role in their lives and becoming healthy.

Reclaiming Our Identity to Become the "Elder You Were Meant to Be"

Alaska Native older adults beginning their healing journey say that they are assisted by cultural motivations such as family member influence and learning from the experiences of those who came before them. They also recognized their desire to become a role model and having a spiritual/religious presence in their lives as important factors in their recovery. A primary reason why these factors served as motivations for recovery was that, when present in an older adult's life, they appeared to have enabled them to age successfully and to teach, guide, and give back to others. Elders will share the specific moment they made the conscious decision to stop drinking, and they viewed this as a healthy step toward fulfilling their personal dreams as they age. They were also able to develop a sense of purpose and become a healthy Elder to serve as a role model for their family and community.

Family Influence

Family support and its role in Elders' journey to wellness may be even more pronounced for Indigenous families [32], including Alaska Natives. Consistent with earlier research [33], Alaska Natives have a desire to create a safe and healthy environment for their family; they discussed their pride in improving their mental health and working toward disengaging in poor health behaviors before their children grew up thus allowing them to live in a healthy home.

Sondra Burman [4] found that in addition to wanting to strengthen relationships with family members, American Indians and Alaska Natives wish to be role models for their family and other community members, which includes not just talking about past experiences with alcohol, but learning and growing from these experiences, and sharing their stories to prevent others from suffering similar experiences. Indigenous Elders also receive support from family and community to engage in meaningful activities [34], such as subsistence activities (hunting and gathering, fishing, berry picking, preparing traditional foods), Native arts and crafts, and tribal leadership, which would not be possible if they were still drinking or suffering from poor health as a result of poor health behaviors.

Role Selection and Socialization

The relationship between becoming an Elder and lifestyle changes are typically understood in terms of role selection and socialization. Role selection occurs when behaviors influence the roles Elders adopt; role socialization occurs when characteristics of the social role adopted influences one's behaviors [35, 36]. For example, an individual will reduce or abstain from drinking while in recovery; however, secure, long-term abstinence requires assuming a role (such as respected Elder) the person believes is incompatible with substance use [35, 36]. Alaska Native older adults also take on socially acceptable roles and acquire responsibilities expected of them by their family and community, paralleling findings of Quintero [37], through a process of role socialization [35] and becoming productive and engaged members of their family and community.

Community and Cultural Engagement

Herzog and House [38] noted the benefits to the broader society from the increased participation of Elders, which is directly related to Indigenous communities and includes engagement in community and cultural events and encouraging the involvement of others. Engagement of others not only improves the overall health and well-being of the family, but also the community. Through these activities, families and communities are able to interact with their Elders, and learn about their own history, language, and culture, which can improve the overall health and well-being of each family member. Also, when Elders are encouraged to engage in these rewarding community-wide activities, and they feel respected and heard. When they are engaging in rewarding activities, these activities and expectations of others replace the unhealthy behaviors that once took priority and encourage them to stay healthy. This engagement is a key predictor of protection from remission [34].

A useful strategy for facilitating health and well-being among Elders is to encourage Elders to participate in activities based on their preferences [38] and interests. For American Indians and Alaska Natives, these preferences can often involve teaching language, Native arts and crafts, volunteering with the school, or serving in a leadership position [39, 40]. A factor enabling Elders to become and remain engaged in their community and assist others is their spirituality, relationship with God, or connection to a higher power [3, 30, 41].

Spirituality

The role of culture and spirituality in sobriety is defined more broadly than religion alone [2, 33, 42] in much of the Indigenous literature. Dustin A. Pardini et al. [43] stated that spirituality and religion may be effective components of mental health treatment because of the positive outcomes associated with spiritual and religious engagement, which can include increased coping, resilience to stress, an optimistic outlook on life, greater perceived social support, and lower anxiety levels [43]; all of these contributed and supported individuals' decision to become healthy.

Mental Health, Indigenous Cultural Generativity, and Successful Aging

Indigenous Elders find meaning and joy when provided opportunities to give back to their family and community, to teach the youth, and leave a legacy to be passed down that will help the families and communities heal and live meaningful and productive lives. These Elders are engaging in generative acts that have clear cultural elements, patterned on being a role model for future generations and, through this, passing on one's culture to the next generation. Elders pass on their knowledge, not as a selfish way to ensure they are not forgotten, but as a way to ensure their family and youth will continue to live with tools and wisdom needed to achieve Eldership.

Earlier in this chapter, I discussed the types of generative acts, and how they are relevant to Indigenous populations. Building upon the literature, James Allen and I have created a term that highlights this unique component of generativity whereby Elders engage in cultural generativity but turn an Indigenous lens on the world. We call this Indigenous cultural generativity.

Indigenous cultural generativity can be defined as "any act of an older adult where they pass on traditional values, subsistence practices, language, beliefs, and any other activity that preserves and passes on the culture of the family and community" ([3], p. 213). Generativity has a focus on individual legacy for the next generation, whereas Indigenous cultural generative acts preserve the history, language, and cultural values and beliefs of an entire, family, community, culture, and way of being for seven generations. Indigenous older adults engage in these acts to ensure their way of life, Indigenous Ways of Knowing and being, the environment, and their family and community are healthy for their children and the children seven generations from today.

In this chapter, I have highlighted the experiences of Alaska Native Elders who maintained sobriety and recovery (physical and mental) by exploring and determining their cultural motivations, also known as engaging in Indigenous culturally generative acts. They are motivated by their desire to care for family and community members, and their wish to be role models and pass on their wisdom and experiences to the younger generations. Families and communities also facilitate opportunities to share and engage with family and community, which are possible through recovery and mental health.

Implications for Research and Practice

I believe this exploration of Indigenous generative acts, or cultural motivations, and their role in mental health among Indigenous Elders, is a first. In this chapter, I have examined what it means for Indigenous Elders to disengage in unhealthy behaviors and establish a pathway to age successfully in order to live the good life [37] and become who they were meant to be. Spicer [13] states that we are "forced to revise our understandings not only of what it means to change behavior, but, indeed, of what it means to be restored to wholeness" (p. 238). By highlighting the lifetime of stories, experiences, and motivations of those who have begun their journey of recovery and the importance of sharing their experiences and motivations with others, I have suggested ways to move Indigenous Elders forward.

These findings and work with Indigenous Elders suggest that mental health research needs to expand from a focus solely on individual recovery to other areas of the individual's life, including their respective roles in family and community life [5] and how shifting the healing from an individual benefit to a family and community benefit may prove beneficial. Both the increasing awareness of mental health problems plaguing American Indian and Alaska communities, and the shift to a positive focus on recovery factors, highlight strengths and resiliency within our Indigenous communities. This heightened consciousness and spirit of self-determination in improving one's health and well-being is a positive force for Indigenous mental health movements rebuilding healthy families and communities.

Further research is needed regarding these initial findings, which can potentially guide treatment approaches focused more directly on strengthening protective resources, promoting recovery [34], and encouraging Elders to share their stories and work in partnership with others to discover their cultural motivations and begin their journey of becoming who they were meant to be.

I view this chapter as the beginning of a discussion I hope can influence future work and research in understanding motivating and maintenance factors that protect the mental health of Indigenous Elders and Peoples and assist them in filling their expected roles and becoming healthy Elders and role models. Figure 1, the journey of "Becoming who I am meant to be," points out that many Indigenous Peoples experience early life adversity, which impacts their lives to some degree. As they age, these early experiences may result in maladaptive behaviors, including substance misuse, abuse, or self-harm, all of which prevent them from fulfilling role expectations or achieving Eldership. As Indigenous people age, they experience turning points in their lives, which can include the birth of their first child or grandchild, being treated as an Elder in their community, or near-death experiences. Or they may realize their current lifestyle will not enable them to become an Elder and have the opportunities their Elders did with them when they were young. Many reach a turning point, and, through these motivations and learning from others, wishing to share their knowledge, they are able to reconnect to their Indigenous family and community, resulting in a healthy and positive identity that was lost earlier in life due to adversity. Reconnecting to Indigenous identity, sharing that journey, and seeing their experiences helping others overcome challenges and find meaning in life, as well as engaging in cultural activities, gives Indigenous Elders their generative acts and behaviors, and thus they attain Eldership. This knowledge can guide development of culture-specific mental health treatment approaches, and more broadly, prevention strategies for all ages. This intergenerational healing can result in pride and improved mental health for Indigenous Peoples of all ages.

References

1. Braveheart MD, Lemyra M. The American Indian holocaust: healing historical unresolved grief. Am Indian Alaska Native Mental Health Res. 2000;8(2):60–81.
2. Napoleon H. Yuuyaraq: the way of the human being. Fairbanks: Center for Cross Cultural Studies, University of Alaska Fairbanks; 1991.
3. Lewis JP, Allen J. Alaska Native elders in recovery: linkages between indigenous cultural generativity and sobriety to promote successful aging. J Cross Cultural Gerontol. 2017;32(2):209–22.
4. Burman S. The challenge of sobriety: natural recovery without treatment and self-help groups. J Subst Abuse. 1997;9:41–61.
5. Etz KE, Arroyo JA, Crump AD, Rosa CL, Scott MS. Advancing American Indian and Alaska Native substance abuse research: current science and future directions. Am J Drug Alcohol Abuse. 2012;38(5):372–5.
6. Mohatt GV, Hazel KL, Allen J, Stachelrodt M, Hensel C, Fath R. Unheard Alaska: culturally anchored participatory action research on sobriety with Alaska Natives. Am J Community Psychol. 2004;33:263–73.
7. Mohatt GV, Rasmus SM, Thomas L, Allen J, Hazel K, Hensel C. "Tied together like a woven hat:" protective pathways to Alaska Native sobriety. Harm Reduction J. 2004;1(10):1–10.
8. Whitesell NR, Beals J, Big Crow C, Mitchell CM, Novins DK. Epidemiology and etiology of substance use among American Indians and Alaska Natives: risk, protection, and implications for prevention. Am J Drug Alcohol Abuse. 2012;38(5):376–82.
9. Albertsen K, Borg V, Oldenburg B. A systematic review of the impact of work environment on smoking cessation, relapse and amount smoked. Preventive Med. 2006;43(4):291–305.
10. Beattie MC, Longabaugh R. Interpersonal factors and post-treatment drinking and subjective well-being. Addiction. 1997;92:1507–21.
11. Bond J, Kaskutas LA, Weisner C. The persistent influence of social networks and Alcoholics Anonymous on abstinence. J Stud Alcohol. 2003;54:579–88.
12. Mohatt GV, Rasmus SM, Thomas L, Allen J, Hazel TB, Marlatt GA. Risk, resilience, and natural recovery: a model of recovery from alcohol abuse for Alaska Natives. Addiction. 2007;103:205–15.
13. Spicer P. Culture and the restoration of self among former American Indian drinkers. Soc Sci Med. 2001;53:227–40.
14. Kotre J. Outliving the self: generativity and the interpretation of lives. Baltimore, MD: Johns Hopkins University Press; 1984.

15. Erikson EH, Erikson JM. The life cycle completed: extended version with new chapters on the ninth stage of development. New York: Norton & Comp; 1997.
16. Fisher BJ. Successful aging, life satisfaction, and generativity in later life. Int J Aging Human Dev. 1995;41:239–50.
17. Baltes PB, Baltes MM. Psychological perspectives on successful aging: the model of selective optimization with compensation. In: Baltes PB, Baltes MM, editors. Successful aging: perspectives from the behavioral sciences. Cambridge: Cambridge University Press; 1990. p. 1–34.
18. Schoklitsch A, Baumann U. Generativity and aging: a promising future research topic? J Aging Stud. 2012;26:262–72.
19. Vaillant GE. Generativity: a form of unconditional love. In: Post SG, editor. Altruism and health. New York: Oxford University Press; 2007. p. 219–29.
20. Erikson EE, Erikson JM, Kivnick HQ. Vital involvement in old age. New York: W.W. Norton; 1986.
21. Keyes, C. L. M., & Ryff, C. D. (1998). Generativity in adult lives: social structural contours and quality of life consequences. In D. P. McAdams, de St. Aubin E. (Eds), Generativity and adult development: how and why we care for the next generation (227–263). Washington, DC, US: American Psychological Association, xxiv, p. 511.
22. McAdams DP, de St. Aubin E. A theory of generativity and its assessment through self-report, behavioral acts, and narrative themes in autobiography. J Personality Social Psychol. 1992;62:1003–15.
23. Snarey J. How fathers care for the next generation. Cambridge, MA: Harvard University Press; 1993.
24. Warburton J, McLaughlin D, Pinsker D. Generative acts: Family and community involvement of older Australians. Int J Aging Hum Dev. 2006;63(2):115–37.
25. Kane R. From generation to generation: thoughts on legacy. Generations. 1996;20:5–9.
26. Manheimer RJ. Redeeming the aging self: John Kotre, George Drury, and cultural generativity. J Aging Stud. 1995;9(1):13–20.
27. de St. Aubin E, McAdams DP. The relations of generative concerns and generative action to personality traits, satisfaction with life, and ego development. J Adult Dev. 1995;2:99–112.
28. Peterson BE, Smirles KA, Wentworth PA. Generativity and authoritarianism: implications for personality, political involvement, and parenting. J Pers Soc Psychol. 2007;72:1202–16.
29. Jones BK, McAdams DP. Becoming generative: socializing influences recalled in life stories in late midlife. J Adult Dev. 2013;20:158–72.
30. Lewis J. What successful aging means to Alaska Natives: exploring the reciprocal relationship between the health and well-being of Alaska Native Elders. Int J Ageing Soc. 2014;3(1):2160–1909.
31. Chen S-T. Generativity in later life: perceived respect from younger generations as a determinant of goal disengagement and psychological well-being. J Gerontol Psychol Sci. 2009;64B(1):45–54.
32. Walters KL, Simoni JM, Evans-Campbell T. Substance use among American Indians and Alaska Natives: incorporating culture in an "Indigenist" stress-coping paradigm. Public Health Rep. 2002;117(Suppl. 1):S104–17.
33. Hazel KL, Mohatt GV. Cultural and spiritual coping in sobriety: informing substance abuse prevention for Alaska Native communities. J Community Psychol. 2001;29(5):541–62.
34. Moos RH. Theory-based processes that promote the remission of substance use disorders. Clin Psychol Rev. 2007;27:537–51.
35. Watson AL, Sher KJ. Resolution of alcohol problems without treatment: methodological issues and future directions of natural recovery research. Clin Psychol Sci Pract. 1998;5(1):1–18.
36. Yamaguchi K, Kandel DB. On the resolution of role incompatibility: a life event history analysis of family role and marijuana use. Am J Sociol. 1985;90:z1284–325.
37. Quintero G. "The lizard in the green bottle: 'Aging out'" of problem drinking among Navajo men. Soc Sci Med. 2000;51:1031–45.

38. Herzog AR, House JS. Productive activities and aging well. Generations. 1991;15(1):49–55.
39. Lewis J, Boyd K. Reconceptualizing long term care in rural Alaska. IHS Primary Care Provider. 2012;37(2):12–44.
40. Lewis J, Boyd K. Forward steps and missteps: what we've learned through the process of conducting CBPR research in rural Alaska. J Indigenous Res; 2013. http://digitalcommons.usu.edu/kicjir/vol2/iss1/3.
41. Lewis JP. Successful aging through the eyes of Alaska Native Elders. What it means to be an elder in Bristol Bay, AK. Gerontologist. 2011;51(4):540–9.
42. Brady M. Culture in treatment, culture as treatment. A critical appraisal of developments in addictions programs for indigenous North Americans and Australians. Soc Sci Med. 1995;41:1487–98.
43. Pardini DA, Plante TG, Sherman A, Stump JE. Religious faith and spirituality in substance abuse recovery. Determining the mental health benefits. J Subst Abuse Treat. 2000;19:347–54.

Jordan P. Lewis is Unangax (Alaska Native) and an enrolled member with the Native Village of Naknek, Alaska. As a cross-cultural community psychologist, his research explores the role of culture in the aging process and how it impacts whether or not individuals are able to age successfully despite sociocultural challenges in rural Alaska. His research links issues of Alaska Native aging and community health and the current cultural dynamics of Alaska Native communities.

Dr. Lewis is a Fellow with the Gerontological Society of America, and he received the Rural Health and Aging Research Award from the American Public Health Association. He has received research funding from the National Science Foundation and National Institutes of Health. Jordan has contributed to *The Gerontologist, The Journal of Cross-Cultural Gerontology,* and the *International Journal of Circumpolar Health.* Jordan is a faculty member at the University of Minnesota Medical School, Duluth campus, and the Memory Keepers Medical Discovery Team.

Ka Huri Te Ao, a Time of Change: Māori Mental Health and Addiction in Aotearoa, New Zealand

Terry Huriwai, Kahu McClintock, and Rachel McClintock

The experience of colonial contact for Māori in Aotearoa, New Zealand has been associated with loss of culture, dislocation, and deprivation [1]. Like other Indigenous Peoples, Māori continues to fare poorly on many social indices, including employment, education, housing, and health [2]. Mental health remains one of the greatest reported health risks to Māori [3–7].

The Ministry of Health, Aotearoa (2015) reported that Māori adults were more likely than non-Māori to be hospitalized (over three times as likely) or die (over two and half times as likely) as victims of violence. The Ministry of Health [2] further stated that with regard to mental health, that Māori adults were more likely than non-Māori (one-and-a-half times as likely) to score high to very high probability of having an anxiety or depressive disorder. This disparity was found to be larger in males; the rate at which Māori males scored high to very high probability was double the rate of non-Māori.

It is our belief that the involvement of *whānau* (family) is essential to address the difficulties these rising statistics reveal. *Whānau* involvement in decision-making processes as well as improving access to both a clinically and culturally capable workforce is seminal to addressing mental health disorders [5, 8].

Whānau remains the foundation of Māori society. It is central to the well-being of Māori both individually and collectively and a principal source of security and identity [9, 10]. Traditionally, *whānau* are those who are bound together as an extended family based on common descent and shared reciprocity, obligations, responsibilities, and aspirations [10, 11].

A contemporary term, *kaupapa whānau,* describes *whānau* as not necessarily linked by *whakapapa* (genealogy) but as a social system and or collective associate

---

T. Huriwai · K. McClintock (✉) · R. McClintock
Consultant Researcher, New Zealand
e-mail: terry.huriwai@outlook.co.nz; kahu.mcclintock@outlook.com; rachel.mcclintock@outlook.com

D. Danto, M. Zangeneh (eds.), *Indigenous Knowledge and Mental Health*,
https://doi.org/10.1007/978-3-030-71346-1_12

for a commonly valued purpose that also reflects traditional *whānau* responsibilities and obligations [10].

Whānau Ora

In Aotearoa, the Ministry of Health [12] plan, *Rising to the Challenge the National Mental Health and Addiction Service Development Plan 2012–2017* (SDP), requires that a Whānau Ora approach be undertaken when working with Māori. The SDP also states that Whānau Ora initiatives require priority action to help cement and build on gains in resilience and recovery for Māori [12]. Thus, *whānau ora* is a strategic direction, an outcome, a policy imperative, and a way of working. Whether it is a direction or a way, the focus is on Māori *mana motuhake* (autonomy), collaborative working (partnership), and taking a systems approach where the collective is the prime focus not the individual.

This innovative development plan supports realizing *whānau* potential, the collective aspirations of the *whānau,* and building on the strengths and capabilities present within *whānau* [13]. Whānau Ora as a strategic direction and as a way of working explicitly recognizes that:

- *Whānau* is a collective entity.
- *Whānau* has a capacity for self-determination.
- *Whānau* is affected by intergenerational dynamics including colonization and historical trauma.
- Māori cultural values, principles, and experiences are to be prioritized.
- There are positive roles for *whānau* within society.
- The approach can be operationalized across a wide range of health, social, and economic sectors.

A Whānau Ora capable workforce, that is, a workforce able to work with the *whānau,* is located in a range of disciplines and contexts, including community work, social work, nursing, public health (including health promotion), and youth justice. It means irrespective of role and context we are working collectively to contribute to improving shared outcomes for Māori [9]. A Whānau Ora capable workforce goes beyond crisis intervention and symptom relief to building skills and strategies that contribute to maximizing positive outcomes, in other words, well-being. [9]. Special skills are required that include:

- ascertaining *whānau* aspirations;
- mediating *whānau* tensions; and
- brokering opportunities for *whānau* to ensure *whānau* have access to the best possible services and resources [9].

In order to collectively contribute to positive outcomes for *whānau,* it is important for mental health and addiction services to establish reciprocal relationships with *kaupapa* Māori services (services that are governed by Māori, delivered predominantly to Māori, and use Māori knowledge and skills in the delivery of their service), providers dedicated to Whānau Ora, and agencies where *whānau* present, for example, government health and social services. Currently, many service providers and commissioners of services operate in a siloed approach; therefore, taking a collaborative approach with others from different services and sectors to contribute to a shared outcome, that is, a Whānau Ora approach, can be daunting.

Pātaka Uara: Whānau Ora in Action

Pātaka Uara is an example of a Whānau Ora practitioner model based on *te reo me ona tikanga* (language, values, beliefs, principles, and practices). Some of the principles included within this model, and detailed in the example[1] below, include *whakapapa* (genealogy), *whanaungatanga* (building relationships with *whānau*), *manaakitanga* (care and support), *ūkaipōtanga* (secure sense of identity), *kaitiakitanga* (stewardship), *kotahitanga* (solidarity), *wairuatanga* (spirituality), and *rangatiratanga* (self-determination) [14].

Working with the Whole Whānau

A Māori family of four (mother, father, and two sons under 11 years of age) residing in Tauranga, a city on the East Coast of the North Island of New Zealand, accessed a local Whānau Ora service. The father came from a tribe further down the East Coast of the North Island (Ngāti Porou) and the mother came from a tribe located in the far north of the North Island (Te Rarawa). While this family lived in a region they did not *whakapapa* to, they still maintained strong links to their *tūrangawaewae* (place of belonging), particularly the tribal region of Ngāti Porou. They regularly participated in events which were Māori-centered, and Māori culture and protocols were demonstrated. The *whānau* accessed a Whānau Ora service in Tauranga because it was based in the city they lived. They wanted the service to assist them with their sons' anger issues, as well as to support their *whānau*. This matched with a Whānau Ora approach, which works with the whole *whānau* instead of only with the boys in isolation from their parents.

[1] This example was originally adapted with permission from "A Mental Health and Addiction Framework, A Whānau Ora Approach" by Te Rau Ora, 2014, Wellington, New Zealand: Author. Copyright 2014 by Te Rau Ora..

Whanaungatanga: Making Connections

In line with Māori cultural practices, the Whānau Ora service first established a good rapport and engagement with the *whānau* (a process of *whakawhanaunga).* As the supporting case manager was from the same tribe as one of the parents, it meant there was a connection between the *whānau* and services, a shared tribal history, that preceded their meeting. This assisted to make the establishment of trust and *whanaungatanga* (a sense of connection) with the whole *whānau* easier.

Ūkaipōtanga: Security and Stability

The Whānau Ora services learned from the *whānau* that when the boys were younger, their mother had been too ill to care for them and their father became her carer. At that time the boys were placed in the care of a trusted family elder—their maternal grandmother. While the boys received good care at their grandmother's and appeared to be coping well, their preference was to be with their mother, who they missed. When their mother's health improved, the boys returned to the care of their parents. In the 2 years before the *whānau* meeting with the Whānau Ora service, the boys developed issues with anger. A link was made between the boys' behavior and their mother's absence from home because of study commitments as well as their resentment from being away from their parents when they were younger. The boys questioned why they had not lived with their mother at that time.

Manaakitanga: Supportive Care

The mother of this family self-referred her *whānau* to this *kaupapa* Māori service in order to gain assistance and support. The staff at this service were able to use *manaaki* to build rapport and trust with this *whānau*, and ultimately help them. During this time all of the *whānau* members were physically well and the parents were engaged in either full-time work (father) or full-time study (mother).

Kotahitanga: Reconnecting

Resolution was made possible through mediation and support. The supporting case managers helped the sons to discuss and understand why they were separated from their parents in the past and what was currently happening. This process included facilitated discussions between the boys and their parents, their mother in particular.

Talking things through and getting support was healing for the boys, who were able to gain a sense *kotahitanga*.

Wairuatanga: Spirituality

The Māori cultural practice of opening and closing each *hui* with *karakia* (reciting prayers, a spiritual process which manages and uses the *taha wairua*/Māori spiritual dimension) was a normal part of interactions between the *whānau* and the services. The *karakia* were often led by the boys, who can speak *te reo* fluently.

Rangatiratanga: Autonomy

This family was supported by this Whānau Ora service for 9 months. By the end of their time with the service, the family identified that they no longer needed help; the boys were doing well at school and fully active in sport again and were content at home.

Māori practitioners, whether involved clinically or in support roles, have endorsed the Whānau Ora process, as described in this study at Pātaka Uara, saying they are more likely to build respectful and trustworthy relationships with *whānau* that ensures quality engagement and ultimately contributes to better health outcomes [15].

Young People and their Whānau

Improving the delivery of mental health services to young Māori and their *whānau* has been identified as a priority in several studies [6, 16]. Parental involvement in the assessment and treatment processes is thought to be essential to this development [5, 8]. Positive contact for parents with Child and Adolescent Mental Health Services (CAMHS) is more likely to influence ongoing dealings with the service that leads to better mental health outcomes for their children [17, 18].

Studies with Māori parents and young people who accessed CAMHS identified that they desired a Māori workforce with cultural capacity and capability [5, 8]. *Whānau* and young Māori valued information about options for both cultural and clinical pathways for support, as they saw this helping with better engagement and participation. They felt Māori working in this space would work to enhance the quality of the relationship between *whānau* and CAMHS [5, 19].

Furthermore, parents wanted CAMHS to factor in the appropriate time and space for real communication, one that valued partnership, relationships, responsibility, and reciprocity with *whānau*. They viewed this as essential to ensuring that positive engagement and participation that would influence better health outcomes [5].

McClintock et al. [5] found that having a workforce appropriate to the Aotearoa context, with *te reo me ona tikanga* and culturally competent health professionals, was an important aspect to ensuring improved health outcomes for Māori who access CAMHS. Likewise, they found that correct and timely information regarding medication and its benefits were further viewed as seminal to assist understanding and therefore compliance with medication regimes offered by CAMHS [5]. Successful access, engagement, and participation of Māori with CAMHS were also deemed more likely to occur when *whānau* involvement was encouraged and valued. A process of engagement and participation, founded on cultural respect, partnership, reciprocity, and commitment is therefore valued [5, 8].

Although this framework of service improvement has been offered to services to champion *whānau* aspirations, sadly, implementation continues to be minimal as services prefer to stay focused on a clinical approach. Managers within CAMHS have reported being pressured by their service to meet key performance indicators that place little value on *whānau* culture. Improving outcomes for Māori who access CAMHS will remain a challenge if it continues to ignore the relevancy of culture.

Mental Health Outcome Measurement: Hua Oranga

A number of national health policies in Aotearoa have endorsed the planning and delivery of effective and culturally relevant treatment practices that promote cultural and clinical competency in the delivery of services for Māori. These directives also include the use of culturally relevant assessment tools and outcome measures [20–22]. Outcome measures are critical to the development of quality mental health services and to their continuous improvement [23]. Assessment and outcome information collected, if fully utilized, can inform the construction and delivery of effective care and treatment plans thus ensuring high-quality services that contribute to better health outcomes [23].

Hua Oranga is a Māori mental health outcome measure for use with Māori that incorporates a holistic method of outcome assessment founded on an existing framework of health and well-being, the *whare tapa whā.* This framework encompasses four dimensions: *taha wairua* (spiritual), *taha hinengaro* (cognitive and emotional), *taha tinana* (physical), and *taha whānau* (family and relationships) [24]. From a Māori perspective, constructing a measurement around the model involves assessment of these four dimensions and taking account of the perspectives of three key stakeholders: the *tangata whaiora* (consumer), *whānau,* and the clinician [24].

Participation in the Hua Oranga

The administration of the Hua Oranga outcomes tool encourages a partnership approach between clinicians, *tangata whaiora,* and *whānau.* In this partnership approach, goals are negotiated using the results from the completed individual Hua Oranga schedules (see Appendix). Clinicians see discussing strengths essential to this process: first, so that the *tangata whaiora* does not feel *whakamā* (ashamed) and, more important, to build on positive experiences and skills of the *tangata whaiora* [19]. The clinicians are adamant that respect for the *tangata whaiora* is essential for a successful partnership leading to improved health outcomes [19].

Benefits of the Hua Oranga

The Hua Oranga provides support and a starting point for developing Māori *tikanga* (values and beliefs) treatment plans based on *kawa* (protocols), and including *wairua* (spiritual dimensions), *te reo Māori* (Māori language), and *karakia* (prayers). Clinicians, *tangata whaiora,* and *whānau* also view the Hua Oranga as support designed to identify needs and areas of improvement. Engagement with *tangata whaiora* and *whānau* is deemed essential to ensuring a collaborative partnership approach to developing care plans [19].

A review of the plan is recommended at 6 weeks, 3 months, or both, depending on the needs identified as part of the collective treatment plan. Assessments are expected to show progress toward a desired outcome, as a result of the collaboration and partnership. Reviews also allow an opportunity to celebrate achievement and to set new goals [19].

Hua Oranga Case Study (See Footnote 1)

This example has been provided by MOKO Māori Mental Health Services (MHS), Whitiki Maurea, the Mental Health and Addiction Services of the Waitemata District Health Board (DHB).

Referral History

At the beginning of 2014, a man (BG) experiencing first-time psychosis presented to the Waitemata DHB MHS. Reasons for BG's psychosis included increased drug use (cannabis), discord with his partner, and increased paranoia—specifically that his neighbors wanted his cannabis plants. BG's *whānau* was initially resistant to the involvement of MHS; BG's wife thought he had transgressed *tapu* (restricted protocols concerned with preserving life). Before coming into contact with MHS, BG had tried seeking help through a *kaumatua* (Elder), who had carried out a *whānau* blessing in an attempt to rectify the transgression.

When BG was first admitted to MHS, it was informally into the acute unit. His stay lasted 4 days, after which he discharged himself. He also turned down the medication he was prescribed. Once discharged, BG was followed up by community MHS. Eventually, against his strong wishes and under the *Mental Health Act,* BG was involuntarily committed to mandatory assessment and treatment. At that time, for the first time, BG was introduced to MOKO Māori MHS.

A service cultural assessment tool was used with his consent to determine his knowledge of his *whakapapa* (genealogy). Through this process, MOKO Māori learned that that BG was trying to find out *ko wai ahau*? (Who am I? Where am I from?) to learn who he was and connect to his cultural heritage. BG's mistrust of MHS was evidenced by his anxiety; MHS could take away his autonomy and liberty. BG was more willing to seek help from a Māori MHS like MOKO services because he felt they listened to him and were more understanding than mainstream MHS of his situation.

Whānau

Through discussion with BG, Moko MHS learned that he was a *tamaiti whāngai* (adopted child) who did not have a relationship with his birth family. The only information he knew of his *whānau* was his mother's name from his birth certificate. Recently BG had learned he was born in a home for mothers with unwanted pregnancies. BG also shared that while he had lived in multiple foster homes growing up, he felt the strongest affinity to an area he had worked in as a farmhand—Kaipara, in the far north of the North Island of New Zealand.

Not knowing his family or where he was from made BG feel incomplete and insufficient. He said "I have no legacy Māori to give my *tamariki* (children), although my wife is Māori" ([14], p. 17–18). BG was a father of two and his wife was a member of a tribe located in the north of the North Island of New Zealand (Ngāti Whātua) and another from the Midlands region (Ngāti Maniapoto).

MOKO Services

Moko services followed up with BG, both culturally and clinically. As part of his work with Moko services, BG agreed to participate in the Hōtaka Hauora Māori program. This program is based on the *whare tapa whā* model and uses basic *te reo* (language). As is usual for Moko services, BG, with his wife, was welcomed into the program in a traditional Māori welcome (*pōhiri,* or *powhiri*). A *powhiri* is a timeless Māori approach to engagement which is based on *tikanga* Māori such as *tika* (to be correct), *pono* (honesty), and *aroha* (love). A *karakia* (prayer) was said to open the *hui*, which solidified the understanding of a shared *kaupapa* (purpose) and journey between BG, his *whānau*, and Moko services.

Hua Oranga

BG enjoyed the powhiri and, while sharing his life story, he was comfortable enough to *tangi* (crying release of sorrow). BG's wife shared the positive changes she had seen in him, and that his life was better for coming to MOKO services. While with MOKO services, BG, his whānau, and his clinical team at MOKO services carried out a Hua Oranga interview. Hua Oranga involves gaining the perspectives of *tangata whaiora,* their *whānau,* and the treatment team as part of the assessment process. It promotes collaboration and shared views going forward.

Everyone agreed to support BG to learn more about his whakapapa, his wish not to take medication, to contest his mandatory treatment under the *Mental Health Act,* and work on reducing his cannabis use. With the start of this journey of self-discovery, BG said he was able to stop his cannabis use.

To review BG's progress, 7 weeks later, Hua Oranga was carried out again. Many positive changes had occurred for BG. He was able to be discharged from the *Mental Health Act,* as he was assessed by the clinical team as free of psychosis and no longer manic. With the support of his *whānau,* BG continued to participate in the MOKO services program, attended his first Hōtaka Hauora *reo,* and was working with a *taurawhiri* (cultural adviser) to help him reconnect with his birth family.

> *"Tawhiti rawa tou haerenga ake te kore haere tonu.*
> *He nui rawa ou mahi te kore mahi tonu*
> You have come too far not to journey further.
> You have done too much not to do more!
> *—Sir James Henare"* (as cited in Te Rau Ora, 2014, p. 18)

Although Māori clinicians have embraced the fundamentals as well as the depth of the Hua Oranga, non-Māori clinicians' understanding of the Hua Oranga, especially the *taha wairua,* presents an ongoing challenge. The test is even greater for clinicians who lack an understanding of Māori spirituality. Mental health and addiction services must however provide an approach that culturally resonates with Māori who access their services if they are to contribute to improved Māori well-being.

The Addiction Workforce

In this section, we specifically examine the development of a clinical and cultural capable workforce that contributes to the minimization of addiction-related harm experienced by Māori. Early snapshots of the alcohol and other drug (AOD) treatment sector consistently found the proportion of the workforce who identified as Māori was substantially lower than the proportion of Māori presenting as clients. A similar trend was noticed in the problem gambling workforce. In the 10 years from 1998 to 2008, the proportion of Māori in the AOD workforce appeared to decrease from 25% to 15% [25].

The most recent surveys [26, 27] found Māori make up about 23% of the addiction workforce, 35% of the ICAMHS workforce, 15% of those employed in DHB addiction services, and nearly 32% of practitioners in NGO AOD services. Māori clients accounted for nearly 33% of AOD service provision. Problem gambling services reported that 24% of the workforce was Māori compared to 31% of those presenting at services.

Although there appear to be increasing numbers of Māori identified as working in the addiction treatment sector, there is no indication as to their capacity or competency to operate from a *mātauranga* Māori (knowledge) space or deliver culturally located models, frameworks, and practice.

The addiction workforce, both Māori and non-Māori, continues to call for and require skills and knowledge to work in Māori-responsive ways thus the development of competency frameworks and development programs such as the Takarangi Framework and Huarahi Whakatū.

The most common professional affiliations in the addiction workforce are reported as addiction practitioners/counselors, nurses, and social workers [25, 28]. The "More than Numbers" survey of the mental health and addiction workforce [27] indicates that more than half (62%) of the *kaupapa* Māori addiction workforce had roles in the allied health group, with support workers and nurses comprising only 14% and 6%, respectively.

Tami Cave et al. [29] reported the average age of the Māori addiction workforce was 47 years, with equal representation of male and female workers. The workforce is an aging one and most are employed in NGOs [28, 30, 31]. Moreover, many in the addiction workforce have lived experience from their own addiction issues or those of their *whānau*.

Competent practitioners can contribute to *whānau ora* (well-being) by integrating cultural and clinical elements within their practices. Eileen Britt et al. [32] emphasize that linking *mātauranga* Māori with other theoretical models is possible when the goal is hope, well-being, and transformation. Using resources such as He Puna Whakaata [33, 34] and opportunities such as the inclusion of *manaaki* (care, thoughtfulness) in the new *Substance Addiction Compulsory Assessment and Treatment Act 2017* [35] is a good beginning. Groups like Te Rau Ora can encourage shifts in practice that will support the realization of *whānau* potential, aspirations, and well-being.

An example of shifts in practice is He Puna Whakaata. This resource offers activities that use *mātauranga* Māori and the wisdom and experience of the *tīpuna* as part of a transformative process of healing. The activities draw on motivational interviewing and encourage practitioners to be more aware of and use cultural symbolism, processes, and metaphor to help *whānau* navigate their own path to sustained well-being.

The Whai Tikanga card sort, described in He Puna Whakaata, is similar to the Value Cards Sort used to help people see the differences between their values and their behavior. Whai Tikanga uses values and *whakataukī* (proverbs or sayings) centered in Te Ao Māori. *Whakataukī* are the handed-down "voices" of *tīpuna* and they reinforce the "values" drawn out in the activity.

Traditionally, sayings, proverbs, and various customs were educational devices highlighting and illustrating morals, principles, models, and behaviors to be applied in everyday life—and they were part of the process of enculturation. Many today no longer know, understand, or live the basic values of these traditional values, practices, and experiences. Increasingly some are disconnected or have been excluded from opportunities to grow and develop as Māori. This disconnection and the compromise of these traditional values and knowledge is one explanation for a range of health and social harms.

During the first 6 months of 2017, more than 130 practitioners in a range of AOD, problem gambling, mental health, and social service agencies across the country received the He Puna Whakaata resource, which included a pack of Whai Tikanga cards. Evaluations from the workshops showed that knowledge transfer occurred during the training and the practitioners were grateful for the opportunity to be able to integrate *mātauranga* Māori into their practice. Feedback after the workshops indicated that there were benefits for the practitioners as well as for the individuals, groups, and *whānau* they worked with.

Respondents also noted that sustaining the shifts in practice promoted in He Puna Whakaata requires cultural competence and ongoing reflective practice. Others noted that activities such as the Whai Tikanga cards tended to lead practitioners from concentrating on deficits and problems to aspirational and strength-based approaches. They also enabled the use of Māori-oriented narratives and talking therapies, the exploration of *mātauranga* Māori, and the development of a greater sense of self as Māori. Further evaluation will determine the degree to which skill transfer occurs post-workshop and how to sustain this change in practice.

Conclusion

In this chapter, we have reported on a range of strategies and initiatives to support the Indigenous population of Aotearoa. These initiatives were created to ensure better health outcomes for Māori, and to help them reach their potential through the delivery of effective culturally and clinically appropriate mental health and addiction services. In sharing the intentions and the associated progress of these programs to date, we look for a future that will continue to focus on providing Māori approaches that resonate with the aspirations of Māori.

Appendix: Hua Oranga Schedules

TE RAU ORA
Strengthening Māori Health and Well-Being

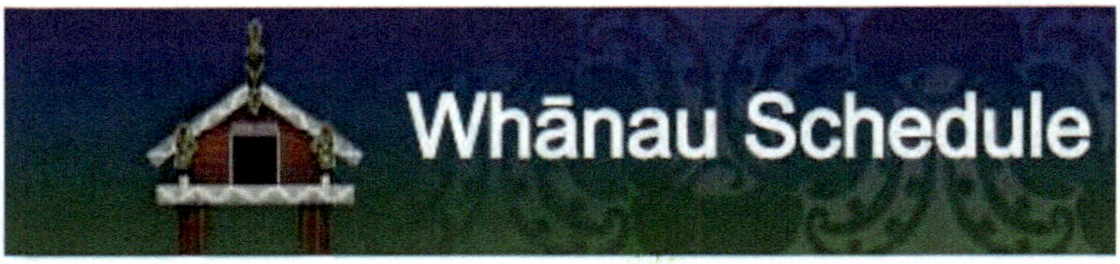

NHI number:
Gender: Male/Female
Date: _ _/ _ _/_ _

Circle the response under each category which best reflects the way you think your relative is feeling.

Wairua

1. I feel that the spiritual health of my relative is extremely good at present
2. I feel that the spiritual health of my relative is good at present
3. I feel that the spiritual health of my relative is just okay at present
4. I feel that the spiritual health of my relative is not good at present
5. I feel that the spiritual health of my relative is very bad at present

Tinana

1. I feel that the physical health of my relative is extremely good at present
2. I feel that the physical health of my relative is good at present
3. I feel that the physical health of my relative is just okay at present
4. I feel that the physical health of my relative is not good at present
5. I feel that the physical health of my relative is very bad at present

Hinengaro

1. I feel that the mental health of my relative is extremely good at present
2. I feel that the mental health of my relative is good at present
3. I feel that the mental health of my relative is just okay at present
4. I feel that the mental health of my relative is not good at present
5. I feel that the mental health of my relative is very bad at present

Whānau

1. I feel that the relationships my relative has with our whānau are extremely good at present
2. I feel that the relationships my relative has with our whānau are good at present
3. I feel that the relationships my relative has with our whānau are just okay at present
4. I feel that the relationships my relative has with our whānau are not good at present
5. I feel that the relationships my relative has with our whānau are very bad at present

TE RAU ORA
Strengthening Māori Health and Well-Being

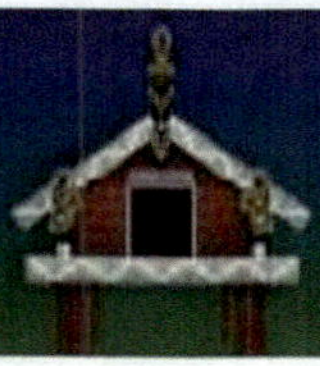

Tangata Whaiora Schedule

NHI number:
Gender: Male/Female
Date: _ _/ _ _/_ _

Circle the response under each category which best reflects the way you are feeling

Wairua
1. I feel that my spiritual health is extremely good at present
2. I feel that my spiritual health is good at present
3. I feel that my spiritual health is just okay at present
4. I feel that my spiritual health is not good at present
5. I feel that my spiritual health is very bad at present

Tinana
1. I feel that my physical health is extremely good at present
2. I feel that my physical health is good at present
3. I feel that my physical health is just okay at present
4. I feel that my physical health is not good at present
5. I feel that my physical health is very bad at present

Hinengaro
1. I feel that my mental health is extremely good at present
2. I feel that my mental health is good at present
3. I feel that my mental health is just okay at present
4. I feel that my mental health is not good at present
5. I feel that my mental health is very bad at present

Whānau
1. I feel that my relationships with my whānau are extremely good at present
2. I feel that my relationships with my whānau are good at present
3. I feel that my relationships with my whānau are just okay at present
4. I feel that my relationships with my whānau are not good at present
5. I feel that my relationships with my whānau are very bad at present

TE RAU ORA
Strengthening Māori Health and Well-Being

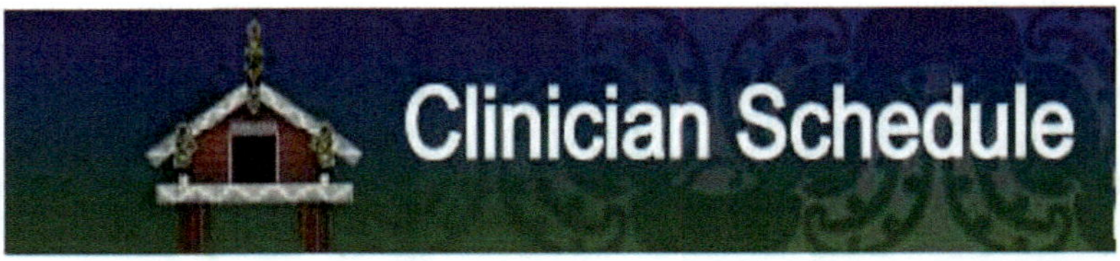

NHI number:
Gender: Male/Female
Date: _ _/ _ _/_ _

Circle the response under each category which best reflects the way you think the tangata whaiora is feeling.

Wairua
1. I feel that the spiritual health of the tangata whaiora is extremely good at present
2. I feel that the spiritual health of the tangata whaiora is good at present
3. I feel that the spiritual health of the tangata whaiora is just okay at present
4. I feel that the spiritual health of the tangata whaiora is not good at present
5. I feel that the spiritual health of the tangata whaiora is very bad at present

Tinana
1. I feel that the physical health of the tangata whaiora is extremely good at present
2. I feel that the physical health of the tangata whaiora is good at present
3. I feel that the physical health of the tangata whaiora is just okay at present
4. I feel that the physical health of the tangata whaiora is not good at present
5. I feel that the physical health of the tangata whaiora is very bad at present

Hinengaro
1. I feel that the mental health of the tangata whaiora is extremely good at present
2. I feel that the mental health of the tangata whaiora is good at present
3. I feel that the mental health of the tangata whaiora is just okay at present
4. I feel that the mental health of the tangata whaiora is not good at present
5. I feel that the mental health of the tangata whaiora is very bad at present

Whānau
1. I feel that the relationships of the tangata whaiora with their whānau are extremely good at present
2. I feel that the relationships of the tangata whaiora with their whānau are good at present
3. I feel that the relationships of the tangata whaiora with their whānau are just okay at present
4. I feel that the relationships of the tangata whaiora with their whānau are not good at present
5. I feel that my relationships of the tangata whaiora with their whānau are very bad at present

References

1. Reid P, Robson B. Understanding health inequities. In: Robson B, Harris R, editors. Hauora: Māori standards of health IV. A study of the years 2000–2005. Te Rōpū Rangahau Hauora a Eru Pōmare: Wellington, New Zealand; 2007. p. 3–10.
2. Ministry of Health. Tatau Kahukura: Māori health chart book 2015. 3rd ed. Wellington: Ministry of Health; 2015.
3. Baxter J. Mental health: psychiatric disorder and suicide. In: Robinson B, Harris R, editors. Hauora Māori standards of health IV. A study of the years 2000–2005. Te Rōpū Rangahau Hauora a Eru Pōmare: Wellington, New Zealand; 2007. p. 121–32.
4. Baxter J, Kingi TK, Tapsell R, Durie M, McGee MA. Prevalence of mental disorders amongst Māori in Te Rau Hinengaro. The New Zealand mental health survey. Aust N Zeal J Psychiatry. 2006;40(10):905–13.
5. McClintock K, Moeke-Maxwell T, Mellsop G. Appropriate child and adolescent mental health services (CAMHS) for Māori: caregivers perspectives. Pimatisiwin J Aboriginal Indigenous Community Health. 2011;9(2):387–98.
6. Ramage C, Bir J, Towns A, Vague R, Cargo T, Niumata-Faleafa M. Stocktake of child and adolescent mental health services in new Zealand. Auckland, New Zealand: The Werry Centre for Child & Adolescent Mental Health Workforce Development, University of Auckland; 2005.
7. Tapsell R, Mellsop G. The contributions of culture and ethnicity to New Zealand mental health research findings. Int J Social Psychiatry. 2007;53(4):317–24.
8. McClintock K, Tauroa R, Mellsop G. Te Tomo Mai, appropriate child and adolescent mental health service (CAMHS) for an indigenous population: Rangatahi (youth) perspectives. Pimatisiwin J Aboriginal Indigenous Community Health. 2013;11(1):125–31.
9. Durie M. *Whānau ora: Flourishing families*. Presentation at APAC forum on quality improvement in healthcare, Auckland, New Zealand; 2013, September.
10. Lawson-Te Aho K. Definitions of whānau: A review of selected literature; 2010. www.familiescommission.org.nz.
11. Irwin K, Davies L, Werata W, Tuuta C, Rokx-Potae H, Potaka P, McCausland P, Bassett D. Whānau yesterday, today, tomorrow. Wellington, New Zealand: Families Commission; 2011.
12. Ministry of Health. Rising to the challenge: the mental health and addiction service development plan 2012–2017. Wellington, New Zealand: Ministry of Health; 2012.
13. Taskforce on Whanau-Centred Initiatives. Whānau Ora: report of the taskforce on Whānau-Centred initiatives. Wellington, New Zealand: Office for the Community and Voluntary Sector; 2009.
14. Te Rau Matatini. A mental health and addiction framework, a Whānau Ora approach. Wellington, New Zealand: Te Rau Matatini; 2014.
15. Te Rau Matatini. November minutes of the advisory to a mental health and addiction framework, a Whānau Ora approach. Wellington, New Zealand: Te Rau Matatini; 2013.
16. Oakley Browne MA, Wells JE, Scott KM, editors. Te Rau Hinengaro—the New Zealand mental health survey: summary. Wellington, New Zealand: Ministry of Health; 2006.
17. Boynton PM, Greenhalgh T. Selecting, designing, and developing your questionnaire. BMJ. 2004;328(7451):1312.
18. Riley SE, Stromberg AJ. Parent satisfaction with services for Medicaid youth at community mental health centres in Kentucky: 2000; 2001. http://www.mhmr.ky.gov/mh/outcomes/files/finalcmhcREPORT.pdf.
19. McClintock K, Sokratov A, Mellsop G, Kingi T. Hua Oranga: service utility pilot of a mental health outcome measurement for an indigenous population. Int Indigenous Policy J. 2013;4(3):1–14.

20. Minister of Health. Te Tahuhu—improving mental health 2005–2015: The second New Zealand mental health and addiction plan. Wellington, New Zealand: Minister of Health; 2005.
21. Minister of Health. Te Kokiri—The mental health and addiction action plan 2006–2015. Wellington, New Zealand: Minister of Health; 2006.
22. Ministry of Health. Te Puāwaiwhero: The second Māori mental health and addiction national strategic framework 2008–2015. Wellington, New Zealand: Ministry of Health; 2008.
23. Mellsop G, Wilson J. Outcome measures in mental health services: humpty dumpty is alive and well. Australas Psychiatry. 2006;14:137–40.
24. Durie M. Whaiora: Māori health development. Auckland, New Zealand: Oxford University Press; 1994.
25. Adamson S, Deering D, Schroder R, Townshend P, Ditchburn M. National telephone survey of the addiction treatment workforce. Christchurch, New Zealand: National Addiction Centre, Department of Psychological Medicine, University of Otago; 2009.
26. Te Pou o Te Whakaaro Nui. Adult addiction workforce: 2014 survey of vote health funded services. Auckland, New Zealand: Te Pou o Te Whakaaro Nui; 2015.
27. Te Pou o Te Whakaaro Nui. Maori adult mental health and addiction workforce: 2014 survey of vote health funded services. Auckland, New Zealand: Te Pou o Te Whakaaro Nui; 2016.
28. Matua Ra<u>k</u>i. Addiction services: workforce and service demand survey 2011 report. Wellington, New Zealand: Matua Ra<u>k</u>i; 2011.
29. Cave T, Robertson P, Pitama S, Huriwai T. He tētē kura: Māori addiction treatment 1980–2008. Ōtautahi, Christchurch, New Zealand: Matua Ra<u>k</u>i; 2008.
30. Ministry of Health. Mental health and addiction: service use 2009/10. Wellington, New Zealand: Ministry of Health; 2013.
31. The Werry Centre. 2010 Stocktake of infant, child and adolescent mental health and alcohol and other drug Services in new Zealand. Auckland, New Zealand: The Werry Centre; 2011.
32. Britt E, Gregory D, Tohiariki T, Huriwai T. Takitaki mai: a guide to motivational interviewing for Māori. Wellington, New Zealand: Matua Raki; 2014.
33. McLachlan A, Huriwai T. He Puna Whakaata: therapeutic activities to guide change. Wellington, New Zealand: Te Rau Matatini; 2016.
34. McLachlan A, Wirihana R, Huriwai T. Whai tikanga: the application of a culturally relevant value centred approach. N Z J Psychol. 2017;46(3):46–54.
35. Te Rau Matatini. Manaaki: Mana enhancing and Mana protecting practice. Wellington. Wellington, New Zealand: Te Rau Matatini; 2016.

Terry Huriwai (Te Arawa, Ngāti Porou, and Tainui descent) has worked in the addiction sector in one role or another for the past 30 years. Was the Addiction lead for Te Rau Ora, where the main goal is to enhance the capability of those working with Māori impacted by substance misuse, gambling, and the various coexisting health and social conditions that often go with them. His role also allowed him to support the integration of Māori knowledge and skills as an everyday part of practice. To achieve this, Terry takes every opportunity to share knowledge at local, regional, and national levels—to influence and shape practice and service delivery to enhance Māori well-being. Terry has publications in gambling, alcohol, and other drug and workforce development.

Kahu McClintock (Waikato/Maniapoto, Ngāti Mutunga, and Ngāti Porou) holds a variety of academic qualifications; including a Diploma in Nursing (Psychiatric), a Higher Diploma in Teaching, a BEd, a MPhil (Māori), and a DPhil (Psychiatry). She has worked in research and evaluation for over 20 years, in the health and disability sector for nearly 30 years, and with Māori communities for over 45 years. She has a special focus on Māori health research, rangatahi (youth) mental health and well-being, and Māori health outcome measurement. Kahu currently sits on the Waikato District Health Board Iwi Māori Council and the Research and Evaluation Team, Waikeria

Ara Poutama Corrections Facility She previously completed terms on the Waikato District Health Board Monitoring Performance Committee, the National Ethics Advisory Committee, and Te Whakakitenga o Waikato (Waikato-Tainui tribal council).

Rachel McClintock (Waikato/Maniapoto, Ngāti Mutunga, and Ngāti Porou) has worked in research for close to 10 years. She has a background in Kaupapa Māori community-based research and evaluation, with experience of research with Māori whānau (families) and communities; across areas such as youth development, mental health and well-being, gambling, palliative care, intergenerational communication, and suicide prevention. She holds a BSocSc (Psychology) and a Masters of Public Health.

I Remember Who I Am: Deg Xit'an Athabascan Perspectives on Wellness

LaVerne Xilegg Demientieff and Patrick Frank

Mother Nature Taught Native Dancing

After reading about the creation of the world in a Native legend, I wondered how the Creator made man ... a man who learned how to Native dance. Sitting under a tall spruce tree meditating one late evening in April, the answer came to me.

Soft, sporadic gusts of wind whistled along the hillside. Listening intently with eyes closed, I heard the distant coming of soprano spirits, high above the trees like a band of swiftly flying pintail ducks, passing in an instant. Next alto sounds from a remote distance approached quickly, whipping the treetops as they passed.

The serenading of tenors began nearby and resonated through the trees rapidly then was gone. Last the vibrant tremors of base, slower in movement, sent waves of peacefulness through me, bouncing at ground level all around me. The Great Orchestrator of creation was replaying ancient melodies from my ancestors' songbook, guiding the singers around me in perfect harmony.

As the force of the wind swept over and around me, I had a visitor. I felt something brushing lightly against my left arm. Startled, I opened my eyes to see who was trying to get my attention. To my surprise it was fingerlike spruce branches swaying to the catchy beat of the wind.

Then I understood how man learned to Native dance! Elders often say, "Observe nature quietly for she is your teacher." Long ago my forefathers had similar experiences, sitting in the woods on windy days while opening their hearts to nature. They patiently observed trees swaying gently under light gusts of wind and moving more rapidly when stronger blasts whipped through the forest.

The movement of sturdy spruce trees was the men dancing, strong and proud. The women were the birch trees gracefully swaying to the soft tune of ancient music. The children were the small willows, flexible, innovative, with an essence as free as the wind. The wise Elders were the gigantic, wrinkled, cottonwood trees with branches waving proud signs of approval. The unseen sap was the spirit of all life, the ancestors, a connecting vibrancy of the universe.

L. X. Demientieff (✉)
Social Work Department, University of Alaska Fairbanks, Fairbanks, AK, USA
e-mail: lmdemientieff@alaska.edu

P. Frank
Anchorage, AK, USA

D. Danto, M. Zangeneh (eds.), *Indigenous Knowledge and Mental Health*,
https://doi.org/10.1007/978-3-030-71346-1_13

On a dark, windy evening under the trees, I'm still. I listen. I remember days when Native People were in tune with nature, in tune with their heritage, a people who danced to the ancient melodies drummed by the Great Creator.

I remember who I am.

——Patrick Frank, Deg Xit'an Elder

In this chapter, we present possibilities and hope for healing and wellness through cultural and ancestral knowledge. Highlighting and focusing on the strengths of people can be a very powerful perspective and tool. Focusing on the problem, or problematizing, is far too common in helping professions and can be very detrimental. Smith [1] says,

> The "Indigenous problem" is a recurrent theme in all imperial and colonial attempts to deal with Indigenous peoples. It originates within the wider discourse of racism, sexism and other forms of positioning the other. Its neatness and simplicity gives the term its power and durability. Framing "the … problem," mapping it, describing it in all its different manifestations, trying to get rid of it, laying blame for it, talking about it, writing newspaper columns about it, drawing cartoons about it, teaching about it, researching it, over and over …. how many occasions, polite dinner parties and academic conferences would be bereft of conversation if "the Indigenous problem had not been so problematized?" (p. 94)

When we focus on the problem, those in the helping field unknowingly create pessimistic expectations and predictions about the clients we work with, and the client also begins to internalize these negative labels [2]. Over time, this is damaging to both the helper and the client. It is essential to acknowledge that every person, family, and community has strengths and every person, family, and community deals with challenges. That is just human nature. We can shift is our lens to magnify and focus on what is working, especially what has worked for people culturally and traditionally. Deg Xit'an Athabascan teachings highlight an understanding of how our thoughts and energy work in the world. Elders share that putting out negative thoughts, feelings, and actions into the world not only hurts others but comes back on you as well. You cannot heal by fighting off grief or trauma with anger or with negative thoughts or force; you have to do this with love, compassion, and forgiveness in relation to all things. This is what I have learned from my Elders.

Deg Xit'an Athabascan People

The "I" in this chapter is LaVerne Xilegg Demientieff. Patrick Frank is my coauthor and uncle. My uncle has helped me to remember who I am as a Deg Xit'an Athabascan woman. He has been an integral part of my healing and he has taught me important concepts and values related to the seen and unseen world, sharing and caring, and the natural way our people show compassion and love for all things. Without him, this chapter could not have been written.

The perspectives and examples shared in this chapter mainly come from the Deg Xit'an People, Elders, and culture bearers who shared their knowledge with me during focus groups for my dissertation on Deg Xitan wellness. *Xisrigidisddhinh* (I am grateful). *Dogidinh* (thank you) for your contributions.

The Deg Xit'an People are river people, very spiritually connected, and strong in mind, body, and spirit. The people come from a culture rich with traditions, customs, and knowledge that have been passed on orally from generation to generation for thousands of years. Yale anthropologist Cornelius Osgood described the Deg Xit'an People as peaceful people (1959). The Deg Xit'an People are the smallest in population of the 11 Athabascan groups located in Southwest Alaska on the lower Yukon and lower Innoko Rivers. The four main Deg Xit'an communities are Holy Cross, Anvik, Shageluk, and Grayling. These rural communities are accessible only by plane, boat, or snow machine. The population estimates for all Deg Xit'an People are unknown. A significant number of Deg Xit'an People live in the larger urban cities of Anchorage and Fairbanks. Many of the Deg Xit'an People currently living in urban communities do so for reasons that include being close to medical care, employment, and educational opportunities, or to be near other resources and activities. Many of these individuals often return home to their rural communities to subsist off the land, visit family, and to attend major events such as births, deaths, and traditional ceremonies, and some still own land or homes or have fish camps in and nearby these communities. Deg Xinag is the language spoken (see Fig. 1); currently, there are a handful of fluent speakers remaining and the work toward reclaiming and revitalizing the language is strong.

This chapter is an opportunity to share information on wellness and resilience from the perspective of the river people, the Deg Xit'an People of Southwest Alaska, and encourage mental health and health care providers to explore and incorporate the benefits of culture with their clients and incorporate compassion, connection, curiosity, ceremony, and community as part of their healing work.

Our Elders tell us stories and share Traditional Wisdom about how to live a good life. Our ancestors used this cultural knowledge and wisdom on a daily basis to live in harmony with the world around them and nurture wellness within the community. Deg Xit'an Elder, Jim Dementi, shared with me his understanding of wellness: "It's just the way we live our lives" (personal communication, n.d.). This is a very simple but also a profound statement. Remembering who we are as Native People, gaining knowledge about how our ancestors understood the seen and unseen world, and learning about and participating in traditional practices can be an empowering process that connects us to each other, creates a sense of belonging and pride, and teaches us how to heal and regain balance in our lives. The pain, shame, and grief perpetrated on Native People through colonization forced cultural knowledge and wisdom, language, spirituality, traditions, and ceremonies under the table to protect the people from harm by colonizers and also to keep the practices safe for future generations. Deg Xit'an Elder Pat Frank shared with me, and often shares with others, that it is time to put these things back on the table—take them out, let them be seen, let them guide us, let them be shared and taught to future generations—because

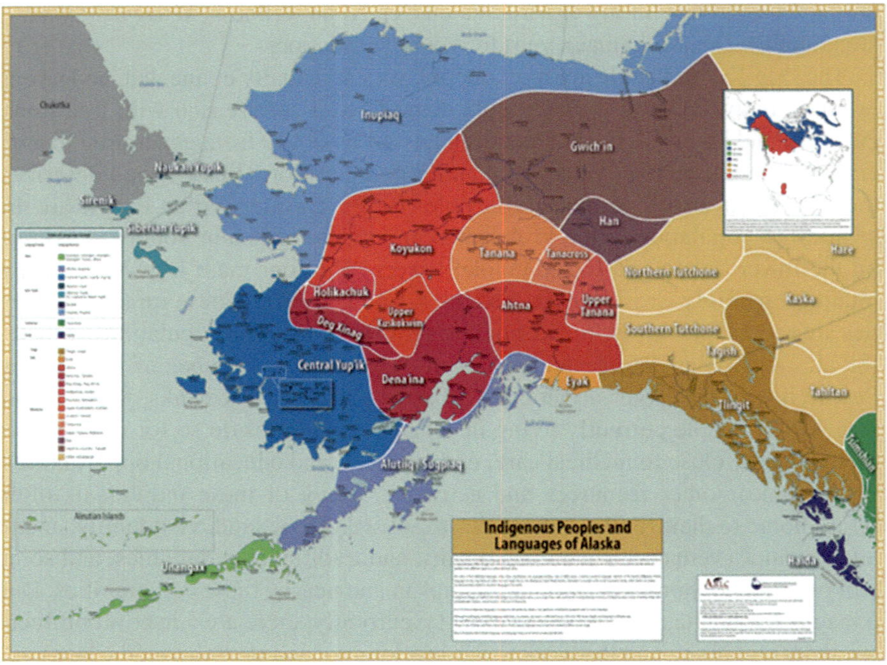

Fig. 1 Indigenous Peoples and Languages of Alaska [3]. Michael Krauss, Gary Holton, Jim Kerr, and Colin T. West. Used with permission from Alaska Native Language Center and UAA Institute of Social and Economic Research. Online: http://www.uaf.edu/anla/map

that is what is going to create healing and power in our people (personal communication, February 2018).

During a social work conference in Anchorage, Alaska, in 2017, University of Alaska Fairbanks (UAF's) Vice Chancellor for Native Education very powerfully stated in a presentation on healing, "All you have to do is be who you are" (E. Peter, NASW-AK Conference, October 2017). Be who you are. For people who have lost so much for "being who they are," this statement can bring feelings of anxiety and fear because Western institutions still often do not embrace or incorporate diverse worldviews. However, if you are able to embrace this act of being who you are, it will also bring about liberation and freedom from shackles of historical trauma and grief and transform the individual and these institutions for the better.

In my own wellness and healing journey, it took me a long time to understand the significance of the phrase "be who you are." I started to wake up to this in my early 20s when I took a Deg Xinag Athabascan language class at the UAF, facilitated by a Deg Xit'an Athabascan language professor, a non-Native linguist, and co-taught by about six Elders from our region in Alaska. My own grandparents, maternal and paternal, died when my parents were young, so I did not know them and was not told much about them. It was a wonderful experience to be with these Elders, some of whom I had never met and others I had not seen since I was young. I introduced myself to these Elders as I had been taught, listing the names of my parents and grandparents on both sides of the family. As I did that, the Elders began to make the connection, and once they did, it was like a puzzle piece fitting nicely into its spot and the bigger picture emerges. My uncle taught me that once the ancestral connection is made, the Elders look at me and see my parents or grandparents when they talk to me, the ones they knew and loved. In a way, I become them, and the Elders will treat me well to show respect for those they knew.

This class was my first introduction to the Deg Xinag Athabascan language, which has only a handful of fluent speakers left. My parents were raised partly in the Catholic mission in Holy Cross and did not grow up speaking the language, so my siblings and I did not learn. This experience was a pivotal point in my healing and wellness journey. The class was held in one of the Elder apartments at UAF and we learned the language through hands-on activities like making moose soup together, going on nature walks, and playing games. The Elders lovingly embraced me. They told me they were proud of me; they told me that I sounded good and that speaking Deg Xinag was in my blood. They also shared stories of my grandparents that I never knew. After each class, I would be inspired and invigorated and would share what I learned of the language with my mother. She would try to guess what I was saying and many times was correct. This was powerful because she was remembering a time when her parents talked to her in Deg Xinag when she was very little. Growing up in the Catholic mission in Holy Cross, my mother lost the ability to speak the language. She was so happy that I was learning the language and sharing it with her—it strengthened our connection and grounded us in our culture. The safe and loving space that these Elders created is a good cultural example of trauma-informed care. This is where healing begins. The walls of colonization in my mind and spirit started to break down as I learned about who I am as a Deg Xit'an woman through the language learning process. What I know now is that these Elders were modeling for me how to be a good Tea Partner (discussed in the following sections) and human being; they offered me connection, compassion, and love, as Elders do. The Deg Xit'an way, which values reciprocity and balance, is for me to offer my knowledge of this to others and to the next generation to come.

The Deg Xit'an Wellness Journey

As I journeyed through my doctoral dissertation on wellness among the Deg Xit'an Athabascan people, I learned more and more about our cultural traditions and the influence of our cultural traditions on our health and well-being through conversational focus groups with Elders and culture bearers. What I learned is that for many Indigenous People seeds are planted early on in a person's life in the form of stories, experiences, and modeling about how to be a Deg Xit'an person. The Deg Xit'an Wellness Journey created from my dissertation work with Elders and culture bearers tells a story about the themes that emerged from the conversational focus groups related to wellness. The themes include cultural and traditional practices; traditional values; embracing challenges by remembering who we are; and Deg Xit'an beliefs and action recommendations. The Deg Xit'an Wellness Journey description is highlighted below.

> The Deg Xit'an, Athabascan people of Southwest Alaska have been taught traditional values and how to be in relationship with the physical and spirit world through the cultural practices modeled by our Elders, parents, and community leaders and seeds for wellness are rooted within us. When we know who we are and where we come from as Deg Xit'an People we are better able to embrace life's challenges. Our ancestors have taught us that the challenges we face in life are viewed as gifts that lead to growth, wisdom and resilience. When discussing wellness and wholeness among Deg Xit'an People the Elders and culture bearers remind us that the Deg Xit'an beliefs about how to live and be in the world give us insight and direction and lead us back to our cultural practices where we are able to live our values and the journey continues. The Tea Partner traditional practice is one example of how wellness was infused into the Deg Xit'an way of life" ([4], p. 103).

The following are highlights from each of the four themes in my doctoral dissertation study on Deg Xit'an Wellness [4].

Cultural and Traditional Practices

Our values are embedded through the lived cultural practices and way of life modeled by Elders, parents, and community leaders. The cultural practices include preparing for the future, transmitting culture and language, and building physical, social, mental, and spiritual strength.

Preparing for the Future

Participants discussed the cultural practice of preparing for the future as an integral part of the Deg Xit'an way of life. It was a matter of survival. The people prepared from day to day, season to season, year to year, and for the future generations following. Everything that was done was done in preparation, thinking ahead, and planning for something coming. A male Deg Xit'an Elder discussed the importance of not taking too much from the land so that it will return in the future for you and your children and grandchildren. He said, "We were taught, never over trap a beaver house, I don't know how many lines or houses they would have in your day but they said never to over trap, just get so much out of a house then your line will always be there for you to make a living for your family, and your grandchildren" [4].

Transmitting Culture and Language

Participants discussed the importance of sharing our stories of our people and experiences, especially with young people. Deg Xit'an People have always been an oral society. Stories are how we learn information, values, skills, protocols, lessons, humor, and more. We also have to learn our story to be able to tell our stories. We will not have a culture if we do not tell our stories to others so they can pass them on and on.

Many stories were shared that began with the phrase "I remember …". These stories were shared with expressions of love, humor, sadness, respect, and longing, and mainly with the intent to teach or learn something from the past. Cultural practices emphasize the Deg Xit'an ways of life and how to be human and navigate through life's challenges. One Elder male participant stated, "It's important to remember … the Elders always say, think about the way you live. Remember your people, remember your ways, remember your language, all the stuff … and they say that for a reason. There's a real reason there—that's to survive" [4].

Building Physical, Social, Mental, and Spiritual Strength

An Elder woman participant discussed how strength is gained through cultural practices and through our own feelings of worth and empowerment. She stated, "I think it just boils down to knowing your power … so many of us go through life and we don't know our power, our power to do anything …. be it, refrain from alcohol, be it, getting a degree, or be it, becoming whatever. And I think if people realize they have the power then they'd find the strength cause they have it within them, that's the human way, the human condition. And I think power is all over, that we gain our strength from, and when you look at it culturally all the setting was there, the Native dances, the hunting, the storytelling" [4].

An Elder male participant spoke about getting spiritual strength from nature. "For me it's out in nature. When I go to nature I pray and it fills me up, the power of the water, I go on the water and … sometimes the trees, animals, and the nature reveal themselves to you and I actually feel their power. When I go on the Yukon, I go out there, that's where I fill myself, that's where I get my strength … how I ground myself is I look for water…because I'm from the Yukon" [4].

Traditional Values

We are taught the Deg Xit'an values of respect, relationships, balance and reciprocity, sharing and caring, and happiness and humor, which are deeply instilled within us from the time we are born. These are not all our values but ones that emerged strongly from the discussions.

Respect

The Tea Partner traditional practice emphasizes this value of respect. An Elder male participant said, "What our people designed years ago was a Tea Partner that connects how you treat one another. How the men treat the women. How the women treat the men. How we all took care of one another, even though you're not related" [4].

Relationships

The Deg Xit'an worldview is that the people are in relationship to everything: people, land, animals, water, spirit, and Creator. An Elder woman shared a story about her relationship with the crow. She said, "When they would travel on the water, she would look up at the clouds, and her mom believed that … the crow was very spiritual. She said, we watch for the crow. He's flying along, then he turns over and he drops and they said, when he does it that means drop a pack sack of good luck to me … and he rights himself up and he flies on, so, we would watch for them, watch for the crow. *Yixgitsiy* we called it" [4].

Balance and Reciprocity

An Elder male participant shared an example of how Elders practiced balance and tended to the spirit of the community. "I always look at the Elders and really wise people do the rituals and ceremonies, they were designed by our ancestors. Even though they didn't have a doctorate degree or master degree or anything, they tended to the spirit of the community. If it was too heavy they did things to bring it up, if it was too giddy they bring it down more logically, they balance it all the time, always tending to the spirit of that community. And as Native People we believe in the seen and the unseen and there is a lot of forces that affect the village that are unseen. So, by introducing spiritual, or rituals and ceremonies, they tended to these forces that carried the well-being with the villages" [4].

Sharing and Caring

An Elder woman also emphasized the value of sharing and caring by discussing the Tea Partner tradition. "I think, my mother chose my Tea Partner, because we had a teacher and his wife over there … and she told me, Mr. so and so is your partner, and every time they would have food passed out he would bring me a nice plate of food, which I was very happy for, and then mom would help me fix up a plate to send over to him, so he was a white man, but he was my partner, my Tea Partner, and that's what I remember about that. It was a good way to have friends, and they cared about us and we cared about them, you know" [4]. This memory highlights incorporating non-Native People from outside the culture within the traditional practices. The net connecting people together is cast far and wide.

Happiness and Humor

The value of happiness and humor as discussed by participants held many meanings. It was used strategically to bring joy to the community, to change the energy from negative to more light and positive, to show friendship and love to someone through teasing and joking, to lessen sorrow and grief, and also to tell stories and teach lessons. One Elder male shared the joy the Elders displayed. He said, "The Elders in Holy Cross, when I first went there … they were a happy bunch, I could remember them, I think about them a lot. I think about the village how it was, the two rows of houses, with, an Elder, almost an Elder in every house, when I first went there" [4]. Humor is healing.

Embracing Challenges by Remembering Who We Are

As Deg Xit'an People grow and develop, and as they move through their wellness journey, they encounter life's challenges, including competing values and practices from Western society and various other types of struggles related to isolation and disconnection, identity and belonging, historical trauma and grief, and alcohol abuse and addiction. These struggles sometimes lead to poor health and mental health and can distance the people from their cultural knowledge and practices and create barriers to wellness. Yet, because Deg Xit'an values have been deeply instilled in the person, they do not ever lose who they are as Deg Xit'an People.

Isolation and Disconnection

An Elder male participant shares his thoughts on wellness as stemming from a community coming together. He wants to make sure people do not think we are just all well. He makes the point that we are not well, but that instead of pulling against each other, we should be coming together and helping each other. He states that we need to get back to the old culture—the ways people lived back then—and we need to try to find solutions to this. Depression, addiction, and suicide happen when there is too much isolation and disconnection. To bring this back to the Tea Partner tradition, which is one good potential solution, the Tea Partner is about connection and respect and sharing and caring.

Identity and Belonging

A young male participant talked about his interest and connection to the culture and to wanting to know more and learn more. He stated, "I'm really interested in … I've never actually seen our dancing before, and I don't know if you guys remember how it was done or if you want to bring it back, you know, but, I'd love to see pictures, if anyone has pictures, and you know I never knew who I was on my Deg Xit'an side so, I'm now finally starting to get back to my roots as a Deg Xit'an person, so I really am interested in learning from you guys, you know, if you ever want, if you ever need someone to talk to, or if you want to teach anyone, I'm here. I love to listen to Elders and if anyone has knowledge out there I'm here and I want to learn"

[4]. The young people are energized and open to learning, practicing, and sharing the culture, as well as creating and adding their own unique spin on traditional practices. It is an exciting time.

Historical Trauma and Grief

Historical trauma and grief were discussed by participants as the efforts and impacts of Western society to colonize and assimilate the Native People, in this case, the Deg Xit'an People. They discussed examples related to mass epidemics, missionaries and boarding schools, religion and church, and loss of traditional ways.

Alcohol Abuse and Addiction

Alcohol abuse and addiction came up in the discussion among participants as a very widespread challenge. Another Elder male participant shared his thoughts on getting sober, stating that being sober does not mean being boring, it means starting to live your life. He said, "You tell kids to stop doing destructive things, but you then tell them, here's what you're supposed to do. I remember a couple of times encouraging people that you've got to stop, and we all have to be sober, and when I say sober to anybody they think and picture someone sitting there sober—not smiling not doing anything except stopped, but that's not the way people are. Think about our families, our people—how they go to a dance, have a good time. You can just see them smiling, and dancing, and their spirits, their whole bodies just exploding with happiness, and you can feel it. Mind, body, and spirit, happy and living the way they're supposed to be living. This is the way they were designed to live. This is the way they should live. It's complete—mind, body, and spirit—being … developing, moving, and enjoying … and that's sobering up, but continue on with life. Yeah, get sober, but continue on with your life. So, wellness is the same way" [4].

Deg Xit'an Beliefs and Action Recommendations

In response to generational changes and life struggles, Elders and culture bearers continue to pass on their knowledge and wisdom of what can be done to get the people back to cultural practices that promote wellness and their way of life. These community action recommendations include people coming together as a community, doing things in a good way, and caring for themselves and others. Through the community action recommendations, these shared values are able to emerge and provide the person with a sense of belonging, direction, and purpose. Through these actions, the Deg Xit'an person will be able to return to the cultural practices of preparing for the future, transmitting culture and language, and building physical, social, mental, and spiritual strength, which then models Deg Xit'an values and practices for the next generation, and the cycle continues.

Coming Together as a Community

An Elder male stated, "What I notice about Holy Cross, even up to this day, when someone passes away, when you lose someone among the people, the people band together. They're strong. They support that person's family, and you could see it there, that there's a degree of wellness that I know of, that's when people are well, and, I told the people, you know we get together, only in sad times nowadays. Why don't we get together in good times? You know. Together. Get the people together" [4]. Coming together as a community has so many benefits. It can create opportunities, build connections and relationships, create a sense of pride and belonging, bring joy, teach the culture and language, and spark radical possibilities.

Doing Things in a Good Way

This includes tending to the spirit of the people and community and also being in relationship with the spiritual world and knowing how to keep oneself and others safe from harm. It is important to be aware of the energy, positive and negative, that exists in the world and to understand how to manage it in a good way. Everything in the world has energy. An Elder male participant discussed the importance of clearing out bad energy or spirits when needed, saying, "So, anybody who comes into the building brings different energy. It's all energy, and it could be good energy, bad energy, or something like that but it stays right in the house. We have to clear it out. There is correct protocol to do this, there is always a good way to do things" [4].

Sharing and Caring for Self and Others

Everything should be done within the spirit of sharing and caring for others. They are both essential values as well as practices. The Tea Partner tradition is an excellent example of how sharing and caring was practiced traditionally. An Elder male participant shares that in order to heal and be well we have to share our knowledge and success. We have to "pass it on" and "give it away," he said. "I found out the easiest way to stay sober today is to help another person that needs it … to pass it on to someone else" [4].

As a people, we have to continue sharing our culture, planting those seeds, so when our kids go through challenges they have that knowledge, those values, and the practices to get them through tough times, and to heal and regain balance and wholeness when they find themselves in these difficult circumstances.

The lessons learned from the Deg Xit'an People related to wellness are many. One lesson is that no human or community or culture is perfect, and that ceremonies were created and used because life is challenging and can topple us out of balance. Together, and with love and compassion for each other, we can move through grief, find joy, and create our best lives on this earth.

Awakening the Spirit: The Influence of Culture on Wellness and Healing

Examples of resilience and wellness are rooted in all cultures and communities across Alaska. Society as a whole can learn and gain a lot from the wisdom and practices of these diverse cultures that incorporate into daily living community practices grounded in love, connection, belonging, and healing. Our Indigenous communities experience the highest levels of wellness when we are able to express ourselves as cultural and spiritual beings and when we feel valued by society for who we are as a people. This includes the ability to speak our language, practice our spirituality and traditions, freedom to subsist off the land, and the right to determine our own needs and solutions. Woods et al. [5], in *A Preliminary Report on The Relationships Between Collective Self-Esteem, Historical Trauma, and Mental Health Among Alaska Native People,* share that "Alaska Native individuals who still positively view their heritage and who are still culturally connected (high levels of Collective Self-Esteem) despite historical colonialism and modern day oppression may be less likely to experience distress and depression, which also lowers the likelihood of substance use and suicide" (p. 2).

They go on to say that programs that help individuals become more aware of the positive characteristics and aspects of their heritage, and helping them stay connected with their heritage, might prevent people from experiencing psychological distress and depression.

We as human beings are multidimensional; from an Indigenous perspective, health and mental health are not separate entities to be dealt with or worked on separate from culture, spirituality, family, and community. Cultural traditions around the world have a lot to share with, and teach, the mental health profession. These diverse cultural practices and ceremonies have been brilliantly constructed by our ancestors and incorporate a holistic approach to wellness, to include a deep love for one another, connection, belonging, community, and values such as having a compassionate spirit, reciprocity, and sharing and caring.

Healing often happens alongside remembering who we are as Native People. This is a process with many stages. It includes claiming who we are as Indigenous human beings, claiming our ancestors, learning our stories, songs, and dances, listening to the Elders, learning about lineage and connecting to our relatives, learning about our unique relationship with water, land, and animals, hearing and speaking our language, partaking in traditional practices and ceremonies, and nourishing our spirits with traditional food from the land. In my Deg Xit'an wellness dissertation, one Elder male participant stated, "It's important to remember … the Elders always say, think about the way you live. Remember your people, remember your ways, remember your language, all the stuff … and they say that for a reason. There's a real reason there—that's to survive. So, that's directly from the Deg Xit'an Athabascan people, and other Athabascan Elders" [4].

Some major challenges for Indigenous People are related to historical and intergenerational trauma, and the embodiment of trauma and how it has manifested as illness and addiction. Colonization efforts have created a loss of trust within Indigenous People. Deg Xit'an Elder, Sam Demientieff, shared with me that much that was lost through colonization and historical trauma was related to trust. As helpers, we recognize that trust is essential to healthy relationships. The loss of trust goes very deep and is very difficult to regain, especially with continued oppression and racism (personal communication, 2017).

I have always been interested in the topic of historical trauma because it is part of our story and it has influenced my people and my family and myself. Yet it is only a part of our story. The more important story to tell is our wellness story, our story of resilience. We have a long line of ancestors whose strength, perseverance, knowledge, and love are part of our DNA and the only reason we are here today. I have been blessed that as I was growing up my aunt, Rose Jerue, instilled in me that the women in our family are very powerful and that my ancestors were extremely strong, proud, and determined people (personal communication, n.d.). That knowledge has carried me through many challenges. I have also had the blessing of having my uncle tell me that when I acknowledge my ancestors they stand behind me and with me, so I honor them by acknowledging them (P. Frank, personal communication, n.d.). These sentiments have laid a foundation of resilience and determination in my spirit.

Our culture is powerful and when practiced has the ability to awaken our spirit and open us up to a profound experience of gratitude and joy. Deg Xit'an Athabascan Elder, Sam Demientieff, shared that practicing cultural traditions is often experienced as an "awakening of the spirit." He often lovingly and animatedly tells the story of his father describing how he feels when he starts to sing and dance to the beat of the drum. He said that his father would share that when he begins to dance, it starts slow but you feel the power entering your spirit, it begins to build as you dance harder and sing louder, and this power and energy fills you up. His father described it to him as an "awakening of the spirit," because speaking the language and engaging in our cultural traditions connects our spirit to our ancestors and Creator and fills our spirit with feelings of joy and connection (personal communication, n.d.). I have heard similar stories from other Alaska Native Elders who describe similar experiences of healing, relief, connection, strength, belonging, pride, and love when partaking in their songs and dances with their community. When I hear Alaska Native People singing loudly and dancing hard, and having fun, I have myself felt the overwhelming feelings of pride and connection and deep love for our people. It is as if the spirit comes alive and is filled with purpose and joy. Definitely, something profound is happening. I believe it is a feeling of deep connection emanating from within our cells and connecting us to our ancestors and to the future generation.

Cultural beliefs and practices connect to the wisdom and knowledge about what it means to be human. Indigenous People know how to live a balanced life, which has always included singing, drumming, and dancing; sharing stories, including survival stories highlighting responsibility, safety, and the power of nature and animals; and participating in ceremonies and practices that helped the people move through grief and trauma, as well as to celebrate life. These practices taught about how to live in harmony with nature, animals, and people. Yes, there were challenges, wars, famine, extreme weather, loss, and other issues; however, the ceremonial practices always imparted how to regain balance and connection. More and more of the literature on the positive influence of culture related to health and mental health is emerging …. reclaiming culture, "culture as a buffer" against stress, cultural protective factors, cultural continuity, cultural resilience, and more [6–10]. This is a positive step in the prevention and intervention of mental health challenges and toward restoring wholeness within ourselves and our communities.

There is a movement within the state of Alaska and around the world in which Indigenous People are reclaiming their culture, including language, traditional practices, singing, drumming and dancing, and connecting to their spirit and spirituality. They are remembering and embracing who they are as a people. Community members, young and old, are interested in learning about their culture and language, they are interested in connecting with others from their culture and using that knowledge and those practices to live a healthy life. Walters et al. [11] created a model highlighting the importance of "reconnecting with our original instructions." They wrote:

> Associations between traumatic life stressors and adverse health outcomes are moderated by cultural factors that function as buffers, strengthening psychological and emotional health, decreasing substance use, and mitigating the effects of the traumatic stressors. Although a vast literature considers the interrelationship among stress, coping and health, little empirical research has addressed either the particular culture-specific stressors of AI or the coping strategies and protective aspects of Indigenous culture. (p. 105–106)

Culture embodies beliefs, values, medicine, identity, spirituality, ceremonies, rituals, food, land, water, language, art, music and dance, and other ways of knowing and being in the world. These aspects are found in all cultures around the world; however, the meanings and practices attached to these concepts throughout and within Indigenous communities are very specific to each culture, and that diversity should be recognized and understood by helpers and those interested in being a part of the solution. In the following paragraphs, I have highlighted and discussed four aspects of culture (land, language, medicine, and traditional practices) to give a few examples of the diversity one might see within distinct cultures.

Land

For many Indigenous People all over the world, the health of the land is often connected to the health of the people. The people of an area took care of the spirit of the land and had a strong relationship with the land. There is also a political history, that varies between tribal nations, related to land. That history, incorporates matters such as reservations, Native allotment, the Alaska Native Claims Settlement Act, historical and political removal of Indigenous People from land, sacred and ceremonial sites, and subsistence living and harvesting , all of which varies from culture to culture. Willox et al. [12] highlighted the impact of climate change on people's health and wellness. They wrote:

> For Inuit communities such as Rigolet, land activities such as hunting, fishing, trapping, and foraging for berries and edible and medicinal plants, as well as the ability to regularly and safely travel on the land, sea, and ice, is of the utmost importance to physical, mental, emotional, and spiritual health and well-being. (p. 18)

This deep connection to the earth and place is considered very sacred, and understanding the diversity of meanings attached to land is extremely important. In her "Ingalik" article in the *Handbook of North American Indians*, Snow [13] stated,

> The relationship between the Ingalik and the world of nature was very close. The principal support of human beings was thought to be the various "animal people" on the flesh of which people lived ([14]:115). All these animals required respectful treatment or they would no longer be available for food. The function of "songs" or magical spells, was to bring into equilibrium the conflicts that existed among the worlds of the spirit, nature, and society. The songs created good relations between the Ingalik and the spirits of the fish and food-giving mammals. (p. 607)

Ingalik was a term used to refer to Deg Xit'an People. It is a derogatory name that was used for many years and has since been replaced with the accurate name of the people, Deg Xit'an. Advocating for the use of correct names of people and places is an essential part of the healing process. The practice of having good relationships between spirit, nature, and society can still be seen today in the way people hunt and harvest food, care for animals and nature, and tend to the spirit of the people and community. Snow's referral to "magical spells" is likely the observation of the Deg Xi'tan people's close connection to spirit and understanding of energy in the universe.

Language

Language includes our stories, medicine, spirituality, and knowledge of who we are as a people. While sitting in a language revitalization gathering in Fairbanks, Alaska, I heard one Elder Athabascan woman share that when she hears the language spoken it is like hearing birds singing. I found this statement very moving and I believe it highlights the deep connection we have to the language. Indigenous People's experiences and relationship to language are very specific, depending on many factors, including political history, time of first contact and colonization efforts, and boarding schools and missionaries or government efforts to remove children from Native homes and place them in non-Native homes. All of the Indigenous languages in Alaska are endangered. As with many other languages spoken around the world, there is not a homeland to return to where people are speaking the language if we as Native People do not reclaim it. There were punishments for generations of children who spoke their language, which had numerous impacts, one being that it created trauma around the language. There are strong efforts to reclaim and revitalize Indigenous languages all over the world. Hallett et al. [7] shared their research conducted among Canada's First Nations communities and found that those communities where a majority of members reported a conversational knowledge of a First Nations language also experienced low to absent youth suicide. By contrast, those communities in which fewer than half of the members reported conversational knowledge, suicide rates were six times greater. There is very little other research published on the connection between language and health, but we know the link is profound; therefore, much more work in this area should be done.

Medicine

My uncle, a Deg Xit'an Elder and cofounder of the wellness and healing group "Returning to Harmony," often reminds me and also shares with others that we have to recognize the power and impact of both the seen and the unseen world in our lives if we are to know how to help others (P. Frank, personal communication, n.d).

Medicine in a variety of cultures can include Traditional Healers, medicine men and women, shamans, spiritual healers, seers, plants, animals, food, and spirit. I recently heard a Yupik Elder in Alaska refer to medicine in reference to the healing stories we share with each other. Bassett et al. [6] highlighted findings from a study with Traditional Healers. They state,

> According to the healers we interviewed, culture is the primary vehicle for delivering healing. The overarching principle articulated here, that "culture is medicine," means that connecting with one's culture has both protective and therapeutic value, promoting both resilience to and recovery from traumatic events. The details of treatment will differ depending on the cultural specifics related to one's culture; however, the principle of culture as medicine is the same across Native cultures, according to the healers we interviewed. Thus, indigenous means of treatment through culture may include any or all of the following: language, traditional foods, ceremonies, traditional values, spiritual beliefs, history, stories, songs, traditional plants, and canoe journeys. Connecting Native patients with their Native culture promotes better health outcomes. (p. 25)

The Healers in the Bassett et al. [6] study gave advice for working with Indigenous People more effectively. They encouraged clinicians to build trust and advised that they needed to have Native Healers on hand and to have visible Native symbols present. Showing inclusion, and having spiritual healing discussed by Healers is extremely important for clinicians to accept and understand. Elders spoke with me about Healers and what they were taught growing up:

> "It's a hard thing … to deal with that trauma … that's an ongoing trauma." "Many people are torn between being told not to talk about what happened or you will be hurt and that it is important to talk about to heal from it." Another Elder male participant shared,

> "Sometimes it's hard to talk about traditional medicine or traditional ways because they were told it was not good, you know." An Elder woman made a similar statement, saying, "It makes me think that now. A lot of the time, when I was growing up, we're not supposed to talk too much about everything." She went on to say, "… not to spill everything out and talk too much because we could get hurt by it." An Elder male shared his thoughts on this topic of talking or not talking and he stated, "We've got to start talking about it. Who else is going to help these young people if we don't start talking about it, so even if I get reprimanded I'm not going to be quiet anymore" ([4], p. 88–89).

The use of traditional medicine is one aspect of Indigenous culture that is still "under the table." There is still fear and misunderstanding about what it means to be a Healer or to use various types of traditional medicine for healing. There are many ways to heal and people need options. We need to bring this out from under the table to the top of the table and use our traditional tools appropriately and as needed. I am grateful to South Central Foundations, Alaska Native Medical Center in Anchorage, Alaska, for opening up a Traditional Healing clinic that incorporates various types of Traditional Healing, including hands-on healing, Traditional Counseling, and a Traditional Healing garden that grows medicinal plants. It is a step toward awareness, acceptance, and healing.

Traditional Practices

Traditional practices, ceremonies, and rituals are very specific to each Indigenous group and community. Below I will share three Alaskan examples of ceremonies that build connection and strength in communities and support the resilience and wellness of the people. These are the Potlatch, Naming ceremonies, and Tea Partner ceremony [15].

The Potlatch is a traditional practice that can be found among many groups within Alaska. Potlatches include community celebrations or coming together in times of tragedy and healing. The Athabascan memorial Potlatch is a traditional practice that pays respect to those that have died and is a process for healing from grief for the family with the community. The family and community prepare together for 1 year or more for a memorial Potlatch to say the final goodbye; throughout the year food is hunted and gathered, beading and sewing occur, and songs are created. This grieving process is not done alone; instead, it is done with the community and is a very powerful process for sending the deceased away in a good way and healing from the loss together. During the Potlatch, the family gives away many gifts to the community for all their support and together the people eat food from the land, and sing and dance together, sometimes for days. The families are held up by the community in their time of grief and loss [18].

Naming practices occur in many cultures in Alaska. A Yupik example would be when an Elder woman's husband passes away, a newborn baby in the family or community will be named after the Elder who passed. In a spiritual way, this child is now the husband of the Elder woman and will grow up with the responsibility to help her when she needs it, packing water or wood, hunting for her, and so on. In turn, the Elder woman will knit socks or sew warm clothing for the child as he grows. This reciprocity ensures connection, support, and a loving tie to one another, and new relatives are created, strengthening the community as a whole.

The Tea Partner tradition is a Deg Xit'an Athabascan custom that is another example of a cultural practice leading to individual and community wellness. In the Deg Xinag language, the term *sixoldhid* is used to describe this tradition, which means "my friend" or "my partner." This traditional practice is like a community-based, culturally grounded "safety net," where individuals create connection, resources, mentorship, share knowledge, stories, and humor, and provide and receive support over a lifetime. The overall intent is to help each other to survive and thrive in a challenging and ever-changing environment, to nurture and promote health and wellness, and establish continuity for future generations. In this traditional practice, a Deg Xit'an man or woman is partnered with another person of the opposite sex, often from a differing community, usually older or younger, and sometimes with someone from outside of the culture. Elders or parents in the community, through a variety of ceremonial processes, connect partners together; and these partnerships last a lifetime and are considered an honor to be a part of. These connections are not romantic; instead, the partnership is meant to be a lifelong friendship (some view the role as a godparent), to create a network or web of support across communities. One could have several partners across communities. The spirit of the Tea Partner meant that you share your best food with your partner, for example, king salmon, moose, *vanhgiq* (fish ice cream), and that you help them and offer them support when they come to your community, and that you gift them with things you make, such as beaver mittens or a warm marten hat—and, in turn, they will share their catch with you. It is all about sharing and caring for others, about reciprocity and balance, and survival. You can imagine the strength that this creates because of these connections. The Tea Partner tradition was closely associated with Deg Xit'an community Potlatches and Mask Dances. Your partner was someone you would honor throughout their lifetime and in turn they would honor you.

There are so many more beautiful examples of cultural practices within our communities that highlight connection and belonging and strengthen our communities. We can and should learn from these practices and implement them into our healing strategies. Today, these practices may not be exactly done in the way our ancestors carried them out, because we live in a different time and there is a protocol to consider. However, the spirit of these traditional practices is what can be shared, with the understanding that for each community the practice and ceremonies may differ and incorporate Sacred Knowledge and processes that are not shared outside of the community. Indigenous Knowledge and practices offer significant insights into the importance of creating solutions, programs, and policies that incorporate within them ways to build connection, show compassion, and nurture strengths of both the individual and the community together. It is important for mental health and health professionals to recognize the diversity within experiences as they work with distinct groups of people who are either connected or not connected to their culture and traditions.

Alaska Native cultural and traditional practices such as the Tea Partner, the memorial Potlatch, Yupik Naming, Whaling Festivals, and numerous other ceremonies are all traditional Indigenous practices that promote and nurture connection and belonging among the people in a multitude of ways. As we continue to advance in a technological society, we also have to remember that culture is dynamic, not static. It is changing and growing with us. Cultural traditions, created with the loving minds and spirits of our ancestors, have remained in the world because they work, are useful, and guide us toward balance and harmony. Our ancestors laid this foundation and prepared us for our journey.

> Culture is an ever evolving process for Indigenous people that is based on traditional values and helps people to establish an identity and a sense of belonging in the world, describes the origin of a people through an oral tradition of legends, songs and stories; and defines people's understanding of why things happen and what they can do to make change. ([6], p. 23).

"I Remember Who I Am"—Reclaiming Our Power

My own healing and wellness journey are both personal and collective. It can be no other way. Since my introduction to learning my language in my early 20s, and feeling the power of the Elders' love and support, I have sought out numerous opportunities to spend time and learn from my Elders and community. Most recently, I have taken trips back to Anvik and Holy Cross, Alaska, my ancestral homelands. These trips have connected me spiritually to who I am as a Deg Xit'an woman in this world. Below is an excerpt from a journal I kept during a trip to Holy Cross in 2017, after being gone for 38 years.

> The first day I came to Holy Cross the Chief told me, *Welcome to Holy Cross, Welcome back .... I mean welcome home!* It's hard to put into words what that meant to me. *Xisrigidisdhinh* is the word that I learned that means I am grateful. I think this captures how I feel. The first day back I also found my dad's miniature cache, cabin, and fishwheel in the visual display case at the school. I was so surprised to see them there and so in awe since my dad has been gone, passed away, for almost 20 years. The school I am staying in was built over the old Catholic Mission, which both my parents attended when they were little. It has been surreal, profound, emotional, and wonderful to be here in my ancestral homeland with so much history of my parents and people. When visiting the gravesite, my sister, nephew, and I found the graves of our Grandpa Stanley Demientieff and Great Grandpa Ivan Demientieff, and Grandma Edith Bifelt, and we paid our respects to my Aunt Marie Alexi and Uncle Claude Demientieff and Aunt Martha among others. I see the Catholic Church next door to the school and know that my great grandfather helped build the original church. I have met numerous cousins and kin and have had the pleasure to meet loving and wonderful people. We hiked up to the cross on the hill and enjoyed beautiful views of the community and the Yukon and Innoko rivers and valley. I got to feel the spirit of the land and community. I continue to learn about and remember who I am as a Deg Xit'an person and a Frank (Modiak) and Demientieff family member. The language work I have been a part of over the years has always led me home. I am so passionate about learning the language because the more I learn the language I am also learning about my culture, history, family, traditions, protocol, and so much more. I am remembering who I am!

Elders Teach Us and Model Love and Compassion

Elders can help us to remember who we are as a people. I am fortunate to teach social work classes with Elders as co-instructors. What I have learned is that Elders create a space for students and myself to be who we are, to be cultural and spiritual beings in the classroom, to connect what we are learning with what is happening in the context of our communities. Elders draw on their experiences, they relate the learning to their people, communities, and culture, and they share what is important and relevant with love and compassion.

A Yupik Elder from Bethel, Esther Green, tells the students regularly that, "Learning is healing. As we expand our knowledge of the world we also learn about ourselves, we grow and heal." This is not something you might necessarily hear in a Western classroom but it is taken very seriously in this classroom, where students are getting an education mainly to create a better quality of life for their people. Another teaching she has shared with students is that "When we focus deeply on something, focus really hard, it becomes a part of us." For me, this Elder is telling me that when I pay attention, when I work hard, when I take the time, that whatever I am doing and learning or focusing on will become a part of me. It also reminds me that if I am focusing on positive thoughts, that will become a part of me, and when I focus on negative thoughts, that also will become a part of me. So, what is it that I want to become a part of me? So what is it that I want to focus on? The Elders help us recognize and remember that as we heal and become more balanced, we will be stronger and can help at a higher level (personal communication, n.d).

An Inupiaq Elder, and co-instructor in the social work department, Elizabeth Fleagle, tells the students that she loves them and misses them when they are away. What a beautiful way to create a safe space of love and belonging in the classroom. Her joy in life is contagious, and I am grateful for her mentorship and modeling of love and compassion in the classroom (personal communication, n.d). Athabascan Elder Howard Luke often reminds us to "take care of our luck." Teaching us that what we do in the world always comes back around to us. Sharing with others and doing things in a good way will eventually find its way back to us (personal communication, n.d). Two Deg Xit'an Athabascan Elder family members have taught me that we have to include "spirit" in all that we do. The seen and the unseen both impact us every day (P. Frank and S. Demientieff, personal communication, n.d.).

This same Deg Xit'an Elder has shared with me also that when a person is healthy, the spirit is round and soft and smooth, and when there is an imbalance and trauma and unhealthiness, the spirit can be seen as jagged and pulled apart, and that this is very physically visible (S. Demientieff, personal communication, n.d). We have to take care of the spirit. I have quoted these Elders because their wisdom is so deep and loving, and the wisdom of Elders can be taken in so many ways. I often have my own interpretation of what Elders share, and someone else might have a different interpretation, which is also true. That is the beauty of listening to Elders … you take away a message that is meant just for you.

It is good to start and end any new endeavor by honoring our ancestors, our creation, acknowledging how all things in the universe are connected, and the importance of remembering who we are as a people. Through this act of remembering, the healing journey begins and we can then light the way for others to follow.

Moving Forward in a Good Way

Five important concepts that professionals in the field of mental health and beyond can take away from this paper as something to consider, reflect on, and integrate into practice are compassion, connection, ceremony, curiosity, and community. I believe that discussions and teachings on trauma-informed care or healing-centered care in all disciplines should include these Five Cs.

Compassion

The concepts and practice of compassion and love are often missing or underused in work with people in the helping profession. Indigenous Elders often show deep love for people, even if they do not know them. When the impacts of trauma on the brain, body, and behavior are understood, we are able to have more compassion and patience, which builds a sense of safety and trust. Love is an essential part of that process.

Connection

Cultural practices within Indigenous communities often incorporate connection at the highest levels: connection to spirit, land, people, and so on. Connection is built into the fabric of the community, creating a foundation of strength and a collective safety net, as in the examples I have discussed in this chapter. The mental health of Indigenous People, and people in general, is complex. One component can be linked to feelings and experiences with connection and disconnection in many facets of life. Continued inequality and oppression on all levels are also major factors impacting mental health. Many challenging life issues, including depression, addiction, anxiety, and suicide, are related to disconnection with family, community, culture, ceremony, spirituality, and society. Add to that the crushing weight of racism, discrimination, institutional racism, and oppression, and mental health becomes very complex for Indigenous People. The unfortunate irony is that the people who need the most connection in their lives, because of their addiction or anger or depression, have the least connection with others. That is why we have to work even harder to find ways to show that connection and compassion and love. The question many people ask is, how do we help build that positive connection? Many Alaska Native Elders and culture bearers hold ancestral knowledge of cultural practices and traditional ways that have been passed on for hundreds and thousands of years, and they are willing to share if people want to listen. These practices should not be seen as remnants or notions of the past; they should and can be reclaimed and practiced in a way that makes sense in the world we live in today. These practices are based on 10,000-plus years of evidence and are considered best practices.

Ceremony

Ceremony has been discussed as a component essential to individual and community wellness, building resilience, and bringing balance back into our lives. Ceremony is important for healing, not just individually, but collectively. According to Athabascan Elder Wilson Justin, one important reason Indigenous People are still here today, despite all of the attempts to eradicate and colonize our culture and people, is because we had ceremony, and the reason ceremony works is because ceremony is about connectivity…a spiritual sense of belonging (personal communication, March 21, 2018). Ceremony links us to the spirit and our ancestors and generations coming. I believe we can incorporate ceremony in multiple ways in work within the field of mental health. One example is through self-regulation and co-regulation practices that help us to regulate our emotions and bring us back into balance, as well as enhance self-awareness, self-care, and community care.

Curiosity

Curiosity is about understanding the whole person, the multifaceted and complex human being who influences the world with their actions and who in turn is influenced by the world, including the past, the present, and the future. We have to be critical thinkers and explorers as we work toward healing and wellness with individuals and communities. Asking questions about what happened is essential. As is asking questions about what is strong with you, what is going well, what is beautiful. Curiosity is about being committed to lifelong learning. It is super exciting to imagine all that we do not know about the world and can learn as we grow and heal together.

Community

Community is essential, as healing and wellness happen within our relationships. Elders shared with me many examples of how our communities came together for celebration and in times of hardship. Our people do things together, such as fishing, berry picking, and other activities. This is also how we have survived and thrived. Elders shared that more positive wellness gatherings need to occur where the people can have fun, laugh, and learn from each other in healthy ways.

The health and mental health field as well as other fields and disciplines have an opportunity to learn from local initiatives and about local solutions from a vast number of Indigenous cultures around the world. There is wisdom and medicine in these diverse ways of knowing and being. What our world needs right now is compassion, connection, ceremony, curiosity, and community to make it through these challenging times. Connecting with and learning from our Elders is a good start. We have a bright future. Things are changing and it is going to be a better world. We no longer have to be stuck reliving our past traumas. We have the power within us, in our cells, in our spirit, in our Traditional Knowledge and practices, to be whole and well. We have to start remembering all that we are as a people, all the strength and all the resilience, and believe it.

Conclusion

It is essential to incorporate Traditional Healing, cultural grounding, reflection, and learning about culture into helping organizations that work with Indigenous People as individuals and as a community. We have to provide Indigenous People opportunities and options for healing that they connect to culturally and spiritually. It is time to move our traditions, knowledge, and practices out from under the table and display them openly on the table without fear of disapproval or reprimand. This is who we are. Our traditional practices are part of our DNA, and through them, we model connection, compassion, and ceremony. Let us learn about them and from them and pass them on as gifts to our future generations. One does not do anything successful in life without the support of the people, communities, groups, and agencies around them. "Indigenous therapeutic interventions usually involve the individual, family, and community and healing occurs within the context of the community as a whole" ([6], p. 24). Our efforts toward wellness and healing, small or large, send ripples throughout the present, send ripples into the past, and send ripples into the future, and influences the healing of all people [16].

This chapter is dedicated to my beautiful mother, Alice Frank Demientieff, and maternal aunts (Cecelia Andrews, Rose Jerue, Marie Alexie, Mary Talley, and Mary Turner)—the Franks and Modiaks—who taught me that physical, mental, and spiritual strength runs powerfully through our blood and that I can call on my ancestors anytime and they will be with me and guide me in my life. This work was supported by the Indigenous Substance Abuse, Medicines, and Addictions Research Training program through the University of Washington's Indigenous Wellness Research Institute; as well as the American Indian/Alaska Native Clinical and Translational Research Program through the University of Alaska's Center for Alaska Native Health Research and Montana State University; and funded by the National Institutes of Health IDeA CTRP grant GM115371. *Dogidinh! Xisrigidisddhinh!* (Thank you! I am grateful!)

References

1. Smith LT. Decolonizing methodologies: research and indigenous peoples. New York, NY: Zed Books, Ltd.; 2012.
2. Saleebey D. The strengths perspective in social work practice. White Plains, NY: Longman Publishers; 2002.
3. Krauss M, Holton G, Kerr J, West CT. Indigenous peoples and languages of Alaska. Fairbanks and Anchorage: Alaska Native Language Center and UAA Institute of Social and Economic Research; 2011. Online: http://www.uaf.edu/anla/map
4. Demientieff LM. Deg xit'an Athabascan conversations on wellness: a qualitative study exploring the radical possibilities of relationships (Order No. 10634333). Available from ProQuest Dissertations & Theses Global (2180107801); 2017. https://search-proquest-com.proxy.library.uaf.edu/docview/2180107801?accountid=14470
5. Woods TM, Zuniga R, David EJR. A preliminary report on the relationships between collective self-esteem, historical trauma, and mental health among Alaska Native people. J Indigenous Res. 2011;1(2):Article 1.
6. Bassett D, Tsosie U, Nannauck S. "Our culture is medicine": perspectives of native healers on posttrauma recovery among American Indian and Alaska native patients. Perm J. 2012;16(1):19–27.
7. Hallett D, Chandler M, Lalonde C. Aboriginal language knowledge and youth suicide. Cogn Dev. 2007;22:392–9.
8. Harris E, McFarland J. The assessment of culture as a protective factor among Native Americans: the survey of Nez Perce culture; 2000. https://eric.ed.gov/?id=ED449941.
9. Mohatt N, Henry D, Ching Ting Fok C, Burket R, Allen J. Assessment of awareness of connectedness as a culturally-based protective factor for Alaska Native youth. Cult Divers Ethn Minor Psychol. 2011;17(4):444–55.
10. Walters KL, Simoni JM. Reconceptualizing native women's health: an "Indigenist" stress-coping model. Am J Public Health. 2002;92(4):520–4.
11. Walters KL, Simoni JM, Evans-Campbell T. Substance use among American Indians and Alaska natives: incorporating culture in an "Indigenist" stress-coping paradigm. Public Health Rep. 2002;117(s1):s104–17.
12. Willox AC, Harper SL, Edge VI, Landman K, Houle K, Forde JD. The land enriches the soul. On climatic and environmental change, affect, and emotional health and well-being in Rigolet, Nunatsiavut, Canada. Emot Space Soc. 2013;6:14–24.
13. Snow JH. Ingalik in subarctic. In: Helm J, editor. Handbook of north American Indians. Washington: Smithsonian Institution; 1981. p. 602–17.
14. Osgood C. Ingalik mental culture. New Haven: Yale University Publications in Anthropology; 1959.
15. Demientieff L. Cultural strength and resilience. Article in Commentary, Newsletter of the Association of Alaska School Boards; 2018. https://aasb.org/cultural-strength-and-resilience/.
16. Duran E. Healing the soul wound. New York, NY: Teachers College Press; 2006.
17. Kawagley O. Alaska native education: history and adaptation in a new millenium; 2006. http://ankn.uaf.edu/curriculum/Articles/OscarKawagley/yer.html
18. Madison C. Hitting sticks, healing hearts (Videorecording). Manley Hot Springs, AK: Rivertracks Productions; 1991.

LaVerne Xilegg Demientieff is Deg Xit'an (Dene) and her family is originally from Holy Cross and Anvik, Alaska. She currently resides in Fairbanks, Alaska, and is working as an Associate Professor for the University of Alaska Fairbanks, Bachelor of Social Work program where she has taught since 2006; she is also a licensed master social worker through the State of Alaska. LaVerne is a statewide trainer on the topics of historical trauma and historical wellness, adverse childhood experiences, resilience, trauma-informed care, and healing-centered care. LaVerne is very active in learning and teaching her Deg Xinag languageand facilitates a weekly Deg Xinag language learning group. LaVerne's research interests focus on exploring how cultural and traditional practices contribute to individual, family, group, and community resilience, health, healing, and wellness, specifically with the Indigenous People of Alaska. She is also interested in studying the connection between language and well-being.

Patrick Frank is a Deg Xit'an Athabascan Elder storyteller, writer, herbalist, and traditional consultant. As a Native Family Systems facilitator for over 25 years, he also served as an adjunct faculty member for the University of Alaska's Rural Human Services Program for 5 years on campuses in Fairbanks, Anchorage, Bethel, and Sitka. Patrick has facilitated workshops focusing on individual, family, and community wellness to over 35 communities in Alaska, including six regional health corporations. A Vietnam veteran, he also served on his regional profit and nonprofit corporations as an executive board member.

Part V
Integrating Indigenous and Western Approaches

Traditional Aboriginal Healing in Mental Health Care, Western Australia

Jocelyn Jones, Hannah McGlade, and Sophie Davison

The Aboriginal[1] concept of health is "holistic, encompassing mental health and physical, cultural and spiritual health" ([1], pp. 19). Traditional Healers have extensive knowledge passed from generation to generation and are able to interpret symptoms and provide Traditional Healing treatments such as bush medicine and spiritual healing. In Australia, Traditional Healing practices remain predominant in the more remote areas of Australia. Aboriginal healers of the Anangu Pitjantjarjara Yangkunjatjara lands in Central Australia are called *Ngangkari,* a Pitjantjara word meaning "Traditional Healer." Traditional Healers have diverse roles. In the Kutjungka region of the Kimberley (Western Australia, or WA), the *Mapan* have been described as "protectors of their people's health, their ability to diagnose the sources of an illness offers security and comfort, their protective role reinforces desert health beliefs and their importance of cultural gatekeepers to those beliefs" ([2], p. 234). Franks, a Ngangkari from Central Australia, noted that "Ngangkari work with the spirit, our work is to touch and heal people, to bring their spirits back" ([3], p. 147). "Ngangkari learn from other Ngangkari. We are taught a long heritage of traditional healing. There are Ngangkari men, women and children. Ngangkari speak many different languages and dialects. Ngangkari become Ngangkari because

[1] For the rest of this chapter, when we speak of Aboriginal people, we include those who identify as Aboriginal and Torres Strait Islander.

J. Jones (✉)
National Drug Research Institute (NDRI), Faculty of Health Sciences,
Perth, Western Australia
e-mail: J.Jones@curtin.edu.au

H. McGlade
Curtin Law School, Faculty of Business and Law, Perth, Western Australia
e-mail: Hannah.Mcglade@curtin.edu.au

S. Davison
Department of Psychiatry and Clinical Neurosciences, University of Western Australia,
Perth, Australia
e-mail: sophie.davison@uwa.edu.au

D. Danto, M. Zangeneh (eds.), *Indigenous Knowledge and Mental Health*,
https://doi.org/10.1007/978-3-030-71346-1_14

somebody else has given them the power" ([3], p. 148). Langton argues that in many areas of Australia, "Aboriginal men and women turn with great confidence to traditional healers to maintain their wellbeing" ([4], p. 2).

In South Australia, Ngangkari Healers work alongside Western medical professionals in hospitals providing "complementary" treatment to medical care [5]. According to Langton, "Healers understand that western medical treatments should be used by Aboriginal patients, and often explain to them that they should go to the clinic or stay in hospital and not fear doctors and nurses" ([4], p. 1). "Traditional healers see their role as complimentary to western medicine we didn't see any conflict with our style of healing and the whitefella doctors that come in because that kind of doctor does operation and so on, I give healing treatments to many children and adults. If anyone is sick and in need of help. I help them" ([3], p. 79). "People still got sick and still needed to see Ngangkari. Doctors can work with open sores and put medicine in and heal them, whereas Ngangkari work with the invisible, and with the spirit. We used to say, 'Yes, they're giving them medicine for the sicknesses that they see, but Ngangkari are working differently. We're working with the invisible, with what we can see with our Ngangkari eyes.' So we worked separately, in the clinic or in the camps, yet the two styles of healing were working together really well" ([3], p. 35).

Aboriginal People and Mental Health

According to Parker and Milroy [6], mental illness was present in Aboriginal culture before colonization but was likely to have been a "rare" occurrence (p. 121). The far greater prevalence of mental illness among Aboriginal communities today "is a reflection of the significant disruption to Aboriginal and Torres Strait Islander society and has a strong context of social and emotional deprivation" (p. 121). High rates of psychological distress and mental health problems relate to the disproportionate number of Aboriginal people who are exposed to social, historical, and economic risk factors for mental illness [6]. The high rates of mental health problems can be understood in the context of the impact of colonization: trauma, loss and grief, separation from families and children, dispossession, and loss of culture and identity. To this list should be added the impact of social determinants, including factors such as homelessness, poor education, consequential unemployment, stigma, racism, ongoing grief and losses, and life stresses [1].

Aboriginal people experience higher rates of mental health problems than other Australians do. Available national figures show that Aboriginal people report 2.7 times the rates of high and very high psychological distress, compared to other Australians, with nearly a third of Aboriginal adults reporting high or very high levels of distress [7]. Aboriginal females reported experiencing greater levels of stress (38.4%) than Aboriginal males (26.7%) between 2014 and 2015 [8]. This significant increase in stress was caused by a range of factors such as overcrowding in their homes and unemployment [8]. Both Aboriginal males and females died from intentional self-harm at a rate two times that of the non-Aboriginal population [9]. Aboriginal people are twice as likely to die from suicide. This disparity in suicide rates is particularly alarming for the 15–19-year-olds, with suicide rates of Aboriginal young women 5.9 times greater than for their non-Aboriginal counterparts. Similarly, suicide rates are 4.4 times greater in males in this age group [10].

National figures show that Aboriginal people present to mental health services at higher rates than other Australians do [10]. General practitioners manage mental health problems for Aboriginal Australians at 1.2 times the rate for other Australians, and specialized community mental health services report that Aboriginal Australians have four times the rate of service contact than other Australians. Nonetheless, it is difficult to quantify whether service use is as high as the underlying need [10]. Aboriginal and Torres Strait Islander people coming into prison who have mental health problems are less likely to have sought help outside than non-Aboriginal prisoners. The WA Aboriginal child health survey found that despite the high proportion (24%) of Aboriginal children at high risk of clinically significant emotional and behavioral difficulties, very few had had contact with mental health services [11].

While alarming, these statistics may not tell the whole story. The "pioneer psychiatrist" Mark Sheldon describes the Western model of psychiatric assessment as "culturally inappropriate" (Sheldon cited in [12], pp. 260–261). Based on his work with the Ngangkari Healers of the Western Desert, Sheldon recommends the combination of Aboriginal Traditional Healing approaches with Western clinical techniques. In earlier research, Vicary and Westerman (2004) similarly argue that Aboriginal People's mental health problems will often "manifest themselves, spiritually and culturally and therefore can only be resolved in this manner" (p. 4). Their research concluded that there were a number of features of depression in Aboriginal people that did not conform to mainstream diagnosis, requiring a blend of Western and Aboriginal models of diagnosis and treatment.

Culturally appropriate explanation of the framework of social and emotional well-being (SEWB) is regarded as critical to Aboriginal peoples' understanding of health and well-being. The SEWB is considered a "multidimensional concept of health," a concept that includes mental health and wider aspects of well-being, such as connection to country, culture, spirituality, ancestry, family, and community [13]. The social determinants of health interact with Aboriginal cultural and spiritual dimensions. These factors include poverty, unemployment, housing shortage, educational disadvantage, race discrimination, exposure to violence, trauma and stress, and other socioeconomic factors.

Access to Culturally Appropriate Mental Health Services

Qualitative evidence indicates that a number of barriers make it difficult for Aboriginal people seeking help with mental illness to engage with mainstream services. Reasons for this include lack of trust in the mainstream system [14]; a mismatch between mainstream services' conception of mental health and the holistic Aboriginal concept of social and emotional well-being, lack of Aboriginal community involvement and consultation in developing services, poor cultural understanding by service providers, and stigma and racism [15].

Wright (2014) reports that Aboriginal people with mental illness experience "double discrimination," living with both the stigma of mental illness and racism because of their Aboriginality (p. 244). Aboriginal caregivers, in the context of mental illness, reported frequent instances of "racism, alienation and social inequality" (p. 248). For most participants, their experiences with hospitals were negative and they reported psychiatric hospitals to be "unfriendly and scary" places (p. 250). Vicary and Westerman [16] carried out research with Aboriginal people in Perth and the Kimberley. They reported that many Aboriginal people were fearful of Western mental health services and practitioners (p. 7).

Delivery of culturally appropriate mental health services are outlined in a number of guidelines, principles, and legislation for Western Australia. The Royal Australian and New Zealand College of Psychiatrists acknowledges there is a need for a broader understanding of mental health within Aboriginal communities. This must be achieved within a holistic construct of social, emotional, cultural, and spiritual well-being. The recognition of Traditional Healers is outlined in the Ethical Guideline 11 of the Guidelines and Principles for Aboriginal and Torres Strait Islander Mental Health. It highlights that it is important for psychiatrists and psychiatric trainees to:

> [R]ecognize that Traditional Healing practices of Aboriginal and Torres Strait Islander people may have much to offer in the treatment of mental health and social and emotional problems; seek out and utilize Aboriginal and Torres Strait Islander expertise including traditional and contemporary practitioners. ([17], p. 3).

An Aboriginal Human Rights Framework

It is also important to recognize that these rights of Aboriginal mental health patients are significant human rights. The United Nations Declaration on the Rights of Indigenous Peoples [18] promotes the collective rights of Indigenous people and includes the fundamental rights to nondiscrimination and self-determination. It includes Article 23, recognizing Indigenous peoples' right to development, particularly the right to be actively involved in developing and determining and administering their own health programs. According to the UNDRIP Article 24, Aboriginal Peoples have the right to traditional medicines, to keep their own traditional health practices, and to have access to health services without discrimination.

The Committee on Economic, Social and Cultural Rights (CESCR) has further considered Aboriginal peoples' right to health in General Comment No. 14 (2000), finding that Aboriginal people have the right to specific measures to improve access to health services and care, which should be culturally appropriate and take into account traditional practices and medicines, and that states should provide resources for Indigenous peoples to design, deliver, and control services. Other international instruments that recognize Indigenous peoples' right to equality of access and self-determination in health care include Article 25 of the International Labour Organisation (ILO) Indigenous and Tribal Peoples Convention, 1989 (No. 169). Under ILO 169, Indigenous people must be allowed access to health care services and should also be provided with resources to design and deliver the services. The training and employment of local community health workers is also supported. The importance of Aboriginal peoples' human rights in mental health context is strengthened in Australia by the *Gayaa Dhuwi (Proud Spirit) Declaration,* which aims to improve the mental health of Aboriginal and Torres Strait Islander peoples by supporting Aboriginal leadership in mental health systems [15]. The statement promotes a balance between clinical and culturally informed mental health system responses to mental health problems in Aboriginal and Torres Strait persons, including providing access to cultural healing.

The Mental Health Act 2014 (WA)

The *Mental Health Act 2014* (WA) sets out the legal responsibilities of services to provide culturally appropriate mental health care and treatment to Aboriginal people (*Mental Health Act 2014* (WA), s. 81, s. 189).

The *Mental Health Act 2014* (WA) Charter of Mental Health Care Principles is a right-based set of principles to which all mental health services must have regard. According to Principle 7, practitioners and mental health services must provide treatment and care to Aboriginal people that is appropriate and consistent with the patient's cultural and spiritual beliefs and practices. They should also, if possible, have regard to the views of their families and significant members of their communities, including Elders and Traditional Healers, and Aboriginal or Torres Strait Islander mental health workers.

In addition, the *Mental Health Act 2014* (WA) (Sections 81 and 189) sets out the requirement for mental health professionals to collaborate with Aboriginal mental health workers, Elders, and Traditional Healers when assessing and treating Aboriginal people. Section 81. Examination of person of Aboriginal or Torres Strait Islander descent states that:

> To the extent that it is practicable and appropriate to do so, the examination of a person who is of Aboriginal or Torres Strait Islander descent must be conducted in collaboration with—(a) Aboriginal or Torres Strait Islander mental health workers; and (b) significant members of the person's community, including elders and traditional healers [and,]
>
> Section 189. Provision of treatment to patient of Aboriginal or Torres Strait Islander descent.
>
> To the extent that it is practicable and appropriate to do so, treatment provided to a patient who is of Aboriginal or Torres Strait Islander descent must be provided in collaboration with—(a) Aboriginal or Torres Strait Islander mental health workers; and (b) significant members of the patient's community, including elders and traditional healers.

The legal requirements adopted in the 2014 legislation are clearly in response to the concerns articulated over some time that the provision of mental health care and treatment to Aboriginal people needs to be culturally secure and nondiscriminatory.

The Standards for Clinical Care of the Chief Psychiatrist of WA also include a standard for Aboriginal Practice. It states that all services and clinicians must recognize the potential value of Traditional Healing practices in the treatment of mental health and social and emotional problems ([19], p. 6). They should understand the mental health implications of the history of contact between Aboriginal communities and Australia's mainstream society and acknowledge that understanding of mental health within Aboriginal communities involves a holistic construct of social, emotional, cultural, and spiritual well-being.

Overall, these statements and legislation all demonstrate that an intended effect of the new provisions of the WA *Mental Health Act* in 2014 was to ensure that voluntary and involuntary Aboriginal mental health patients have Aboriginal mental health workers or Traditional Healers or both involved in their treatment. This reflects the demands of Aboriginal People worldwide and the commitment of the government to an accessible, effective, and nondiscriminatory health care system.

To assess the effectiveness of the 2014 changes to the WA *Mental Health Act,* we examine the experiences of mental health practitioners, patients, and Traditional Healers as related to implementing the Act.

A Case Study: The Wungen Kartup Specialist Aboriginal Mental Health Service

The Wungen Kartup Specialist Aboriginal Mental Health Service (SAMHS) is a specialized mental health service that provides best practice mental health care to Aboriginal people across the Perth metropolitan area and regional WA. The philosophy of SAMHS is to operate with cultural integrity and provide a "whole of family," spiritual, and holistic approach to service delivery. It utilizes the services of Traditional Healers in conjunction with non-Aboriginal (Western) mental health care to provide Traditional Healer treatments.

We interviewed the SAMHS health service providers and patients who have used the services of Traditional Healers. We interviewed the SAMHS health service providers and patients who have used the services of Traditional Healers. Three major themes were identified from the interviews: cultural safety, implementation of the *Act*, and positive outcomes.

Cultural Safety

There was significant concern from health service providers about cultural safety for Aboriginal patients. Participants acknowledged that Aboriginal patients should have a better level of care and improved access to service, including workers who are "empathic and experienced in working with our people, who are wanting to help our people." There was some frustration at the lack of cultural security for Aboriginal people: "There's only so much you can shake your head … so many times before it gets stiff and my neck got stiff a long time ago" (Male 01).

Many services and non-Aboriginal staff "don't really listen to our families" and were dismissive of Aboriginal families who were caring for family members by not engaging respectfully. Limited service was reportedly provided to Aboriginal people, and medical interactions were reported as lacking in empathy and compassion: "There's very different models of care being delivered to Aboriginal and non-Aboriginal clients and that … is so obvious" (Male 01).

The need for more Aboriginal people trained and working in mental health was regarded as critical.

Some opposition to the *Act* requirements was reported. For example, some mainstream psychiatrists were reportedly unwilling to refer patients because they did not believe that Aboriginal culture was relevant to treatment. Their attitude was "it's just mental illnesses and should be treated as that." Others did not believe Aboriginal Healers could assist Aboriginal patients and were dismissive of the role of Traditional Healers. An SAMHS service provider reported that there was a lack of understanding and interest in traditional Aboriginal healing, with the misunderstanding that a Healer may even be detrimental to the patient: "…if the client was psychotically unwell and had a religious component to their illness I wouldn't put them in front of a priest (Male 02)."

There was a reluctance to engage in Traditional Healing because of concern that a Healer would advise patients against medication, and this fear appeared unfounded, as no Aboriginal Healers had advised patients against taking medications. When there was a working relationship between Healers and psychiatrists it was regarded positive: "I've never come across any issues where doctors and healers disagreed or anything like that they seemed to always work together in that way (Female 01)."

Unfortunately, according to reports, because of a lack of understanding of the wider societal factors or determinants and cultural awareness, Aboriginal patients could even be blamed for their mental health. "There's a lot of people out there who don't know, and they don't mix with Aboriginal people, they don't have Aboriginal friends." Prejudice and ignorance were also reported: "I've worked with nurses who have referred to culture as mumbo jumbo and voodoo stuff … palmed it off as not relevant (Male 01)."

A lack of knowledge on the part of non-Aboriginal staff was linked to lack of cultural awareness training—doctors working with Aboriginal people "…have never done a cultural awareness training and only have been in Australia for two or three years, straight from England … yet they're the case managers of our people…." (Male 01).

SAMHS staff reported that there was some resistance to cultural awareness programs conducted by Aboriginal staff, and frustration with lack of cultural competency of doctors and resistance to the *Act* provisions came from psychiatrists who were "…not long on these shores and still [haven't] learnt how our mob are." Some overseas-trained staff had experience in regional Western Australia and became too confident, thinking "they're a full bottle working with our people." One health provider was ascribed high-level cultural engagement skills because he worked with Aboriginal people; however, in his view, it was the development and commitment to a respectful relationship with Aboriginal patients that was the key to positive engagement.

The Implementation of the *Mental Health Act 2014*

The SAMHS reported their success in meeting the needs of Aboriginal people came from "knowing your clients, knowing your community and understanding Aboriginal ways and the Aboriginal world." (Male 04). They reported that patients were more comfortable using their service, which employed Aboriginal workers and had positive outcomes. Notwithstanding their ability to deliver culturally appropriate service, the SAMHS were not being consulted to assist in the provision of services according to the *Act:* "To this date, I don't think we've ever been phoned to actually ask, do we have access to a Traditional Healer or do we have access to significant community members that could represent that particular client" (Male 02).

Non-Aboriginal mainstream clinical staff, who may not have made appropriate efforts to meet the requirements of the *Act,* appear to have "bypassed" its provisions. There was no funding attached to implement the *Act* provisions, and, while there had been some interest in establishing a database of Traditional Healers before the *Act* came into force, there was an assumption that SAMHS would have an advisory role about the *Act* implementation.

According to a health service provider, the mainstream mental health services had some general awareness of the *Act* requirements, but the services were not implementing the requirements. Notwithstanding, provisions were significant within the SAMHS, "… it's actually been really beneficial to not only us as clinicians, but also the clients as well and their families …. It's a big aspect of the *Act,* having the Aboriginal clinician there" (Female 02).

The Aboriginal clinician was seen to be advocating, consulting, and providing an important educative role in relation to the *Act.*

One health service provider advised that some mainstream providers were using Aboriginal Liaison Officers to meet the provisions of the *Act,* even though they were not trained Aboriginal mental health workers. This was described as a "battle" SAMHS was having with mainstream services:

> I said to them you're not complying with the Act when you sent one of your liaison officers who is not trained, no idea of what's going on its not in the Act...there is no protection for them should anything go wrong...

The importance of the provision in assessing Aboriginal patients was highlighted through one example provided by an interviewee concerning a misdiagnosis of an Aboriginal woman flown into Graylands Hospital. The hospital contacted SAMHS, who ascertained that her presentation was cultural and not due to mental illness:

> It would have just been a trauma for her getting, boom, on a plane and sent in a place you don't even know, and now I'm labelled because I've been to this mental health ward. All this stigma going around. It was really sad they didn't check with her family before they even put her on that plane.

Another interviewee considered that there were likely many cases of misdiagnosis before the *Act* introduced provisions concerning assessment of patients. These provisions also allowed for Aboriginal health service providers to ".... deter non-Aboriginal mental health workers from going down those paths to protect the clients ..." and especially relevant where non-Aboriginal mental health workers may be "prying" into culturally sensitive matters not within the scope of Western medical treatment.

Positive Outcomes

Aboriginal health providers spoke of the importance of Aboriginal culture to social and emotional well-being and believed that Traditional Healers had a "major role." They reported positive outcomes were evident when Aboriginal Traditional Healers worked with patients and the impact of Traditional Healing was powerful:

> The change is almost immediate. The relief, it's almost like the pressure that weighs fellas down ... is constant and been there for years, and in some cases the instant relief in the 24 hours is massive ... You can't really describe to a non-Aboriginal person the change. It's just remarkable (Male 01)

Another health service provider described the beneficial impact as the patient being treated in a respectful cultural manner "for their whole beliefs and values ... I've seen it make improvements in people and work together with the traditional Western model of health care." The Aboriginal health workers saw Aboriginal Healers and Western medicine as complementary and synergistically aligned.

They described Healers as "specialists in their own rights, and what they do is like any confidential patient doctor ... treatment." Patients reported having weight lifted from them, feeling lighter, better, and more motivated. A Traditional Healer interviewed described his healing as promoting peoples own strengths and relationships: "I know its strengths that we need and a lot of people around. I think it's so important to have families strong with families." His knowledge of healing encompassed physical, emotional, mental, and spiritual levels and was a "journey of trust" between two people.

The provisions of the Act concerning Elders and family helped to build trust and rapport between the service and the Aboriginal patient. This engagement helped clinicians to understand the issues facing Aboriginal patients: "A lot of times ... there is more than mental health going on." Many patients were fearful of mental health services, and the engagement of Elders and family members helped to provide support and allay fears. One patient believed he experienced spiritual or cultural harm, and while the Healer ascertained this was not the case, he continued to treat the patient and helped him feel safer, comforted him, and increased his understanding of his illness.

Family members were both "shocked" and "really happy" to know that Traditional Healing was happening. The use of Traditional Healers can be important also to the patient's family and, if so, it needed to be facilitated: "Otherwise ... in the end you just don't get the trust of the family or the patient. So I think it's very important and also I've seen how it can work for people ... it's a very important part of the process" (Male 05).

It was essential that women Healers were available given that many Aboriginal women have experienced sexual abuse and traumatization. One woman spoke about how the Traditional Healer had a powerful impact on her and had given her peacefulness. She had experienced 20 years of nightmares involving sexual abuse. The healing impact was immediately positive and she reported she had had no bad dreams since the healing took place. She also felt that she had been having "good luck" since the healing and had been living healthier, "And I've been cooking healthy meals every night since it's like I've woken up from a bad dream, bad dreams for 20 years."

Another woman patient reported that she felt it was important that she had also been able to see a woman Healer. She felt that there should be more Healers available and they should include the local Noongar people. She also thought that Traditional Healers "would benefit in other government services like public housing, for example, especially if someone's just moved into a house." According to cultural beliefs, homes may not be suitable following a person's death without proper spiritual and cultural ceremony.

Traditional Healing is very different from Western medicine, and Healers have a different and complementary role to psychiatrists. The Ngangkari Healers' work was concerned with Aboriginal spirituality and it could not be learned through Western psychology. Aboriginal Traditional Healing involved bush medicine, bush tucker, and it was seen as "a big medical certificate in itself." There was a role for male and female Healers; they were people who had knowledge in law and culture. All Aboriginal people should have access to Healers who come from and understand their own country and culture. Healers had worked with Aboriginal patients who had a strong cultural background and those who had not–they had made a positive impact regardless.

Conclusion

Aboriginal health providers, Aboriginal consumers, and their families all reported that Traditional Healers had an important role to play in the care of Aboriginal people with mental health problems and reported positive outcomes where Traditional Healers had been involved. They also reported that the involvement of Elders and Healers improved the trust and rapport with mental health services as well as the assessment and treatment provided by mental health services.

Our exploratory research unfortunately reveals a marked lack of attention to the implementation of the *Mental Health Act* provisions introduced in 2014 to ensure Aboriginal people have access to cultural safety in the assessment and provision of mental health treatment. While SAMHS has promoted the *Act* within its service, and Aboriginal patients of SAMHS were receiving the benefit of the *Act*, mainstream mental health services and hospitals were not yet utilizing SAMHS to undertake assessments or use Traditional Healers. Furthermore, there was no evidence of any system-wide dialog about how to ensure implementation of the important provisions of the *Act*.

Our research indicates a lack of cultural safety for Aboriginal people in the mental health system. While the positive effects of Traditional Healers and the importance of culturally safe assessment are demonstrably clear, it is also clear that many Aboriginal people appear not to receive the benefit of culturally safe mental health interventions. Although the *Act* was changed to incorporate Aboriginal cultural safety, there was little or no consideration given to funding, policy, and oversight to ensure the implementation of the new provisions. The SAMHS has made a concerted commitment to provide culturally safe mental health care, with positive healing outcomes resulting for some Aboriginal people; however, the wider lack of culturally safe treatment of Aboriginal people as required by the *Act* represents a clear breach of the *Act* and, more widely, Aboriginal human rights.

The WA government should require mental health services and Aboriginal people to partner in a system-wide dialog to promote cultural safety and ensure the provisions of the Mental Health Act are implemented. This will assist Western mental health practitioners to better understand the needs of their Aboriginal patients and the adjustments to practices this dictates, including collaboration with Aboriginal Healers. The aim is to establish a research-informed basis for the synergistic collaboration between Aboriginal and Western approaches to mental health services. These developments should lead to Aboriginal people having much better access to culturally safe, responsive, person-centered services provided by a culturally competent and confident workforce. This will also clearly require adequate resourcing, training, and robust monitoring.

Cultural safety for the Aboriginal people is a national priority identified by the Australian Health Practitioner Regulation Agency [20], who "made a commitment to ensuring that Aboriginal and Torres Strait Islander Peoples have access to health services that are culturally safe and free from racism so that they can enjoy a healthy life, equal to that of other Australians, enriched by a strong living culture, dignity and justice" (ref). The MHA (2014) provisions alone have not been sufficient to realize these important objectives, a genuine commitment to Aboriginal health equality lies at the heart of this challenge.

References

1. Swan P, Raphael B. "Ways Forward": national consultancy report on aboriginal and torres strait islander mental health. AGPS; 1995.
2. McCoy BF. Outside the ward and clinic: healing the aboriginal body. J Contemp Ethnogr. 2008;37(2):226–45. Mental Health Act 2014 (WA). https://www.mhc.wa.gov.au/media/1245/mental-health-act-2014.pdf
3. Ngaanyatjarra Pitjantjatjar Yankunytjatjara Women's Council Aboriginal Corporation (NPYWWCAC). Traditional healers of Central Australia. Ngangkari: Magabala Books Aboriginal Corporation; 2013.
4. Langton M. Traditional aboriginal healing practice. In: Healy J, editor. The art of healing: Australian indigenous bush medicine. Victoria: Medical History Museum, University of Melbourne; 2018.
5. Panzironi F. Hand in hand: report on aboriginal traditional medicine. Anangu Ngangkari Tjutaku Aboriginal Corporation; 2013.
6. Parker R, Milroy H. Aboriginal and torres strait islander mental health: an overview. In: Dudgeon P, Milroy H, Walker R, editors. Working together: aboriginal and torres strait islander mental health and wellbeing principles and practice. 2nd ed. Canberra: Department of The Prime Minister and Cabinet; 2014. p. 25–38.
7. Australian Institute of Health and Welfare. The health and welfare of Australia's Aboriginal and Torres Strait Islander peoples 2015. Cat. no. 147. Canberra; 2015.
8. Steering Committee for the Review of Government Service Provision (SCRGSP). Overcoming indigenous disadvantage: key indicators 2016. Canberra, Australia; 2016.
9. Australian Bureau of Statistics. Causes of death, Australia, 2017. Cat. no. 3303.0. Canberra: Australian Government; 2018.
10. Australian Health Ministers' Advisory Council. Aboriginal and Torres Strait Islander health performance framework 2017 report. Canberra: Australian Government; 2017.
11. Zubrick S, Lawrence D, Silburn S, Blair E, Milroy H, Wilkes E, et al. The Western Australian aboriginal child health survey: the health of aboriginal children and young people: Telethon Institute for Child Health Research; 2004.
12. Dudgeon P, Ugle K. Communicating and engaging with diverse communities. In: Dudgeon P, Milroy H, Walker R, editors. Working together: aboriginal and torres strait islander mental health and wellbeing principles and practice. Canberra: Department of The Prime Minister and Cabinet; 2014. p. 257–67, Chapter 15.
13. Gee G, Dudgeon P, Schultz C, Hart A, Kelly K. Aboriginal and torres strait islander social and emotional wellbeing. In: Dudgeon P, Milroy H, Walker R, editors. Working together: aboriginal and torres strait islander mental health and wellbeing principles and practice. 2nd ed. Canberra: Department of The Prime Minister and Cabinet; 2014. p. 55–68.
14. Wright M, O'Connell M, Jones T, Walley R, Roarty L. Looking forward aboriginal mental health project final report; 2015.
15. Dudgeon P, Calma T, Brideson T, Holland C. The Gayaa Dhuwi (Proud Spirit) Declaration—a call to action for aboriginal and Torres Strait islander leadership in the Australian mental health system. Adv Ment Health. 2016;14(2):126–39. https://doi.org/10.1080/18387357.2016.1198233.
16. Vicary D, Westerman T. That's just the way he is': Some implications of Aboriginal mental health beliefs. Australian e-Journal for the advancement of mental health. 2004;3(3), 103–112.

17. Royal Australian New Zealand College of Psychiatrists. Ethical guideline 11, principles and guidelines for aboriginal and torres strait islander mental health; 2014. https://www.ranzcp.org/files/resources/college_statements/ethical_guidelines/eg11-principles-and-guidelines-for-aboriginal-and.aspx
18. United Nations. United Nations declaration on the rights of indigenous peoples; 2008.
19. Chief Psychiatrist of WA. Chief psychiatrist's standards for clinical care (standard aboriginal practice); 2015. https://www.chiefpsychiatrist.wa.gov.au/wp-ontent/uploads/2015/12/CP_Standards_2015.pdf
20. Australian Health Practitioner Regulation Agency. Cultural-safety-training-provider-announced; 2019. https://www.ahpra.gov.au/News/2019-07-25-Cultural-safety-training-provider-announced.aspx

Jocelyn Jones identifies as a Nyoongar woman with connections to the land in the southwest of West Australia (WA) (Whadjuk and Ballardong nations) and the Pilbara in the north of WA (Palyku peoples). She holds a PhD and Master's in Applied Epidemiology and was awarded her doctorate in 2018 on "Exploring the Pathways to contact with juvenile justice in Aboriginal and Torres Strait Islander children: developing a strategy for change." Dr. Jones has extensive experience working in health and justice, in both Aboriginal community controlled health services and in senior management positions in the Department of Health and Corrective Services in Western Australia. She is an early career researcher and has made significant contributions to Aboriginal health and social well-being through her work with Aboriginal prisoners and juvenile detainees. She is a current member of the Ombudsman's advisory group and volunteers as an official visitor for the WA Office of the Inspector of Custodial Services. She is a coauthor of several recent publications on Aboriginal women and children, including "Australian Aboriginal Women Prisoners' Experiences of Being a Mother: A Review," in the *International Journal of Prisoner Health* (2018).

Hannah McGlade is Associate Professor with Curtin Law School and a member of the UN Permanent Forum for Indigenous Issues. Admitted to the West Australian Supreme Court as a barrister and solicitor in 1996, she holds degrees in law and international human rights, (LLB, LLM, Ph.D). Dr. McGlade is an experienced tribunal member, her academic and research career has focused on justice for Aboriginal people, race discrimination law and practice, Aboriginal women and children, family violence, and sexual assault. As a member of the Mental Health Tribunal in WA, Dr. McGlade reviewed many cases of involuntary mental health care for Aboriginal people and advocated for the implementation of the cultural safety requirements of the law.

Sophie Davison is the Deputy Chief Psychiatrist of Western Australia and also works clinically for the State Forensic Mental Health Services in Perth Western Australia. She is Adjunct Senior Lecturer at the University of Western Australia and at the University of New South Wales. Her research interests are in the mental health of prisoners. She completed her training and advanced forensic psychiatric training at the Maudsley Hospital and Institute of Psychiatry, King's College in London, UK, and has worked in a number of clinical forensic mental health settings. She has published on the topic of women's mental health, drug addicts in police custody, offenders with personality disorder, prisoner mental health, and the mental health of detainees under anti-terror legislation. She has experience in preparing psychiatric reports for the Courts, including the UK Court of Appeal, and human rights cases involving the mentally disordered. Dr. Davison is also the Director of Advanced Training in Forensic Psychiatry in Western Australia.

Integrating Indigenous Healing and Western Counseling: Clinical Cases in Culturally Safe Practice

Teresa Beaulieu and Allison Reeves

Research has shown that effective counseling interventions for many Indigenous Peoples infuse Indigenous worldviews, values, and practices into treatment. Research has also shown that the use of only mainstream or Western therapeutic interventions has often proved ineffective for Indigenous clients, as indicated by an under-usage of services and high dropout rates. In response, many scholars working in Indigenous mental health have called for an integration, or harmonization, of Indigenous healing approaches and Western therapeutic frameworks in counseling. However, clear examples demonstrating the effectiveness of successful integration are required to guide mainstream Western psychology toward culturally safe practice in this regard. This chapter presents the background and context for an integrative healing movement, as well as case studies of integration grounded in examples from two counseling settings in Toronto, Canada, where these authors have worked providing mental health care. This chapter identifies obstacles to, and the facilitation of, counseling environments which support the work of Indigenous Healers, Elders, and counselors, and discusses next steps for the successful practice of integrated mental health counseling.

Indigenous Peoples of North America have had systems and practices in place to address and ensure the health and well-being of communities for generations. As with all populations, Indigenous Peoples encountered a diverse range of physical and mental health problems prior to contact [1], and Indigenous groups had comprehensive systems and methods in place for healing. However, with the arrival of European colonizers and the enduring and devastating impacts of colonial policies, the nature, etiology, and occurrence of such health problems transformed

T. Beaulieu
Weaving Wellness Centre, Toronto, ON, Canada

A. Reeves (✉)
Department of Psychology, University of Guelph, Toronto, ON, Canada
e-mail: allison.reeves@guelphhumber.ca

D. Danto, M. Zangeneh (eds.), *Indigenous Knowledge and Mental Health*,
https://doi.org/10.1007/978-3-030-71346-1_15

substantially. In addition to the introduction of new infectious diseases through colonization, such as influenza and tuberculosis, legislated efforts at cultural genocide by colonial governments have had severe and long-lasting impacts on the mental health of many Indigenous peoples today.

Although Indigenous populations represent a small percentage of Canada's total population, Indigenous communities experience a wide range of health problems at disproportionately higher rates than non-Indigenous peoples. While much variability and diversity exist within Indigenous families, between rural and urban groups, and across First Nations, Inuit, and Métis communities in Canada, general trends continue to indicate substantial health inequities. Physical health ailments representing serious chronic diseases, including heart disease, cerebrovascular disease, diabetes, cancer, and AIDS, are issues of current concern in many communities [2, 3]. Mental health challenges are also seen in many communities in the form of higher rates of depression, anxiety, and other psychiatric disorders, suicide, self-injury, substance abuse, violence, and trauma [4–6].

As with all population health trends, these findings should be contextualized with an understanding of historical and social trends. First settlers to North America in the sixteenth and seventeenth centuries were aided in their survival in large part by Indigenous Peoples, who assisted with navigating new climates and environments [7]. In time however the governing European authorities began to see the "Indians" as an impediment to new immigrant settlements [1]. The enforcement of colonial policies to "manage" the Indigenous Peoples throughout contact was oppressive, racist, and paternalistic. Two notable pieces of legislation, the *British North America Act of 1867* and the *Indian Act of 1876*, enabled the Canadian government to classify Indigenous Peoples as wards of the state, to determine who could identify as "Indian," to eradicate Indigenous forms of governance, to secure title to the land and its resources, to force Indigenous Peoples off their traditional lands and onto designated "reserve" lands, and to restrict and control essential components of healthy living, such as access to food, recreational activity, and the practice of cultural customs and traditions—including the use of healing practices and ceremony [1, 3, 8]. In essence, the principal goal of this legislation was the assimilation of Indigenous Peoples to Euro-Canadian beliefs, customs, and values.

One pronounced and grave example of legislated assimilation is the establishment of the residential school system in the late 1800s. This was an effort by the Canadian government, with the assistance of Christian institutions, to assimilate Indigenous children into the dominant culture. Children were forcibly removed from their homes, separated from their families, and enrolled in these institutions. The curriculum included training in academics, domestic tasks, and manual labor, as well as indoctrination into Christian values [8, 36]. Indigenous languages and spiritual practices were denounced and specifically targeted for eradication in these schools, as they were perceived as a principal vehicle for the transmission of Indigenous cultures. Rampant physical, psychological, and sexual abuse was well documented through the national Truth and Reconciliation Commission (2008–2015), which heard from more than 6000 witnesses who were affected by this multi-generational assimilation policy [36]. Children also experienced malnourishment, neglect, inadequate medical care, and high rates of child mortality related to medical crises such as tuberculosis. Residential schools began to close their doors in the mid-twentieth century because of financial constraints and growing awareness among the population of the depraved conditions of the schools. The government then changed its welfare policy toward mass adoption of Indigenous children into non-Indigenous families; commonly referred to as the "Sixties Scoop," this practice lasted well beyond that decade. The last residential school closed its doors in 1996, and the thousands of court cases against the government by survivors and their families led to the largest class-action lawsuit in Canadian history [36] and the establishment of the Truth and Reconciliation Commission.

The attempt to fully assimilate Indigenous Peoples into the dominant culture in residential schools was unsuccessful, and many families and communities were able to maintain ties to culture, language, and land. However, as a result of the intergenerational effects of trauma, many communities experienced lasting psychological and spiritual wounds. Also, the graduates of the residential school system often found themselves on the periphery of two distinct worlds, ill-equipped to navigate either completely. Survivors noted an inability to thrive in mainstream culture thanks to a fractured educational experience and ongoing racism in the dominant culture. Those who lost their language struggled to return home to build a life in their community. The effects of these colonial efforts have had long-lasting impacts on individuals, families, and communities as a whole. Indeed, the deleterious effects of European settlement in Indigenous lands across the continent are well documented in the psychological literature (see, for instance, [9–11]) and across health disciplines. As Canada moves toward reconciliation, turning our gaze toward healing is paramount.

Healing Perspectives

Indigenous Medicine

While Indigenous approaches to healing were driven underground by Canadian legislative acts that banned cultural ceremonies in the twentieth century, Indigenous knowledges and practices continued to be passed down through the generations. Indigenous Elders, often viewed as the bearers of cultural knowledge and tradition, have played a pivotal role in the transmission of Indigenous cultures, and in the practice of Indigenous healing. The revitalization of Indigenous healing practices and community-based approaches to healing over the past 50 years speaks to the undeniable strengths of Indigenous communities in Canada in surviving assimilationist policies aimed at cultural genocide.

As we have noted, significant diversity exists among First Nations, Inuit, and Métis peoples, and the hundreds of communities that exist across Indigenous Nations. While recognizing this diversity in worldviews and practices, scholars and

Healers have also highlighted several important over-arching similarities. Central values that comprise Indigenous worldviews include the importance of relationship and the role of family and community; an emphasis on holism and balance between the sacred aspects of the self (physical, emotional, mental, and spiritual); and a recognition and respect for the interconnectedness of all things in the natural world, including plant and animal worlds, ancestral and spiritual worlds, and the cosmos [6, 12, 13, 37].

One of the most commonly identified defining features within Indigenous conceptions of healing values and health is the notion of holism and balance. An individual is viewed as consisting of four sacred parts of self, including the physical, emotional, mental, and spiritual, and it is the balancing of these aspects of the self that constitutes well-being [3, 37]. If one of these dimensions is out of balance, the remaining three aspects of the person will be impacted, and the person may become unwell. For instance, if an individual is not eating healthy foods or is not eating routinely, her mental and emotional health may become compromised by malnourishment and life stress. In this view of the self, these dimensions of health are not viewed as independent entities, but as interconnected elements that together comprise an individual's health. It is for this reason that some Indigenous Healers struggle to define mental health concretely because mind-body dualism is not a concept that is readily found within many Indigenous cultures historically [14].

Another important healing value is the centrality of spirituality and spiritual health in Indigenous conceptions of wellness. As noted, spiritual health is one of the dimensions of well-being and it represents a central tenet in Indigenous healing. All things in creation evolved through spirit and heal through spirit; the human condition is interpreted through spiritual understandings of existence, and Healers use spiritual relationships in their helping work and in order to make meaning of illness [9, 15]. In some cultures, illness is thought to originate in spirit and is indicative of spiritual disconnection. In these cases, healing therefore takes place through spiritual reconnection [9]. These are but a few examples of the critically important nature of spirit as an aspect of overall health and wellness. However, a focus on spirituality is often absent in Western mental health practices [13, 14], suggesting that Western mental health interventions lack balance in caring for the sacred aspects of self. While healing through the spiritual dimension is unique for each individual, generally individuals derive healing from relationships to Creator or Gitchi Manitou (the "Great Spirit" in Anishnawbe cultures), to ancestral spirits and spirit guides, and to one's own spirit.

Indigenous medicine also includes a diverse system of practices for healing [1], including the use of plant medicines and hands-on medicines for curing illness and treating physical wounds and injuries. As in all Indigenous cultures around the globe, plant medicines have been used in healing for generations; in fact, as much as 80% of the world's population relies on herbs for their primary health needs [16]. Other practices to heal the sick body include curing ceremonies, bone-setting, massage, and the removal of disease objects [1]. Spiritual ceremonies are facilitated by Healers and or Elders in the community; the type of ceremony performed depends on the nature of the problem presented by the individual who is in need. There are numerous Indigenous ceremonies that Indigenous practitioners may prescribe to address the healing needs of an individual. Ceremony is often embedded within other medicinal practices, such as talk therapy with Elders, counselors, and Healers, and hands-on medicine. These are only a few examples of the vast array of healing modalities used across Indigenous cultures. As Garrett and Wilbur [17] note, "Medicine is everywhere. It is the very essence of our inner being; it is that which gives us inner power. Medicine is in every tree, plant, rock, animal, and person. It is in the light, the soil, the water, and the wind... There is medicine in every event, memory, place, person, and movement. There is even Medicine in 'empty space' if you know how to use it" (p. 197–8).

We have offered a brief overview of Indigenous models of healing and practices. Next, we consider Western approaches to mental health service provision.

Western Mental Health Services

Many Indigenous individuals and communities possess strengths and community-based healing approaches that prevent or remedy mental health problems. However, the vast majority of available mental health services in Canada are rooted in a Western paradigm and approach to health. The majority of Indigenous Peoples who seek help for mental health problems are therefore sent to Western mental health service providers. Western counseling services vary considerably in theoretical orientation, framework, and technique; for instance, therapies may include a focus on cognitive restructuring, unearthing social oppressions, improving communication, solving problems, building self-esteem, managing trauma and grief, and gaining self-awareness of thoughts, feelings, and the body. In the following section, we consider the fundamental assumptions behind the models of health that have dominated the field of Western psychology and psychotherapy throughout the twentieth century.

The notion of mental health and mental illness in a Western context tends to be defined in relation to disorder; that is, the absence of disorder is often an indicator of good mental health. The field of psychotherapy and psychology have been largely informed by psychiatry's dominant text on disorders, the *Diagnostic and Statistical Manual of Mental Disorders* (DSM), currently in its fifth edition. This text is so central to the profession of mental health in North America that many insurance providers in the United States, and some in Canada, will not offer financial coverage for mental health services if clients are not first diagnosed with a DSM disorder. Within this diagnostic text, each mental disorder is conceptualized as a clinically significant behavioral or psychological syndrome or pattern that occurs in an individual and that is associated with present distress or disability [18]. A variety of concepts are used in the assessment and diagnosis of mental health issues, including distress, dysfunction, disadvantage, disability, inflexibility, irrationality, etiology, and statistical deviation. In this regard, mental health challenges are assessed through a pathological lens where the location of the disorder lies within the individual, often has a biologically based etiology, and represents a deviation from a population "norm."

Within Western mental health practice, a practitioner may spend time evaluating and assessing the client's cognitive and personality features through the use of psychodiagnostic tools and using interventions that are designed to facilitate individual change. As in the practice of physical medicine, where the disease is confirmed through lab tests, psychodiagnostic tools are used to determine the presence of psychological "disease." Treatments focus on finding cures rather than on helping individuals find meaning in their suffering, or on seeking to understand the underlying imbalance, unlike some Indigenous approaches that prioritize wider contexts of understanding and healing of the "whole" person and community [19]. In Western practice, the goals for change focus on the individual client, as opposed to other units (for example, family) or systems (for example, the Canadian child welfare system) the client may be influenced by, and which may be contributing to mental health distress [20].

Western psychology and psychotherapy also values and prioritizes evidence-based practice. Evidence-based practices are forms of treatment that use an empirical base of evidence to document their efficacy. These practices tend to be seen as most "valid" in terms of therapeutic approaches and are often employed on this basis in managed care settings. There are some challenges in determining the evidence base of Indigenous medicine, including the often inappropriate use of a Western research paradigm and the potential clash with Indigenous community ethics in terms of, to give but one example, documenting sacred practices.

A related concern is the bureaucratization of Indigenous healing methods. As Waldram [21] and Gone [22] note, the institutionalization of Indigenous health practices and services of Healers has the potential to result in the formalized surveillance of Healers and Indigenous health practices, which leads to concerns related to contracting the services of Healers and Elders, remuneration of Healers and Elders, and documentation of Indigenous health practices. In sum, the growing emphasis on empirical validation of therapeutic interventions and practices affects how Indigenous healing practices are perceived by Western health-care systems, practitioners, and government funding agencies, and the formalization of Indigenous medicine will impact its practice.

Lewis-Fernandez and Kleinman [23] note several dominant culture views in North America that influence mental health. These include "mind-body dualism" (the mind and body are separate, with little influence on one another), the "egocentricity of the self" (people are individuals and are not affected by the web of relationships around us), and the view that culture does not influence our biology, among others. Western mental health systems look to scientifically informed approaches that strive for an "objective" and "value-free" encounter between practitioner and client, and which tend to result in the client being seen through a pathological lens. Despite technologically sophisticated medical practices and forward movements in health care, many patients have reported feeling alienated from their health-care professionals, who now seem more technicians than Healers [24]. This contrasts starkly with the holistic, socioculturally informed, and wellness-based conceptions and approaches to health and healing that are integral to many Indigenous cultures [13].

In order to assist in the healing work, any counseling endeavor with those who have experienced mental health issues must consider the specific value systems and unique culture(s) of the client; the most appropriate ways of dealing with various mental health challenges in a dominant culture context, for instance, might not be entirely appropriate or ideal for members of other cultures [25]. Accordingly, Stewart [11] noted that most mental health services in urban areas have not been adapted to meet the needs of Indigenous clients. This lack of cultural appropriateness of services has resulted in lower rates of mental health service use as well as higher dropout rates from counseling among Indigenous Peoples [26–28]. The use of Western approaches to healing with Indigenous clients has indeed often proved ineffective, as indicated by an under-usage of services, high dropout rates, and Indigenous Peoples' reports of low quality of care and services received [26–28]. Numerous scholars have offered potential explanations for why Western approaches to healing have proven ineffective, including the absence of an Indigenous worldview and conception of health [11], culturally insensitive practitioners [9], and difficulties in establishing trust between the client and practitioner [10]. To tailor and enhance counseling services for Indigenous Peoples, researchers, administrators, and practitioners alike have begun to call for an integration, or harmonization, of Indigenous and Western approaches to healing (see, for example, [1, 9, 29]).

The Integrated Healing Movement

In the following section, we review the movement toward integrating Indigenous and Western paradigms and practices of healing. We outline the rationale for integration and its merits. We also consider the various pathways through which integration may occur, including training epistemologically hybrid practitioners, integrating mental health programs, and the harmonization of healing paradigms and services.

Rationale for Integration

For many decades, Western mental health systems have failed to adequately serve Indigenous Peoples' needs [11, 26, 36]. Studies that consider attitudes of Indigenous clients toward Western mental health services have noted that participants lack confidence in Western mental health services and that some use these services only as a last resort [14, 28]. Also, fostering or strengthening spiritual identity and spiritual relations with other beings (for instance, Creator and ancestral spirits) has been identified as a core component of healing for many Indigenous peoples [12, 13, 22]. This understanding has been absent from Western treatment models, which tend to fragment medical, psychological, and spiritual healing approaches. Integrating Indigenous medicine and healing with Western mental health services would provide a more holistically oriented approach to health and wellness that would better serve Indigenous Peoples. It is likely that if Indigenous approaches to healing were made available in Western mental health or counseling settings, Indigenous clients interested in pursuing Indigenous medicine may be more likely to access these services. If Indigenous clients see Western practitioners working collaboratively with Indigenous Healers and Elders in these settings, obstacles related to developing trusting relationships between client and counselor may be assuaged.

While Indigenous healing systems, including the services of Healers and Elders, continue to be accessed and identified as a successful option for healing [12, 29, 30], relying solely on Indigenous Healers and Elders for treatment is no longer a viable option. Among the primary obstacles to accessing the services of Indigenous helpers are the cost and accessibility of Indigenous medicine [30]. Additionally, given the complexity of health challenges among many Indigenous communities today, and mental health challenges in particular, the singular use of Indigenous medicine may not be adequate to address contemporary health needs.

Interestingly, many Indigenous clients who use both Indigenous and Western services simultaneously often fail to inform their helpers of their multiple service use [3]. Multiple service use potentially poses a risk when one considers the possible negative interactional effects between Western and Indigenous medicines, including opposing treatment approaches and differing care instructions. Developing systems in which both Western and Indigenous practitioners work collaboratively could provide the client with clearer treatment guidelines and a greater range of treatment options, presumably increasing the retention rate of Indigenous clients. Centralized systems would also allow for communication, case consultation, and treatment planning between helping professionals, which would decrease the chance of a client receiving contradictory treatment.

Finally, an inspiring motivation for the integration of Indigenous and Western healing paradigms is that these approaches have the potential to complement one another and to enhance the healing process. A study by McCabe [13] identified 12 therapeutic conditions that facilitate the successful implementation of Indigenous Healing methods. Several of these conditions, such as empathy, genuineness, acceptance of the client, readiness to heal, and trust and safety, also represent the core conditions of many Western psychotherapies. Given the congruence between these models of healing, some of the foundational elements for an integrated approach are already in place. Psychologists working in Indigenous community contexts have noted that all healing approaches (including Western approaches) offer value to clients, and that Indigenous clients, who often present with complex challenges related to a history of oppression, can benefit from complex solutions [1, 9, 10]. If Western mental health services and Indigenous medicine can work together in a hybrid model, this harmonized healing approach for clients, families, and communities may be more effective than any one approach alone.

Levels and Forms of Integration

Epistemological Hybridism

In Eduardo Duran's groundbreaking text *Healing the Soul Wound* [9], Duran outlined the philosophical tenets of what he refers to as "hybrid psychotherapy." He stated that the term "hybrid" emerged from postmodern thinking, and referred to the idea that there can be two or more ways of knowing, and that these different views can exist harmoniously with one another. He noted his belief that the mental health profession must transcend the practice of culturally sensitive psychotherapy and engage in what he calls "epistemological hybridism," which is the ability to think or see the truth in more than one way ([9], p. 14). Duran notes that practitioners adopting an epistemologically hybrid stance take "the actual life-world of the person or group as the core truth that needs to be seen as valid just because it is. There should never be a need to validate this core epistemology or way of knowing by Western empiricism or any other validating tool" (2006, p. 14).

Embracing and practicing hybrid psychotherapy means that a mental health practitioner commits to creating space for the expression of diverse forms of knowing and healing while being able to accept the client's beliefs, perspectives, and experiences as legitimate, valid, and authoritative sources of truth and knowledge. This approach to integration allows both the practitioner and client to explore the client's worldview and to identify the healing needs and preferred methods or strategies for healing work. It is this collaborative and conceptually flexible space which allows for the co-occurrence, integration, and acceptance of both Western and Indigenous healing knowledges and practices.

Importantly, Duran [9] wrote that objectives and definitions of healing in Western and Indigenous paradigms are related: the meaning of the term psychotherapist is "soul healer," and the task of the soul healer is to help individuals overcome psychopathology, or "soul suffering." Duran noted that the primary objective for all helpers is to recognize and "engage in the healing tradition that is part of our genetic memory and be true to that tradition" ([9], p. 44). Although this notion of a genuine alignment between Indigenous and Western paradigms of healing may be ideal, it is unlikely that the Eurocentric model of healing will be abandoned by the disciplines of Western psychology and psychiatry. While training programs may work to ensure that practitioners develop the appropriate skills to be culturally sensitive or competent, this is still fundamentally different than a practitioner who is epistemologically hybrid and is able to accept multiple forms of knowing and healing as valid and legitimate.

One challenge within the integration discourse is whether mental health interventions (such as cognitive therapies and Indigenous ceremony) can be used conjointly if integration at a paradigmatic level has not occurred. For instance, Western practitioners, as part of culturally sensitive training procedures, are instructed to be open to client worldviews and values related to healing, and the possibility of working or consulting with Healers and Elders [20, 29]. However, simply because a practitioner refers a client to the services of an Indigenous Healer, or communicates with a Healer from time to time, does not necessarily mean that the clinician is practicing as an epistemologically hybrid practitioner, where Indigenous medicine is viewed as equally legitimate as Western medicine. Even Western practitioners who refer Indigenous clients to Indigenous Elders, Healers, and counselors may continue to take a stance of Western elitism [31].

This type of criticism and skepticism of Indigenous healing methods has, of course, been present throughout history. The maltreatment of Indigenous Healers and Elders began with European contact in the late fifteenth century [3] and has continued to date with ongoing Eurocentric epistemological racism. Although the Western mental health system and its practitioners have made strides in terms of acknowledging and validating diverse systems of knowledge and healing, some authors have commented that Indigenous health practices continue to be stigmatized and viewed as "magical," irrational, and illegitimate forms of healing [3, 32]. Given the relative newness of the integrative healing movement, questions about how paradigms of healing may be integrated in practice remain, and combined interventions continue to be experimented with.

Program-Level Integration

It has become a commonplace recommendation that Western practitioners remain open to the possibility of referring, consulting, or collaborating with Indigenous Healers and Elders (for example, [20, 29, 33, 34]). Referring a client to an Indigenous Healer without the establishment of a formal relationship between the Healer and clinician however likely does not capture the true spirit of integrative helping. Consulting with Indigenous Healers and Elders to learn of a client's cultural background, developing a culturally informed understanding of the presenting psychological issue, and collaborating with Healers in the design of a treatment plan (such as incorporating the use of ceremony as part of a client's healing work), better represent an integrated approach to treatment and healing.

A study by Shore, Shore and Manson [29] identified how Western mental health practitioners and Indigenous Healers can establish collaborative working relationships. The study outlined how Western and Indigenous helpers work together to serve Native American war veterans in a culturally competent care model. In order to begin working relationships, psychiatrists made multiple trips to the community to meet with community figures, members, and Healers. The psychiatrists, with the aid of a cultural informant who was part of the clinical team, attended community events such as powwows and Indigenous ceremonies. Participating in such events allowed the psychiatrists to come into contact with Healers and demonstrate an interest in Indigenous activities and culture. Thereafter, the psychiatrists continued to have ongoing meetings with Healers and collaborated on models of healing, perspectives on symptoms, the development of treatment plans, case consultation, and mutual referral. This form of integrated care proved effective for client retention and in the reduction of symptoms.

Another example of integrated mental health services relates to the Knaw-chi-ge-win mental health program on Manitoulin Island in Ontario [30]. Knaw-chi-ge-win services are coordinated by two regional Indigenous health organizations, which place an emphasis on community-based Indigenous approaches to care. The Knaw-chi-ge-win core team is made up of professionals working in the areas of psychology, nursing, and social work, as well as a coordinator of Indigenous Healing services who has expertise in the area of Indigenous medicine and healing. The core team is also complemented by consultants who possess expertise in the areas of psychiatry and Indigenous healing, and who visit monthly. The core team's home office is centrally located within the region, and satellite clinics are located throughout the seven First Nations on the island; clients can access services either through the home office or the various clinics. Services are provided within a holistic Indigenous framework that recognizes the sacred aspects of the self (physical, emotional, mental, spiritual) and considers client context (cultural, historical, and socio-economic factors). At intake, the client is assigned to the most suitable health-care provider(s) (for example, nurse, psychologist, Healer). The healing team coordinates specialized care for the individual and team members attend psychiatric consultations and Indigenous Healing services with their clients to ensure continuity of care and a collaborative approach to healing.

To evaluate the Knaw-chi-ge-win program, Maar and the research team (2009) conducted focus groups with community service providers and interviewed clients. Their study found that in order to effectively integrate Indigenous and Western healing services, the health-care professionals needed to accept and have an in-depth understanding of both paradigms of healing. One clinician noted that it can indeed be challenging to fit the paradigms together when one of them is poorly understood ([30], p. 7). The inclusion of Indigenous medicine in the program and the training given to staff in this approach removed the "mystique" of Indigenous medicine and eased integrated practice (p. 7). Clinicians reported that they were more comfortable referring clients to Indigenous services once training in this healing approach was given and protocols for Indigenous Healing practices had been established. Other evaluation results indicated that the Knaw-chi-ge-win program improved the cultural safety of services, increased access for clients to receive care in an Indigenous language, decreased stigmatization in using Indigenous medicine, improved quality of illness management, reduced wait time, and reduced number of patient admissions to acute care psychiatric hospitals, among other benefits. Challenges included a lack of stable funding for Indigenous health services and a lack of qualified mental health professionals in the area.

In this section, we have reviewed epistemological hybridism and integration in services and programs as distinct aspects of integration. In the following case studies, we describe examples of integration on the paradigmatic level, the clinic level, the program level, and the individual practitioner level.

Clinical Cases in Integration and Harmonization

In addition to collaborations at the program level similar to those described in the case examples of the Knaw-chi-ge-win program and the promotion of mental health among war veterans, we (Beaulieu and Reeves) have also worked in psychological roles within health programs in the Toronto area that integrate at the paradigmatic, program, and practitioner levels. Integrated health programs have begun to emerge over the past 20 years, and Toronto has seen the rise of several community-based health and resource centers designed by, and for, Indigenous clients from the "roots up." Aboriginal Services at the Centre for Addiction and Mental Health (CAMH) and Anishnawbe Health Toronto (AHT) represent two community health centers that offer access to a diverse range of health-care practitioners, including psychiatrists, psychologists, nurses, Healers, Elders, and medicine people. In this section, we describe harmonized mental health care for clients at these agencies.

Aboriginal Services, Center for Addiction and Mental Health

Chapter coauthor Tera Beaulieu is of Métis, Hungarian, and Ukrainian ancestry and is currently completing her PhD in clinical and counseling psychology at the Ontario Institute for Studies in Education (OISE) at the University of Toronto. Beaulieu learned of her Indigenous ancestry as a young adult and spent the better portion of 10 years on a learning and healing journey to reconnect with her Indigenous lineage, culture, and community. Parallel to this personal journey was Beaulieu's academic and clinical training journey. Over the past 10 years, Beaulieu has held administrative and clinical roles in several of the programs at CAMH, including the Youth Addiction and Concurrent Disorder Service, the Aboriginal Engagement and Outreach Program, the Women's Program, the Psychological Trauma Program, and, most recently, Aboriginal Services.

CAMH is located in Toronto, Ontario, Canada, and is the largest mental health teaching hospital in Canada. CAMH is a leader in research innovation and is fully affiliated with the University of Toronto; it is also a Pan American Health Organization/World Health Organization Collaborating Centre. CAMH provides a full range of hospital and community-based services, including inpatient and outpatient care and services for children, youth, families, and adults. Speciality clinics serve individuals with diverse mental health and addiction issues, including anxiety and depression, substance use, psychosis, and concurrent disorders, among others.

Established in 2000, Aboriginal Services (ABS) at CAMH provides culturally safe clinical and Indigenous health care using a holistic approach that is based on Indigenous values, beliefs, and traditions. Serving individuals who self-identify as First Nations, Inuit, or Métis, the program focuses on taking care of the spiritual, emotional, physical, and mental health needs of its clients. ABS's client population comprises individuals from the urban Indigenous community of Toronto as well as communities throughout Ontario and abroad. Clinical offerings include outpatient groups, individual therapy, and Indigenous Healing services, with support being offered to Indigenous inpatient clients throughout the hospital. The team is comprised of Indigenous social workers, an occupational therapist, and a Healer, with allied health support from various other disciplines, such as psychiatry. Clients who access the service may present with a range of concurrent mental health and substance use issues, including complex intergenerational trauma.

ABS clinicians collaborate to identify holistic healing and treatment plans that focus on spiritual, emotional, physical, and mental wellness. Clinical interventions offered are founded on Indigenous worldviews and values, including Indigenous Knowledge systems and healing practices, and are culturally integrated alongside mainstream interventions. In 2016, ABS at CAMH established an on-site Sweat Lodge for Indigenous clients to access as part of their healing and treatment journey; it was the first hospital in Ontario to do so. Also on site are an Indigenous medicine garden and sacred fire pit where ceremonies may be held throughout the year. ABS practices self-determination in service design and delivery, and aims to use promising and wise practices in its clinical programming to address the diversity of issues that have affected Indigenous people's health and well-being. In the following vignette, coauthor Tera Beaulieu describes her personal experiences working as a clinician and administrator in various CAMH programs to design and deliver clinical services for First Nations, Inuit, and Métis peoples.

Vignette 1 *My learning journey and immersion into Métis culture, community, and Indigenous Knowledge systems paralleled the beginning of my master's program in clinical and counseling psychology at OISE-University of Toronto. At the time, I had learned of my Indigenous ancestry but did not have a thorough understanding of my ancestral community or culture. I set out on a healing journey in which I researched my ancestral lineage and the historic Métis communities that my family originated from (Qu'Appelle, Saskatchewan, and St. Laurent, Manitoba). I also contacted the Métis Nation of Ontario and the Toronto and York Region Métis Community Council to establish connections and begin to develop a sense of community within urban Toronto. Part of this process entailed developing relationships with Indigenous Knowledge Keepers, both First Nations and Métis Elders and Senators, who supported and nurtured me along my pathway of healing.*

As I began to learn about Métis culture, spirituality, and healing, I was simultaneously learning about Western approaches to mental health and healing through my academic program. I spent as much time as possible with Indigenous Knowledge Keepers as I could, attending teaching circles, ceremony, and engaging in my own ceremonial and healing work, while also engaging in psychotherapy with Western trained health-care professionals. As I learned and experienced diverse approaches to health and healing, my worldview and framework for understanding knowledge systems and healing processes took shape synergistically: my lived experience as a Métis woman, alongside participating in Indigenous healing and Western health care, informed the development of my epistemologically hybrid approach to health, well-being, and healing. For instance, as I began to work with clients of various ethnic and racial backgrounds, I would often conceptualize their health and healing needs from a holistic lens that accounted for their mental, emotional, physical, and spiritual well-being. As I began my PhD in counseling and clinical psychology, I continued to meet with Indigenous Knowledge Keepers, both to learn about Indigenous approaches to healing and well-being, such as the use of sacred medicines and the transformative properties of Indigenous ceremony, and to deepen my understanding of spirituality and how it relates to mental health.

A great deal of my clinical work during my early training was with non-Indigenous individuals. Despite this, I would often share with them my approach and understanding of health and well-being, including my assumptions and biases regarding spirituality. I would frequently introduce the concept of a Medicine Wheel to discuss the different aspects of the self (mental, emotional, physical, and spiritual) and how imbalance in different areas of one's life can impact overall health. I kept Indigenous medicines and ceremonial items in my offices at all times (next to the "coping tools box" on my desk), both for my own spiritual health and well-being and for my clients'. I also maintained a strong focus on self-care practices and regularly engaged in my own healing and ceremonial work. As I progressed in my practice through my PhD training and began to conduct psychological assessments that surveyed symptomatology and psychological functioning, I also attempted to assess and conceptualize psychological presentations from a spiritual lens. This meant attempting to understand specific symptoms from a spiritual/cultural perspective, and also coming to understand mental health distress and unwellness as a spiritual imbalance and or wound. I regularly consulted Indigenous Knowledge Keepers to discuss clients' psychological presentations and to conceptualize treatment and healing plans. This activity, on occasion, included attending ceremonies with Indigenous clients to complete a spiritual consultation whereby the respective Indigenous Knowledge Keeper would provide a spiritual explanation (or diagnosis) with spiritual and ceremonial prescriptions being given as part of the client's treatment and healing plan. In the beginning, it often took great effort and time to consolidate the different perspectives and approaches that I was practicing (that is, Western and Indigenous frameworks) as part of an epistemologically hybrid practice. However, I learned early in training and clinical work that I could not divorce myself from, or "turn off," my Indigenous worldview and lens regarding psychological health. Instead, I chose to share this with both my non-Indigenous and Indigenous clients and invite them into a process of co-constructing and understanding their mental health functioning and well-being.

In my position with Aboriginal Services (ABS) at CAMH, I supported the program and staff with a review of its clinical programming. As noted above, clinical offerings included outpatient therapy groups, individual therapy, and Indigenous Healing services, with support offered to Indigenous inpatient clients throughout the hospital. The team was comprised of Indigenous social workers, an occupational therapist, and a Healer, with support from allied health professionals in areas such as psychiatry. At the time I was engaged with the program, the clinical team had expressed interest in further defining the therapeutic goals and milestones of their therapy groups, and was looking for a clearer articulation of how Indigenous healing and knowledges intersect with the Western clinical elements of their programming (for example, with the cognitive-behavioral interventions that are used in Western groups). The discussions that ensued included the importance of ensuring that Indigenous Knowledges and healing practices are valued equally, are as readily accessible, and comprise a proportionate share of the programming in comparison to Western interventions. For instance, all ABS clients would be offered, in addition to standard group therapy offerings, Indigenous healing services if the clients were interested and the services were appropriate (for example, unless medical complications prevented them). Indigenous ceremonies, such as sweats and full moon ceremonies, would be offered on a monthly basis for Indigenous clients at CAMH to access, with additional culture-based groups being developed and offered as part of the program (for example, teachings and drumming circles).

Also, the epistemological foundation of each of the standard group offerings in the service was altered to be rooted in Indigenous worldviews and Indigenous Knowledge systems. For instance, all "groups" were run as "circles," with Indigenous teachings guiding the formation and operation of the circle. Each circle included an opening and closing prayer, drum song, and purification ceremony. The content for most circles would include a cultural integration of both Indigenous and Western knowledges and practices. For example, clinicians might introduce the concept of a substance use continuum to discuss various degrees of substance use but would contextualize the discussion of why Indigenous Peoples have used substances within the historical narrative of colonization. Another example would be a circle focused on coping tools that included a discussion of holistic coping strategies and detailed examples of spiritual and/or cultural coping tools for clients to use. Additionally, certain circles might be strictly dedicated to ceremonies or Indigenous teachings by the Healer, or other Knowledge Keeper working with the service, to support clients in achieving therapeutic and developmental milestones in their healing. It was obvious that the ABS clinicians had embraced an epistemologically hybrid praxis in their clinical work, which significantly influenced program-level integration.

In my work with ABS, I was also asked to lead the cultural adaptation of a mainstream trauma and substance use treatment. In its clinical program review, ABS staff had identified as a priority the addition of a trauma treatment to its clinical offerings. The ABS clinical team participated in a training session of the mainstream cognitive-behavioral treatment and piloted a cycle of the treatment with ABS clients with minor cultural adaptations made, such as including an opening and closing prayer, drum song, and purification ceremony. Following the completion of the pilot cycle, I met with the ABS team to debrief their experiences facilitating the group and ask for their perceptions of the challenges and strengths of the treatment. ABS team members reported that, overall, clients benefited from the treatment; however, they felt that significant adaptation work was required to ensure that the materials were culturally relevant and safe for First Nations, Inuit, and Métis people. For instance, team members noted challenges with the literacy level required for handouts, the abstinence-oriented approach of the treatment, and the overall tone of treatment (for example, deficits-based, focusing on pathology and problems). The cultural adaptation process consisted of ABS team members, including the Healer, participating in weekly meetings in which the Western treatment materials were reviewed in detail. The cognitive-behavioral interventions and treatment materials that the team felt were most appropriate and relevant for Indigenous Peoples were retained, with additional suggested edits put forward by team members. Treatment materials were then recreated, with the new culturally adapted content integrated into preexisting materials, such that the adapted content became more culturally relevant for First Nations, Inuit, and Métis people, and increasing the level of cultural safety for clients. Additionally, new materials, including exercises and handouts, were created by the ABS team, and new culturally specific examples, skills, and strategies were identified. Circles dedicated to Indigenous teachings and ceremony were also built into the program to address certain healing needs, such as a doctoring ceremony to heal trauma wounds.

At the end of the cultural adaptation process, it became apparent that the ABS team had created substantially new content, so much so that the groundwork for a new trauma and substance use treatment had been completed. As a result, I turned my attention to focusing on developing additional materials to bolster the new clinical treatments. Although the cultural adaptation process was challenging, the journey of examining a mainstream treatment, and attempting to integrate Indigenous Knowledge and Healing practices into it, was enlightening. The challenges that emerged related to the cultural adaptation of treatment materials, including issues related to the cultural appropriateness, relevance, and safety of materials for Indigenous peoples, highlighted the need, and resulted in, the development of a new clinical intervention that is grounded within Indigenous knowledge systems. The development of innovative and culturally founded treatments, led by Indigenous Knowledge Keepers and health professionals, is a promising practice for addressing the mental health and healing needs of First Nations, Métis, and Inuit people.

Anishnawbe Health Toronto

Chapter coauthor Dr. Allison Reeves is a registered clinical and forensic psychologist in Ontario. She joined Anishnawbe Health Toronto (AHT) in 2011 as the program coordinator for a province-wide cultural safety training program developed by AHT. This program trained health professionals and post-secondary students in the health professions in culturally competent health service delivery for Indigenous clients. Dr. Reeves then transitioned into the role of psychologist on staff at AHT after completing her licensing exams. She continued in this role for the following 4 years.

AHT is a culture-based multidisciplinary health center that has been servicing the Indigenous community in Toronto since 1989. In the urban city of Toronto, there exist numerous Indigenous individuals representing various Nations and Indigenous affiliations, varying in socioeconomic, linguistic, and cultural backgrounds. AHT offers health and well-being services in various Indigenous languages and offers clients a sense of Indigenous identity as well as a place to engage in physical, emotional, spiritual, mental, and social healing. This facility offers Indigenous cultural teachings, ceremonies, access to Elders and Healers as well as mainstream Western health-care services. The facility also exposes clients to social justice issues facing Indigenous peoples through Anishnawbe teachings on the political, social, and economic histories of Indigenous peoples in Canada, and therefore serves an additional role in community empowerment [38]. The mental health services offered at AHT place Indigenous culture and traditions centrally by using a client-centered, strength-based approach to assist in healing [35].

AHT offers primary care services (general practitioners, physiotherapy, chiropractic, nursing, and others) at the Waash-Keshuu-Yaan[1] unit. AHT also has social workers who offer housing supports for clients in search of stable housing and who help connect clients to outside health services. AHT houses a learning center where young adults who have not yet obtained their high school diploma can work toward this. For individuals struggling with addiction issues, AHT offers a day treatment program at the Chayuuwaytim unit that involves both Indigenous medicine and Western addiction mental health services.

AHT's mental health services at the Babishkahn unit are built around Indigenous cultural practices. The Indigenous practitioners, including Healers, counselors, and Elders, are employed through stable government funding and stand at the core of the programs. The medicine storage area is plentiful and includes tens of plant medicines used by Healers, much of which is picked by the Healing team in the summertime. Clients can obtain counseling services from Healers and Elders, can be given healing services or medicines from Healers, and can participate in various cultural practices and ceremonies, including community circles, a Sweat Lodge (on-site), a Shake Tent (on-site), and fasting (off-site). Clients can access Western mental health services in addition to Indigenous Healers and counselors at the Babishkhan unit, including counseling, psychology, and psychiatry services.

All staff, Indigenous and non-Indigenous, must complete a cultural competency training module upon joining the organization, and all staff have access to participation in healing activities through the Sweat Lodge ceremony, as well as other ceremonies such as the Shake Tent, fasting in the bush, naming ceremonies, and so on. All staff can also book themselves in to see Healers and Elders at the center for personal support and healing. In this sense, staff are encouraged to take on the challenge of being epistemologically hybrid themselves. The following vignette shares the personal experiences of coauthor Allison Reeves in her experience of working in a harmonized psychology model.

Vignette 2 *As a psychologist who is deeply involved in cultural psychology, I am also personally involved in a continuous process of discovering my own culture and identity. Born in the Toronto area, I was encouraged by my Indigenous Elders*

[1] *Waash-Keshuu-Yaan* is an Anishnawbe term that refers to the deer hide that covers a traditional hand drum. *Babishkahn* refers to the lacing, also made of hide, that holds the hide in place on the drum. The hand drum is sacred in the culture and is seen as having its own spirit. *Chayuuwaytim* translates to "the shadow that speaks wisely" and is the name gifted to the mental health and addiction workers by an Elder.

(Anishnawbe, Haudenosaunee, and Cree) to engage in a lifelong process of self-discovery into my own ancestry and my spiritual path. Under their guidance, I have learned more about my diverse European ancestry, as well as my mother's Afro- and Indigenous-Caribbean ancestry. In sharing my spiritual engagement with my ancestry with my Elders, they interpreted that my blood memory guided me into my psychology work with Indigenous Healers and community members.

My lived experience in Indigenous communities on Turtle Island is varied and includes time in Mi'kmaq communities through my work at Healing Our Nations and my years of working and having close friendships in the Anishnawbe community in Toronto. I attended Anishnawbe language classes, participated in Sweat Lodge and Shake Tent ceremonies, received my spirit name, received cultural gifts and teachings to mark rites of passage in my life (for example, I passed my hand drum along when instructed by my Elder when I became married, and later made a new drum with materials gifted to me by community members), met with Elders regularly for guidance in my life, and sought help from Healers when I was mentally and physically unwell. All of this occurred while I was completing a PhD and post-doctoral fellowship in psychology at the University of Toronto, and carried over into my time working as the psychologist at AHT. In this sense, I learned the practice of Western psychology while experiencing first-hand the emotional, spiritual, and mental health benefits of engaging with Indigenous medicine and culture-based healing.

As the psychologist at AHT, I had the great fortune of working down the hall from four Indigenous Healers who rotated through the program, Elders at the three sites in Toronto, and the eight Indigenous counselors who used Indigenous teachings and approaches in their therapy work. I also had the support of three culturally safe psychiatrists (one of whom was Indigenous) who took historical trauma and family context into account in their work, and a team of social workers who operated from a social justice lens. Our case consultations involved a diverse team of practitioners, and we met regularly, formally and informally, to support one another in client care. These staff interactions were facilitated by the close quarters we shared at the community health center, the natural and friendly collegial relationships among staff, the egalitarian tone among staff (from the Healers to the psychiatrists to the receptionists), the mutual respect shown between practitioners of different schools of medicine, the genuine curiosity among staff about different ways of helping, the commitment to client healing, and, of course, humor. That being said, no workplace is idyllic, and we did have our interpersonal challenges from time to time. But overall, the through-line of commitment to community wellness and prizing Indigenous ways of knowing and healing kept our ship on course.

As a clinical psychologist, my duties included psychological assessment, diagnosis, psychotherapy, research, case consultation, and clinical supervision. Psychological assessment referrals came from external agencies and from other practitioners within AHT. Also, if a practitioner and client felt stuck, they could request diagnostic clarification from me to offer perspective on case conceptualization and some insight into the therapy work. Educational assessments helped clients understand their areas of strength for returning to school or potential cognitive or learning challenges that might require accommodation in post-secondary studies. Disability assessments could provide insight into psychiatric challenges or cognitive issues (for example, posttraumatic stress disorder, fetal alcohol effects, attention deficit hyperactivity disorder, learning or memory challenges) and could help to secure resources such as housing and government support payments for clients in need.

Some clients found these psychological assessment services useful for helping to clarify challenges they had long since struggled with, or for determining next steps in their lives. Some clients were uninterested in Western diagnostics and preferred to opt out of these services, which was their prerogative. When discussing assessment and diagnosis in a culturally safe way, I felt it important to have a lengthy discussion with clients about the benefits of these Western psychological services (for example, in providing access to further helping resources), but also warned about the culture-bound nature of the Western psychological approach. In much of my work with clients, whether through assessment or psychotherapy, we discussed the history of colonization and how it affected their families and communities, the nature of Eurocentric medicine, the veracity of Indigenous Ways of Knowing, and the usefulness of seeing and understanding through multiple frameworks. These discussions would occur over many weeks and clients would oftentimes impress me with their insight into these topics. Others would be less interested in these sometimes philosophical discussions. As one of my colleagues noted, when given the choice between Western and Indigenous services, many of our community members simply say, "Just help me."

As a psychologist, I also met with clients for psychotherapy. I am trained primarily in emotion-focused therapy, feminist therapy, and cognitive behavior therapy. With all new therapy clients, the effort toward building strong therapeutic relationships is always paramount. Through training in feminist therapy and Indigenous ways of knowing, I take on an anti-oppressive lens in my work, which acknowledges social injustices and which promotes egalitarian relationships in therapy, largely through therapist authenticity and self-disclosure. This aligns well with Indigenous epistemologies and teachings around humility and sharing stories. In this sense, I would self-disclose in ways that would let me be seen and known by my clients (for example, by sharing family history, marital status, community involvement). As noted earlier, in my therapy practice, I would also incorporate decolonizing discourse by discussing the shortcomings of Eurocentric worldviews (which have often included racism, sexism, and homophobia, for instance) and by honoring Indigenous cultural knowledges. I would also share with clients that I work with Healers for my own healing, that I participate in ceremony, and that I have benefited from Indigenous medicine generally. I did this in an intentional effort to validate and normalize these varied approaches to care, which in many cases were foreign to Indigenous community members who had previously become culturally dispossessed through colonization.

Throughout treatment, I would check in with clients about their health-related needs and offer to refer them to a Healer or Elder. For those who worked with me and a Healer concurrently, I would honor the Indigenous teachings clients received from Healers in our psychology session, and would reinforce and support those wisdoms. I would also attend community ceremonies with clients, including the Shake Tent ceremony and the graduation ceremony at the Chayuuwaytim unit, where Healers and clients would honor the program participants.

AHT also offers group therapy to clients in the Chayuuweytim unit, and this process is harmonized, since both Western trained addictions counselors and Healers co-facilitate the group. The Western psychoeducational group, which is typically didactic, is adapted to include interactive components, personal sharing, storytelling by the facilitators, the use of metaphor and Indigenous teachings, and Indigenous languages. These programs carry at their core the philosophy of respecting the teachings of all peoples. Practitioners bring in teachings from cognitive therapy, motivational interviewing, mindfulness meditation and Buddhism, 12-step programs, Mohawk teachings, Anishnawbe teachings, Cree teachings, harm reduction teachings, Reiki teachings, Christian teachings, queer theory, feminist theory, decolonizing therapies, and others. Practitioners speak of the synergistic effects of Western, Indigenous, and other therapies, and note that using the best of different ways of knowing and harmonizing can result in a "one plus one equals eight" effect.

My experience in this setting taught me that Indigenous and Western approaches can work together effectively. When the practitioners of different medicines engaged in respectful knowledge sharing, there were rarely conflicts between Western and Indigenous medicines. In cases of questions or confusion, or if clarification was needed from an Indigenous perspective, we would consult with a Healer regarding client care or the appropriateness of the psychological services. If ever a disagreement surfaced between Western approach and Indigenous therapeutic approaches, we would discuss it–the client, the Healer, and I–and we would, each in our own way, consider these varying perspectives and engage in a deeper dialog with one another. Are Western and Indigenous practitioners working together vastly different than psychiatrists and social workers collaborating? Typically, a psychiatrist takes an illness model lens to her work and a social worker takes social determinants and social justice lens to her work; yet these clinicians are always seen working side by side in a Western health-care setting. It seemed from my experience that the necessary ingredients to work in a cross-cultural and cross-disciplinary manner were these three essentials: harmonized services at the programmatic level; healthy relationships involving mutual respect between practitioners, encouraged through the normalizing and equalizing of services at the policy level; and openness to engage in hybrid thinking/feeling/being at the individual practitioner level. I would also add that self-discovery and decolonizing work at the individual level (no matter the practitioner) is also necessary for social justice practice at centeres like AHT.

Throughout my time with the organization, I received many teachings from Joe Hester, the executive director of AHT. He shared his insight that culture and identity are the "sign posts" that walk us through life in a good way—especially when we need healing. Culture teaches us about who we are, our responsibilities, and how we relate to creation. For Indigenous peoples, these sign posts were knocked down and outlawed through colonization. The communities are now rebuilding culture and identity in many ways, and AHT offers one such pathway in an urban context. He notes that when you are exposed to culture, it often strikes a chord and resonates deeply. Suddenly, through cultural engagement, clients experience a place of belonging and community healing. Immersion in tradition and community acceptance is part of the healing journey, and this opportunity to connect is a unique offering at AHT compared to mainstream mental health treatment centeres. He says that, although Indigenous and Western services can disagree at times, with patience and respect, they can work together. He feels that our people deserve the best and that the "best" treatment is a combination of both Indigenous and Western medicines.

Discussion and Concluding Remarks

One of the most obvious challenges related to the integration of Indigenous and Western mental health-care services is the differences in epistemological and conceptual understandings of mental health and healing [22, 32]. As has been outlined previously, significant differences exist between Indigenous and Western paradigms of healing, including an emphasis on holism versus mind-body dualism, the role that spirituality, relationship, culture, and community plays in each paradigm, and the formulation of illness etiology.

This last point raises the issue of both Indigenous and Western practitioners' willingness to collaborate and integrate their services. Indigenous methods for healing are often stigmatized and viewed as illegitimate forms of treatment by many Western professionals [3]. At the same time, the Royal Commission on Aboriginal Peoples [39] illustrated that Indigenous Healers are entrusted with the task of healing in their communities, and for some Healers and Elders, it is Western medicine that has become suspect. As is noted in the RCAP [39] report, Healers and Elders "have seen people become addicted to Western medicines or be subjected to uncomfortable or painful treatments with little or no positive results" (p. 13).

Suspicions and mistrust may therefore impede both groups of helpers in collaborating and integrating their services. Part of this suspicion may stem from a lack of understanding and awareness of the work and approach that each helper takes. Becoming educated about each helper's healing paradigm, approaches, and practices has been identified as a critical task for collaboration and integration. However, practitioners and Healers must be open to developing their own cultural awareness and understanding of each approach, and be willing and interested in integrating their own services.

While developing cultural awareness and providing education about Indigenous practices is important, a key element in the formation of collaborative working relationships is respect. At its core, epistemological hybridism is founded upon the notion that acceptance and respect for diverse realities and ways of knowing and being are paramount. Principal among Indigenous helpers' grievances with the Western health-care system, and its professionals, is a lack of respect for Indigenous

Knowledges and healing practices, and for Indigenous Healers themselves. As was reported to Beaulieu by an Elder who was a participant in her cultural research study, "We're available, our Healers are available, but they have to come to us and ask us in the right way. They have to respect us. They can't just expect something to happen without there being some kind of respectful protocol of how we're going to work together" (2011, p. 165). Practitioners must also be mindful of respecting cultural protocols related to the disclosure of sacred rituals, ceremonies, and teachings. As a result of colonial legislation which outlawed the practice of many Indigenous healing traditions and increased surveillance of Indigenous peoples and communities, much cultural knowledge and tradition was forced underground [40]. Great strides have been taken to protect this knowledge throughout the decades and to also avoid persecution, punishment, or exploitation—both historically and in the present day. We believe the onus falls on Western practitioners and health systems to create the safety needed for practitioners of Indigenous medicine to come forward and collaborate.

Despite the various challenges that exist with respect to culturally integrated care, it is important to not lose sight of the potential significant benefit that may result from the harmonization of these approaches to healing in mental health care. We are encouraged by the success stories from AHT and ABS at CAMH. However, again, the integration of worldviews, knowledge systems, and practices must be founded on values of respect, equality, and reconciliation. In the era of "truth and reconciliation" in Canada, it is important to approach and understand the mental health care of Indigenous peoples within a reconciliatory framework. It is essential to acknowledge these truths: that Indigenous peoples have experienced, and continue to experience, significant health disparities as a result of colonization [1]; that Indigenous peoples have been chronically under-served in mental health care and often receive a poorer quality of care [11]; and that Indigenous clients have been the recipients of imperialistic clinical interventions rooted in Western worldviews, values, and ways of knowing [41]. In order to reconcile these truths and injustices, it is imperative that mainstream health-care professionals not only ensure their practices are culturally safe but are also committed to adapting their services so that cultural integration with Indigenous Knowledge and healing systems is possible. At the core of this practice is the establishment of trusting, mutually respectful, and authentic relationships between Western trained clinicians and Indigenous clinicians and clients. As articulated in the Truth and Reconciliation Commission's final report [36],

> Together, Canadians must do more than just *talk* about reconciliation; we must learn how to *practice* reconciliation in our everyday lives—within ourselves and our families, and in our communities, governments, places of worship, schools, and workplaces. To do so constructively, Canadians must remain committed to the ongoing work of establishing and maintaining respectful relationships. For many Survivors and their families, this commitment is foremost about healing themselves, their communities, and nations, in ways that revitalize individuals as well as Indigenous cultures, languages, spirituality, laws, and governance systems. (p. 20)

The pathway toward enhancing mental health service delivery for Indigenous peoples requires clinicians to embrace a position of flexibility, humility, openness, and a genuine interest in transformative innovation.

Upon release of the Truth and Reconciliation final report in 2015, the Liberal government stated that Canada was committed to a full implementation of the 94 Calls to Action outlined in the final report. This included Canada's adoption and implementation of the *United Nations Declaration on the Rights of Indigenous Peoples* (UNDRIP), and the use of UNDRIP as the framework for reconciliation. The UNDRIP Declaration is made up of 46 articles which pertain to the inherent rights of Indigenous peoples globally. The articles address individual and collective rights related to culture, identity, education, health, employment, language, economic sustainability, Indigenous lands and resources, and self-determination, among other rights. Canada was only one of four nations that initially voted against the UNDRIP when it was first introduced in 2007, in comparison to the 144 states that voted in support of the Declaration. This was due to the refusal of the government of the time to accept a provision related to land rights. It took 9 years for Canada to reverse its standing, and in 2016, Canada declared its adoption and intention to fully implement UNDRIP. As of May 2018, Bill C-262, an act to ensure that the laws of Canada are in harmony with the *United Nations Declaration on the Rights of Indigenous People*, had passed its third reading before the House of Commons. Canada's commitment to the implementation of the TRC Calls to Action and UNDRIP has implications for mental health service design and delivery, and clinicians' individual practice.

Two of the UNDRIP Articles that speak directly to Indigenous peoples' rights to culture, health care, and the use of cultural practices as a means for healing include Article 12 and Article 23:

> *Article 12:* 1. Indigenous peoples have the right to manifest, practice, develop and teach their spiritual and religious traditions, customs and ceremonies; the right to maintain, protect, and have access in privacy to their religious and cultural sites; the right to the use and control of their ceremonial objects; and the right to the repatriation of their human remains.
>
> *Article 23.* Indigenous peoples have the right to determine and develop priorities and strategies for exercising their right to development. In particular, indigenous peoples have the right to be actively involved in developing and determining health, housing and other economic and social programmes affecting them and, as far as possible, to administer such programmes through their own institutions.

The principles of UNDRIP clearly delineate Indigenous peoples' rights to culture and spiritual practices, as well as their self-determination in developing health and other social programs. In addition, TRC Call to Action 22 stipulates that: "We call upon those who can effect change within the Canadian health-care system to recognize the value of Aboriginal healing practices and use them in the treatment of Aboriginal patients in collaboration with Aboriginal healers and Elders where requested by Aboriginal patients."

Taken together, the design and delivery of mental health-care services for First Nations, Inuit, and Métis peoples in Canada are on the precipice of significant and long-lasting change. In order to move forward in allyship, we recommend that

Western mental health services begin with the following recommendations for change at the systemic (national) level, at the health agency level, and at the individual practitioner level:

Systemic Level

- Educate mental health professionals in accredited counseling and psychology programs across Canada in Indigenous mental health and cultural safety.
- Train all mental health practitioners and administrators across mental health delivery programs in Canada in Indigenous mental health and cultural safety.
- Support Indigenous communities to have autonomy in determining their own health priorities and needs and to procure helping services from Western and Indigenous healing services, as communities deem necessary.

Health Agency Level

- Build relationships and collaborate with Indigenous mental health professionals in clinical practice issues, teaching, and research initiatives.
- Engage in consultation with Indigenous community members and Healers to determine if integrated services (Indigenous and Western) would be appropriate in a health organization that serves Indigenous clients.

Practitioner Level

- Complete coursework and specialized training on Indigenous cultural safety and cultural humility, including education on the history of Indigenous peoples, current health needs, and healing approaches of First Nations, Inuit, and Métis peoples.
- Cultural safety training also involves personal reflection of one's social location, as well as personal assumptions and biases related to health services, Indigenous peoples, and culture-based approaches to health and healing.
- Cultural safety training involves intellectual, emotional, spiritual, and relational learning related to allyship.
- Obtain clinical supervision from an Indigenous or culturally safe clinician in order to deepen your practice of cultural humility and cultural safety.
- Be a respectful health-care consultant if your services are requested by the community; engage in sincere relationship building with Indigenous community members, health professionals, and associations.
- Collaborate on treatment and healing plans with Indigenous helpers involved with a shared client's care.
- Where appropriate, engage in a deepening of your own understanding of Indigenous cultural knowledges. This may come in many forms and can be understood as an ongoing learning journey that is personal for each of us. Some examples might include attendance at cultural teaching sessions in the workplace or community, or attending personal teaching sessions with Indigenous helpers.

It is our hope that all clinicians can work toward offering collaborative, harmonized care to Indigenous clients in a manner that promotes optimal healing. To do so, Western mental health systems and practitioners must embody the spirit of allyship and reconciliation in their work, by embracing epistemological understandings of health and well-being from more than one perspective. If mental health care is to be aligned with the needs of Indigenous peoples in Canada, health-care professionals and organizations must understand their ethical and legal obligations to ensure that First Nations, Inuit, and Métis peoples have access to their cultural and spiritual traditions as part of their healing work and journeys. Ultimately, First Nations, Inuit, and Métis peoples must be supported and enabled to exercise self-determination in the development and provision of health and healing services for their people and communities.

References

1. Reeves A, Stewart S. Historical perspectives on indigenous and Western healing in Canada and implications for mental health service provision. In: Stewart S, Moodley R, Hyatt A, editors. Indigenous cultures and mental health counselling. New York: Routledge; 2017. p. 127–40.
2. Reading CL, Wein F. Health inequalities and social determinants of Aboriginal peoples' health. National Collaborating Centre for Aboriginal Health; 2009. http://ahrnets.ca/files/2011/02/NCCAH-Loppie-Wien_Report.pdf.
3. Waldram JB, Herring DA, Young TK. Aboriginal healing in Canada: historical, cultural, and epidemiological perspectives. Toronto: University of Toronto Press; 2007.
4. Health Canada. A statistical profile on the health of First Nations in Canada: Health services utilization in Western Canada, 2000; 2009. http://www.hc-sc.gc.ca/fniah-spnia/pubs/aborig-autoch/index-eng.php. Accessed 10 June 2009.
5. King M, Smith A, Gracey M. Indigenous health part 2: the underlying causes of the health gap. Lancet. 2009;374:76–85. https://doi.org/10.1016/S0140-6736(09)60827-8.
6. Stewart SL. Indigenous mental health: Canadian Native counsellors' narratives. Doctoral dissertation, University of Victoria; 2007.
7. Hill W. Understanding life...what my ancestors taught me through dreams. Pittsburgh, PA: Red Lead Press; 2009.
8. Aboriginal Healing Foundation. A healing journey: final report summary points. Ottawa, ON; 2006.
9. Duran E. Healing the soul wound: counseling with American Indians and other native peoples. New York, NY: Teachers College Press; 2006.
10. Haskell D, Randall M. Disrupted attachments: a social context complex trauma framework and the lives of aboriginal peoples in Canada. Aboriginal J Health. 2009;5(3):48–99.
11. Stewart SL. Promoting indigenous mental health: cultural perspectives on healing from native counselors in Canada. Int J Health Promot Educ. 2008;46(2):49–56.
12. Gone J. The red road to wellness: cultural reclamation in a native first nations community treatment center. Am J Community Psychol. 2011;47:186–202. https://doi.org/10.1007/s10464-010-9373-2.
13. McCabe G. Mind, body, emotions and spirit: reaching to the ancestors for healing. Couns Psychol Q. 2008;21(2):143–52.
14. Vicary DA, Bishop BJ. Western psychotherapeutic practice: engaging aboriginal people in culturally appropriate and respectful ways. Aust Psychol. 2005;40(1):8–19.
15. Koss-Chioino JD. Jung, spirits and madness: lessons for cultural psychiatry. Transcult Psychiatry. 2003;40(2):164–80.
16. Burkhardt MA. Healing relationships with nature. Complement Ther Nurs Midwifery. 2000;6:35–40.
17. Garrett MT, Wilbur MP. Does the worm live in the ground? Reflections on native American spirituality. J Multicult Couns Dev. 1999;7(4):193–206.

18. American Psychiatric Association. Diagnostic and statistical manual of mental disorders (DSM-5). American Psychiatric Pub; 2013.
19. Egnew TR. The meaning of healing: transcending suffering. Ann Fam Med. 2005;3(3):255–62.
20. Constantine MG, Myers LJ, Kindaichi M, Moore JL. Exploring indigenous mental health practices: the roles of healers and helpers in promoting Well-being in people of color. Couns Values. 2004;48:110–25.
21. Waldram JB. Revenge of the Windigo: the construction of the mind and mental health of north American aboriginal peoples. Toronto, ON: University of Toronto Press; 2004.
22. Gone J. Psychotherapy and traditional healing for American Indians: exploring the prospects for therapeutic integration. Counseling Psychologist. 2010;38(2):166–235. https://doi.org/10.1177/0011000008330831.
23. Lewis-Fernandez R, Kleinman A. Culture, personality, and psychopathology. J Abnorm Psychol. 1994;103(1):67–71.
24. Schneider GW, DeHaven MJ. Revisiting the Navajo way: lessons for contemporary healing. Perspect Biol Med. 2003;46(3):413–27.
25. Phiri-Alleman W, Alleman J. Sexual violence in relationships: implications for multicultural counseling. Family J Counsel Ther Couples Families. 2008;16(2):155–8.
26. Harris KM, Edlund MJ, Larson S. Racial and ethnic differences in the mental health problems and use of mental health care. Med Care. 2005;43(8):775–84.
27. Oetzel J, Duran B, Lucero J, Jiang Y, Novins DK, Manson S, et al. Rural American Indians' perspectives of obstacles in the mental health treatment process in three treatment sectors. Psychol Serv. 2006;3(2):117–28.
28. Shah CP. Health status report of aboriginal people in Ontario; 2005. http://www.aht.ca/webfm_send/25
29. Shore JH, Shore JH, Manson SM. American Indian healers and psychiatrists: building alliances. In: Incayawar M, Wintrob R, Bouchard L, editors. Psychiatrists and traditional healers: unwitting partners in global mental health. West Sussex, UK: John Wiley & Sons Ltd.; 2009. p. 123–34.
30. Maar MA, Erskine B, McGregor L, Larose TL, Sutherland ME, Graham D, et al. Innovations on a shoestring: a study of collaborative community-based aboriginal mental health service model in rural Canada. Int J Ment Heal Syst. 2009;3(27):1–12.
31. Gregory D. An exploration of the contact between nurses and Indian elders/traditional healers on Indian reserves and health centres in Manitoba. In: Young DE, editor, Health care issues in the Canadian North, pp. 39–43; 1988.
32. Crowe-Salazar N. Exploring the experiences of an elder, a psychologist and a psychiatrist: how can traditional practices and healers complement existing practices in mental health? First Peoples Child Family Rev. 2007;3(4):83–95.
33. Ellerby JH. Working with indigenous elders. 3rd ed. Winnipeg, Manitoba: Aboriginal Issues Press; 2005.
34. Rayle AD, Chee C, Sand JK. Honoring their way: counseling American Indian women. J Multicult Couns Dev. 2006;34:66–79.
35. Anishnawbe Health Toronto. About Anishnawbe Health Toronto; 2011. http://www.aht.ca
36. Truth and Reconciliation Commission of Canada (2015). Honouring the truth, reconciling for the future: Summary of the final report of the Truth and Reconciliation Commission of Canada. Accessed on June 7, 2021 at http://www.trc.ca/assets/pdf/Honouring_the_Truth_Reconciling_for_the_Future_July_23_2015.pdf
37. Poonwassie A, Charter A. Aboriginal worldview of healing: Inclusion, blending, and bridging. In: Moodley R, West, W (Eds.), Integrating traditional healing practices into counselling and psychotherapy. Thousand Oaks, CA: Sage Publications; 2005. p. 15–25
38. Smye V, Mussell B. The Aboriginal Mental Health Best Practices Working Group. Aboriginal mental health: What works best. Vancouver, BC: University of British Colombia; 2001.

39. Royal Commission on Aboriginal Peoples. Report of the Royal Commission on Aboriginal Peoples (Vol 4): Perspectives and realities. Ottawa, ON: Minister of Supply and Services Canada; (1996).
40. Hill, DM. (2003). Traditional medicine in contemporary contexts: Protecting and respecting Indigenous knowledge and medicine. National Aboriginal Health Organization. Accessed on June 7, 2021 at: https://fnim.sehc.com/getmedia/50ecae25-69f3-4e7a-8483-0be5e65add98/research_tradition.pdf.aspx?ext=.pdf
41. Gone, JP. Psychotherapy and traditional healing for American Indians: Exploring the prospects for therapeutic integration. The Counseling Psychologist. 2010;38(2):166–235

Teresa Beaulieu is completing Doctor of Philosophy in Clinical and Counseling Psychology at the Ontario Institute for Studies in Education at the University of Toronto. She is also a Registered Psychotherapist and is the founder and director of the Weaving Wellness Centre, an Indigenous clinical and consulting practice in Toronto, Ontario. Tera is a citizen of the Métis Nation of Ontario, is past president of the Toronto and York Region Métis Council, and has received several awards for her leadership within the Indigenous community of Toronto.

Allison Reeves is a Registered Psychologist in Toronto and an assistant professor in Psychology at the University of Guelph. Allison's research looks at the impacts of complex trauma in Anishnawbe communities as well as cultural resurgence and healing. Her current areas of interest are in anti-oppressive psychologies and ethnocultural empathy training to reduce racial bias. Dr. Reeves is of mixed descent with European and Caribbean roots.

Part VI
Reconciliation and Mental Health

Reconciliation Social Work: Sustainable Community Development

Cynthia Wesley-Esquimaux and Steven Koptie

This paper draws on the work of social work scholars Michael and Judith Bopp[1] who, together with Phil Lane Jr. of the Four Worlds International Institute, developed 16 guiding principles[2] for Indigenous community development:

> The Sixteen Principles for building a sustainable and harmonious world community emerged from a 40-year process of reflection, consultation and action within Indigenous communities across the Americas. They are rooted in the concerns of hundreds of Indigenous Elders, Spiritual Leaders and Community Members, as well as the best thinking of many non-Indigenous scholars, researchers and human and community development practitioners.
>
> These guiding principles constitute the foundation for the process of healing and developing ourselves (mentally, emotionally, physically, and spiritually), our human relationships (personal, social, political, economic, and cultural) and our relationship with Mother Earth. They describe the way we must work and what we must protect and cherish. [1]

Throughout the narrative, we contrast the *94 Calls for Action*[3] tabled by the Canadian Truth and Reconciliation Commission (TRC) in December 2015 with those 16 principles and ask whether these works can frame new directions for social justice and social work practice. The TRC was established in 2009 and completed its work on truth gathering from survivors of Indian residential schools[4] in June

[1] http://www.fourworlds.ca/who_principals.html

[2] http://www.fwii.net/profiles/blogs/sixteen-guiding-principles-for

[3] http://www.trc.ca/websites/trcinstitution/File/2015/Findings/Calls_to_Action_English2.pdf

[4] http://www.residentialschoolsettlement.ca/Schedule_O-4.pdf

C. Wesley-Esquimaux
Office of the President, Lakehead University, Orillia, ON, Canada
e-mail: cynthia.wesley@lakeheadu.ca

S. Koptie (✉)
Mamaway Wiidokdaadwin, Orilla, ON, Canada
e-mail: mwcbt@banac.on.ca

D. Danto, M. Zangeneh (eds.), *Indigenous Knowledge and Mental Health*,
https://doi.org/10.1007/978-3-030-71346-1_16

2015, and tabled its final reports in December 2015. This left Canadians and the Indigenous population across Canada to take up and implement the 94 Calls to Action on reconciliation and to view through new lenses social justice, child welfare, education, language and culture, health care, and spiritual practices.

We see our own personal knowledge and experience with social justice issues reflected in the 16 principles of practice and the 94 TRC Calls for Action, all of which offer promising approaches for change in Indigenous and mainstream relations. We are calling this approach "reconciliation social work" in order to tie the potential for change directly to the need for better social work relations between Indigenous Peoples and Canadians, especially when it comes to building and sustaining sociocultural understandings. The principles provide an inclusive, ethical, and culturally intelligent framework for establishing collaborative partnerships with the goal of reconciling Canada's colonial injustices against Indigenous Peoples. The Calls for Action specify terms of engagement that can be mobilized by the federal, provincial, and territorial governments, Indigenous Peoples and their governments, Canada's churches, educational institutions, child and family care organizations, and the general population.

Social Work Engagement

A truthful review of the historic patterns of destruction promulgated since contact on this continent, and the consequent devastation of Indigenous social efficacy, which undermined each Indigenous community's social system and ability to maintain its own behavioral and cultural norms and controls, will require multiple layers of action by next generations of social workers tasked to mitigate the damage of colonial practice. Our own experience has demonstrated that social work students are rarely exposed to culturally inclusive curriculum contextualized and taught by Indigenous instructors. There is a need therefore for more Indigenous social work faculty (and the faculty of all disciplines) and educational materials that critically address the collusion of social workers, whether consciously or unconsciously, in Canada's quest to assimilate Indigenous Peoples. Social workers have inadvertently been bystanders, witnesses, and perpetrators of gross human rights violations, most of which remain unresolved if even acknowledged [2–4]. The TRC presented an opportunity to address unfortunate historic and contemporary perceptions about Indigenous Peoples through the development of a "Statement of Reconciliation" by the Deans of Social Work in every college and university, which acknowledge and amend the skewed application of external standards and values long deemed inappropriate by First Nation, Metis, and Inuit peoples.

The influences of colonialism and Indian residential schools on our families and communities means our own lifelong learning processes have been framed by the kind of melancholic journey of self-discovery described by Irihapeti Ramsden in 2002, a Maori nurse who introduced the concept of cultural safety to her profession. However, as Indigenous scholars, we have also experienced unique and rewarding opportunities to participate in the academy through graduate studies in Cultural Anthropology at the University of Toronto and programs such as the Wholistic Indigenous Social Work Practices offered through Wilfred Laurier University in Ontario. Throughout our community service careers, as seasoned community helpers, we have often found ourselves struggling through multiple layers of metaphoric reflections. We have discovered that *wholeness* in social work practice actually means unlearning the impulse of colonial, patriarchal, or hierarchal social work to change others, and adopting a deeper appreciation of the meaning of Indigenous Spirit, Nature, Knowledge, Intellect, and Character, as offered by Absolon in 2009 [5]. It also means allowing and embracing the presence of "good minds with good intentions," from Haudenosaunee teachings,[5] and opening our own practices to cultural transformation. The concept of "holistic," when embedded within reconciliation social work practice, can then become a vital journey of self-discovery, beginning with a personal self-reflective evaluation of our personal Spirit, Nature, Knowledge, Intellect, and Character. This understanding and approach have served to alter and enhance our entire worldview, providing us with a deeper acceptance and cultural regard for those around us, and infusing our community practice with a deeper sense of compassion and inclusion.

Social workers must not only be tasked with engaging Indigenous communities; they must learn to acknowledge that unique Indigenous identities can be formed only through the collective lived experience of their families, communities, and nations. Social workers themselves often have bicultural roles within the worlds they inhabit, and embracing their roles in both worlds can have a positive impact on the wellness and well-being of Indigenous and other cultural communities. Self-identifying influences from our own cultural backgrounds can strengthen our traditional worldviews and lead to reconciliation of different lifeways and practices. Social workers who acknowledge influences from their own cultural backgrounds will feel more compelled and better able to relate to the possibility of transformation in their own and other worlds, even while they serve to promote and protect reconciliation commitments. According to Ramsden [6] and Absolon [5], we can recover cultural safety[6] in our relationships by starting from within and working outward in multiple circles in sacred ways, so we can heal ourselves, our worlds, and our relations.

Principles*: (1)Human Beings Can Transform Their Worlds, and****(16)****Be the Change You Want to See.*

Call to Action:*(18)We call upon the federal, provincial, territorial, and Aboriginal governments to acknowledge that the current state of Aboriginal health in Canada is a direct result of previous Canadian government policies, including residential schools, and to recognize and implement the health-care rights of Aboriginal people as identified in international law, constitutional law, and under theTreaties.*

---

[5] http://www.iroquoiswhitecorn.org/about/good-minds. Retrieved 2 Dec 2015.

[6] http://www.naho.ca/jah/english/jah05_02/V5_I2_Cultural_01.pdf

Contemporizing the Context

Next generations of social workers and Indigenous Healers can employ unique Indigenous perspectives to assist in resolving the intergenerational traumatic impacts of Indian Residential Schools, the (w)recklessness of the Sixties Scoop, and the contemporary cultural devastation institutions like provincial jails and Corrections Canada bring to Indigenous Canada. The justice system has created and sustains what can be referred to as Canada's largest reserve system. The effects are inexorably tied to an increasingly problematic legacy of problem drinking patterns, broken health through systemic diseases, and mental health complications associated with historic trauma, unmitigated stressors, and the intergenerational transmission of unresolved grief [7]. Unrecognized and untreated intergenerational trauma has led to poor parenting, mental illness and general unease, sectorial exploitation, problems with the justice system, and, finally, a repetition of lifelong unwellness and negative behaviors. Marlyn Bennett [2] speaks to how these historic intrusions break the "Circle of Life," the traditional circle of immediate and extended family, community, and nations. Her 2008 report, *Jumping Through Hoops,* chronicles the experiences of families and social workers in the child welfare system in Manitoba, and offers profound insights on the multiple trajectories that devastate Indigenous communities and cripple cultural resilience. The narratives within this study testify to the multigenerational ordeal women have endured to sustain a parental identity, because they are "mothers under siege" from state-sanctioned efforts to destroy a culture. None of the attempts to protect children by saving them from living "like Indians," ranging from the experimentation of reserves, establishing assimilationist residential schools, or perpetual social exclusion and marginalization, have worked—and for good reason. Stolen lands, stolen children, and broken cultural resilience have no place in the twenty-first century. Before a First Nations reemergence is possible, there must be a reframing of the historic common experience and a reassertion of the self-determination needed for the next seven generations. And those two visions must reconcile with each other. The Elders tell us we borrow our time from our children, and we are taught they are born to heal us, so we must recover our internal strengths, protect their well-being ourselves, and promote the wellness of our nations.

Principles:*(6)No Unity, No Development,(8)Justice.*

Call to Action:*(57) We call upon federal, provincial, territorial, and municipal governments to provide education to public servants on the history of Aboriginal peoples, including the history and legacy of residential schools, the United Nations Declaration on the Rights of Indigenous Peoples, Treaties and Aboriginal rights, Indigenous law, and Aboriginal–Crown relations. This will require skills-based training in intercultural competency, conflict resolution, human rights, and anti-racism.*

When we are attempting to locate the genesis of addictions, one significant lapse in historical investigation and contemporary representation is reviewing the improper use and distribution of alcohol [8]. The dangerous drinking patterns generated throughout the settlement period and out of Indian residential school traumas have carried forward into modern forms of substance abuse [7, 9]. Fortunately, historical records exist to enable Indigenous researchers to redefine the use of alcohol as an insidious currency to gain control over trade for goods and resource extraction and the unfettered acquisition of lands in the developing state of Canada [3, 4, 10]. To this day, vast areas of Canada have no system for regulating the use of alcohol, including on dry reserves where under the *Indian Act* it is illegal to buy or sell alcohol, or band councils have decided to ban its use. There, homemade alcohol (homebrew) and its illicit sales continue a pattern of unsafe use of a harmful substance strictly controlled in mainstream Canada. Understanding certain truths help to contextualize the hurt Indigenous Peoples have suffered historically and continue to suffer everywhere in Canada. Even if an individual has somehow personally escaped the ravages of this particular substance, the impact from long-standing addictions unfolding around them throughout multiple Indigenous nations has its own detrimental effects.

The sharing of successful healing narratives will assist in the restoration of well-being, contribute to holistic wellness "on the ground," and help to correct the health disparities that Andrea Smith [11] referenced in *Conquest: Sexual Violence and American Indian Genocide (2005)*. Postcolonial Indigenous scholars must locate and include direct narratives of strength and resistance in their published interpretations of the sociopolitical upheavals within their traditional territories. Equally transformative is a realization that the historical upheavals and injustices that led to internalized self-hatred, and ultimately became interwoven in many generations of First Peoples families, were in fact an external attack [12]. These narratives will guide healing journeys from the despair, hopelessness, helplessness, and oppressive dependency that continue to have an impact on physical, social, mental, and spiritual wellness. Our ancestors had a vision for our survival that was blocked, and these healing narratives will unblock that vision. This purity of historical understanding, which also frames Canada's true identity, was what was meant to constitute and protect the Spirit and Intent of the Treaty relationship and informs the 16 principles and Truth and Reconciliation Calls to Action.

Principles:*(5)Interconnectedness,(8)Justice,(9)Spirit,(10)Morals and Ethics.*

Call to Action:*(19) We call upon the federal government, in consultation with Aboriginal peoples, to establish measurable goals to identify and close the gaps in health outcomes between Aboriginal and non-Aboriginal communities, and to publish annual progress reports and assess long-term trends. Such efforts would focus on indicators such as infant mortality, maternal health, suicide, mental health, addictions, life expectancy, birth rates, infant and child health issues, chronic diseases, illness and injury incidence, and the availability of appropriate health services.*

Fetal Alcohol Spectrum Disorder

Waldrum et al. [13] called for researchers in Canada to address and create holistic healing strategies for the multidimensional and complex biological, environmental, socioeconomic, and cultural determinants of poor health in Indigenous communities. Designing community capacity models to embrace prevention strategies and provide culturally relevant interventions is key to reversing overlapping lifespan problems. For example, improved sociocultural understanding about the treatment of fetal alcohol spectrum disorder (FASD) can present a potential opportunity for "key community workers and members" in Indigenous communities to restore cultural norms that honor all children as gifts of Creation. Indigenous social workers with the support of external allies can address the complex needs of youth living with FASD, and alcohol- or opiate-related neurological disorders and create a powerful model for transformative community development work. Generated through a lens of integrated Western social work practices with Indigenous principles and practices, combined work on FASD and ARND can form the foundation of reconciliation social work practice.

It is critical that social workers understand that less than 1% of the population suspected of having spectrum disorders are actually diagnosed, and this includes individuals from all racial and cultural backgrounds [14–16]. Carolyn Tait [17] also warned of diagnostic inconsistencies that target Indigenous women, their children, and their communities. Even in 2018, there is an ever-present danger of stigmatization, which creates additional burdens for women incapable of acting in their own best interests. Tait [17] warned against maintaining oppressive social work practices that tend to pathologize "Indian health" in order to allow governments to maintain paternalistic control of Indigenous territories. We agree that reliance on nonmedical labeling targets Indigenous women and children without making long-term commitments to addressing the roots of victimization. Tait added that pitting the state against victims does little to address or promote wellness issues, all of which are critical for a healthy pregnancy regardless of race, especially when women are living in poverty. She promoted the transfer of knowledge from "experts" to the community and key community worker training to address unhealthy binge-drinking patterns in communities that misuse alcohol. Knowledge transfer can intercept the intergenerational transmission of trauma and unresolved grief and allow transformative healing of the collective scars of colonization. Her thesis contributed an extremely important argument for workforce development and skills transfer to the community level so that external experts are moved to the periphery and community members become the central carriers and disseminators of knowledge. Their awakened Traditional Knowledge and social consciousness can then be used to directly address and lessen the effects of personal and communal dysfunction.

Principles:*(2) Development Comes from Within,**(13)** Learning, **(14)** Sustainability, **(16)** Be the Change You Want to See.*

Call to Action:*(33) We call upon the federal, provincial, and territorial governments to recognize as a high priority the need to address and prevent Fetal Alcohol*

Spectrum Disorder (FASD), and to develop in collaboration with Aboriginal people, preventive programs that can be delivered in a culturally appropriate manner.

Indigenous peoples and social workers may ask themselves what the potential gain might be by examining past events. The tragic loss of two babies on the Yellow Quill First Nation in Saskatchewan in 2008 because of alcohol-induced behaviors added to the roster of unconscionable stories that painfully remind Indigenous People it is the children who suffer the most. Two small children were dropped in the snow by their father, who had been drinking alcohol, and they froze to death. This horrible event reminded us of the code of silence around unhealthy drinking patterns in Indigenous communities. It is a silence that continues to create pockets of suffering and leads directly to an inability to confront the hurting of children by hurting adults. Hurt people hurt people. These intergenerational roots of self-destructive and self-defeating behaviors continue to adversely impact communities across the country. The missing narrative from the Yellow Quill story is the subtle presence of FASD. There was enough background and visual information available to suspect multigenerational alcohol abuse was present in this family and community, but the media did not raise this.[7] The reality of FASD and now opiate addiction in families remains a complication in the matter of justice sought and the healing required following such traumas. The father was given a 3-year sentence; the mother, pregnant with a third child, was found drinking alcohol with a relative when the story broke and lost her then-unborn child to the child welfare system.

FASD could once again become the sociocultural challenge that will force First Peoples to reexamine their history with alcohol and reintroduce responsible consumption and sobriety to personal, family, and community living. Addressing addictions will be necessary to heal our nations and stop the loss of hope for successive generations. Too many Indigenous people over time have experienced what must have felt like a massive, drunken rampage of recklessness and excess, which in turn caused destruction to crucial segments of our societies. This included babies, youth, parents, traditional caregivers, and even those who sustain the political, economic, and social safety of our territories. Indigenous research goals might encompass the following questions. Is it possible to reverse the impact on families where FASD is generationally entrenched? How many young people are repeating pathological cycles of self-destructive and self-defeating behaviors because of gestational brain damage? Can we reverse our collective failure to protect and advance healthy childhood and the coming of age for all of our youth? Will children already subjected to teratogens (agents of birth defects) in the womb find justice in the reconciliation process? Finally, will dangerous drinking patterns continue to decline, so Indigenous Peoples can return to natural sovereignty?

Now that the "world is watching" how Canada responds to Indigenous Peoples through the 94 Calls to Action tabled by the Truth and Reconciliation Commission in [18], these questions have global implications. The First Peoples of Canada can

---

[7] http://www.ctvnews.ca/reserve-where-girls-froze-worse-than-third-world-1.273793 and http://www.theglobeandmail.com/news/national/yellow-quill-was-so-ripe-for-tragedy/article718139/. Retrieved 24 Dec 2015.

now call upon significant allies to help articulate and transform the experiences of colonization and historic and contemporary trauma. Successive generations of children have been lost to the child welfare system because adults have been unable to assume their traditional roles of preparing them for healthy lifeways. After reading about the Yellow Quill Reserve tragedy, we resolved to develop new workshops to address the question, "Who Is Watching Our Children?" We tested "The Children Are Watching" violence prevention workshops in remote reserves to help communities restore safe and sober homes for child-rearing. The challenge to protect the future of Indigenous Peoples from the debilitating influences of alcohol must be spoken out loud again and again [8]. Our survival as healthy and strong Indigenous peoples requires us to do everything possible to restore to prominence child protection in our homelands, and for all children, everywhere. We can stop the destructive violence—sexual, domestic, social, and economic—by taking action family by family and community by community. Harold Johnson has already begun the process of taking action in Saskatchewan by meeting with individuals and family members, whether they drink or not, to try and stop the destructive cycles of violence within his own and local communities.

There has been a significant weakening of the natural supports and cultural mechanisms of intervention that prevent high-risk behaviors and lead to preventable tragedies. A culture of dependency allows an external locus of control to develop, and this shifts the natural power in families to outside social structures. *TheIndian Act* has always represented the oppressive control that brought confusion and disruption of collective responsibility for the physical, social, mental, and spiritual welfare of Indigenous peoples [19]. Those who honor children as gifts from the Creator are deeply perplexed by the neglect, abandonment, and abject failure to protect children from the cruelest aspects of life. The deep pain of helplessness has replaced sound parenting practices; drunkenness and addiction replaced the care and protection of our most precious gifts from Creation. And the code of silence around the use and abuse of alcohol is broken only by the wail of mothers, grandparents, sisters, brothers, and yes, fathers, when communities face the loss of innocent lives to preventable deaths such as suicide, murder, and accident.

Principles:*(7)No Participation, No Development.*

Call to Action:*(34) We call upon the governments of Canada, the provinces, and territories to undertake reforms to the criminal justice system to better address the needs of offenders with Fetal Alcohol Spectrum Disorder (FASD), including i. Providing increased community resources and powers for courts to ensure that FASD is properly diagnosed, and that appropriate community supports are in place for those with FASD. ii. Enacting statutory exemptions from mandatory minimum sentences of imprisonment for offenders affected by FASD. iii. Providing community, correctional, and parole resources to maximize the ability of people with FASD to live in the community. iv. Adopting appropriate evaluation mechanisms to measure the effectiveness of such programsand to ensure community safety.*

Mobilizing a Strengths-Based Model

A good example of the application of the 16 principles for sustainable community development and several of the 94 Calls to Action is an unpublished project supervised by Dr. Alicia Dunlop in 2003, called "Strengthening the Roots." The project was designed to address homelessness among Indigenous youth aged 15–35 suspected of having FASD. Dr. Dunlop shared Dr. Carolyn Tait's [20] contention that merely giving youth a label of FASD did little to assist them in their day-to-day lives or reverse the trajectory of foster and adoptive care, homelessness, and incarceration. Dr. Dunlop, a psychologist with a specialty in healing from trauma, taught and promoted the "strengths model" developed by Charles Rapp [21] as a useful guide to work with at-risk youth living with FASD. The paradigm shift she encouraged was taking social work practice beyond fixing life-skill deficiencies, and toward creating innovative youth engagement. She saw the need to help youth locate dependable strengths within themselves and to learn how to seek assistance for decision-making from social service guides. This project was reconciliation social work in action and practice because the strengths model focuses on abilities the person already possesses rather than labeling weaknesses and behavioral problems, or identifying deficiencies to fix. Dr. Dunlop held, and additional research has shown, that most youth find ways to survive even though their behavior may be labeled dysfunctional by society [22–24]. Their strength is in their ability to mobilize assets within their immediate living spaces and experiences. What appears to be dysfunctional socialization in Canadian society is actually functional utilization of resources and savvy navigation of social relationships in precarious circumstances. Social workers all too often operate from paradigms learned from white middle-class constructs and Western academia, and from values and standards generally unavailable to kids living on the streets. Most social workers have little exposure to cross-cultural historic Indigenous realities and curriculum, and at most levels of education are lacking guidance on how to mitigate stigma and stereotypes, especially when it comes to Indigenous youth.

Tait also addressed inconsistencies in what is taught to social workers with respect to FASD and youth. FASD is frequently presented as a massive "Indian problem," and this stereotype marginalizes Indigenous young people across Canada [17]. It also perpetuates a legacy of inconsistent social service delivery and prevents modification of the spaces Indigenous youth find themselves in. There is a need to shift the emphasis to helping them locate positive resources or create social niches and groups that have protective qualities. Research has demonstrated that we can help vulnerable youth understand and strengthen their roots and grow up into capable and productive citizens [23, 24]. This requires assertive outreach, engaging youth within the environments that work for them, and not merely waiting for them to attend what are often culturally unsafe adult-based agency spaces. Equally important is the education of community social service providers on the complexity of special needs clientele. When youth are integrated into non-threatening work, play, and living environments, resilience factors they have already developed on the street balance out what are frequently regarded as maladaptive social behaviors. They know what it takes to survive, to work with what they are presented with, and how to work with varying authority figures. Personal and adaptive change can then come from an ecological perspective at the individual, family, and social levels.

Rapp [21] stated that the concept of hope derives from the totality of "willpower and waypower" toward goal achievement. The larger community benefits from inclusive connectedness, adaptive role modeling, and peer support offered as a shared struggle, as opposed to increased isolation and marginalization. Rapp advocated a case management model based on engagement and relationship maintenance, focused on strengths as opposed to pointing out weaknesses, teaching ownership of personal recovery or goal achievement, learning to approach resources as needed, and always renewing collaborative opportunities. This allows gradual disengagement from resources with limitations on what they can provide. Rapp [21] held that diminished progress and failure to follow a healing plan often come from the failure of services to hold parallel visions, philosophies, and action plans. The result is youth falling through gaps, with lapses in accountability on all sides, and shortfalls in the provision of necessary interventions from those tasked with supporting our young people through crisis.

Principles: *(3) No Vision, No Development* ***(15)*** *Move to the Positive,* ***(16)*** *Be the Change You Want to See.*

Call to Action: *(**31**) We call upon the federal, provincial, and territorial governments to provide sufficient and stable funding to implement and evaluate community sanctions that will provide realistic alternatives to imprisonment for Aboriginal offenders and respond to the underlying causes of offending.*

Connecting the Dots

Across Canada, there are numerous inquiries, such as the Ashley Smith case (2008) out of New Brunswick, that have provided evidence of the sad trajectory of youth, especially First Nations and Inuit youth, into negative incarceration experiences. Two other inquiries out of New Brunswick, which also became public in 2008, offered guidance in the use of the "continuity of care" model developed by Dr. Dunlop and Charles Rapp, which they continue to advocate for today and which would also fit a reconciliation social work model. The first inquiry was *Connecting the Dots: A report on the condition of youth-at-risk and youth with very complex needs in New Brunswick*. Released in January 2008 by the New Brunswick Ombudsman and Child and Youth Advocate; it was initiated by a call for the investigation of systemic failures to provide humane care for children with mental health or undiagnosed complex needs. The failure to identify complex needs and implement early interventions can set vulnerable youth on a collision course with maltreatment and human rights violations that all too often carry tragic consequences.

The stories of seven youth in that report mirror the experience too many Indigenous children suffer when jurisdictional battles and failure to collaborate services in their best interests create ordeals that challenge society's claim it cares about the needs of its future generations. This is why today the debate over how Jordan's Principle[8] is interpreted and implemented is so critical to the dialog on social justice, and will influence the direction of a National Child Welfare Reform process.

The Ashley Smith (2008) inquiry into the suicide of a young woman with complex needs within a correctional institution highlighted an unfortunate failure of continuity of care. The needs of children like Ashley often begin with family breakdown, move to child protection issues for maltreatment, to unmanageable youth referred to foster care, to foster care breakdown, to multiple placements, to youth detention, and, finally, to incarceration. This chaotic path is never without the desperation of helpless caregivers trying to act in a youths' best interest, but far too often ends in repetitive patterns of loss, abandonment, and tragedy. This is too frequently the face of youth mental health—a preventable inertia fostering suicide, violence, substance abuse, homelessness, and marginalization. It is these narratives Indigenous social workers know too well. They also recognize the indifferent and dismissive attitudes of a dominant society that fails so many of its own young people. It makes our collective shame in circumstances such as the death of those children at the Yellow Quill First Nation incredibly selfish.

Principles: ***(8)*** *Justice,* ***(10)*** *Morals and Ethics.*

Call to Action: *(1) We call upon the federal, provincial, territorial, and Aboriginal governments to commit to reducing the number of Aboriginal children in care by: i. Monitoring and assessing neglect investigations. ii. Providing adequate resources to enable Aboriginal communities and child-welfare organizations to keep Aboriginal families together where it is safe to do so, and to keep children in culturally appropriate environments, regardless of where they reside. iii. Ensuring that social workers and others who conduct child-welfare investigations are properly educated and trained about the history and impacts of residential schools. iv. Ensuring that social workers and others who conduct child-welfare investigations are properly educated and trained about the potential for Aboriginal communities and families to provide more appropriate solutions to family healing. v. Requiring that all child-welfare decision-makers consider the impact of the residential school experience on children and their caregivers.* ***(27)*** *We call upon the Federation of Law Societies of Canada to ensure that lawyers receive appropriate cultural competency training, which includes the history and legacy of residential schools, the United Nations Declaration on the Rights of Indigenous Peoples, Treaties and Aboriginal rights, Indigenous law, and Aboriginal–Crown relations. This will require skills-based training in intercultural competency,conflict resolution, human rights, and anti-racism.*

---

[8] https://www.canada.ca/en/health-canada/services/first-nations-inuit-health/jordans-principle.html

What Kind of Healing?

We have both worked for close to 40 years in areas of historic trauma, mental health, child welfare, justice, family violence, addictions, and youth with FASD, as well as personal and community counseling and healing. We have long questioned how the richness of past generations, who were able to maintain social cohesiveness, can (re)influence today's healing movements. How can their knowledge and wise practices [25] once again guide the lifeways of Indigenous children and their parents? We need to actively acknowledge and address the cultural shock that followed unrelenting historic trauma and unresolved grief, the legacy of colonial warfare, disease, poverty, dislocation, oppression, forced colonial education, and assimilation since contact [3, 4, 10, 26, 27].

We more recently opted for on-the-ground social and reconciliation work in northwestern Ontario's urban, rural, and remote fly-in Indigenous communities. Five years of living in northwestern Ontario meant combining our forces and giving deep consideration to how colonial practice has sought to destroy and to control, and has altered our own community practice perspectives. It has also strengthened our determination to contextualize, analyze, and strategize a way to mediate the tragic impacts of the current opiate addiction crisis and address the proliferation of opiate harm reduction programs locally and in First Nation communities. On-the-ground reports and conversations suggest that more than 60% of Indigenous community members require harm reduction support because of past opiate pain medication addiction. We believe alcohol, insulin, Suboxone, and suicide are modern representations of new threats to the will to survive for Indigenous Peoples.

Healing strategies for Indigenous people of Canada must promote the transformation of victimization to *survivance* to "victorization" [28, 29] by reconciling multigenerational traumas into a strengths model of healing. The documentation of historic and successful First Nations social, emotional, physical, and spiritual practice is often absent in outsider mainstream research on contemporary Indigenous "disease." A paradigm shift is required to challenge the over-reliance on outside explanations for the perceived cultural and racial inferiority of Indigenous Peoples across Canada. More internal attention and community discussion are necessary to highlight the inherent strengths that have provided historic and contemporary resistance to what was and is for the most part a one-sided Canadian colonization experiment. The role of modern Indigenous scholars will then be to generate a restoration of true identities and powerful representations of the cultural and social humanity of our ancestors.

From an Indigenous perspective, this moral and ethical recovery will remove the burden of being confronted with curative options aimed solely at "Indian problems," which have been viewed through a simplistic and marginalizing lens. Reframing the colonial interpretation of Indigenous health and well-being will then make space for the full recovery of Indigenous worldviews and wise practices.[9] This is essential for

[9] http://c4f.qmts.ca/wp-content/uploads/2014/08/Aboriginal-Community-Development.pdf

building mutual goodwill and accepting the implementation of the Royal Commission on Aboriginal Peoples recommendations and the 94 Calls for Action put forward by the TRC. Reframing research through an Indigenous lens will critically challenge the mythology of the settlement of Canada and will truthfully represent Indigenous voice and place in what has so far been an unfair historical representation.

Principles:*(4)Healing is a Necessary Part of Development,(12)Authentic Development is Culturally Based,(15)Move to the Positive,(16)Be the Change You Want to See.*

Call to Action:*(21) We call upon the federal government to provide sustainable funding for existing and new Aboriginal healing centeres to address the physical, mental, emotional, and spiritual harms caused by residential schools, and to ensure that the funding of healing centeres in Nunavut and the Northwest Territories is a priority. (22) We call upon those who can effect change within the Canadian health-care system to recognize the value of Aboriginal healing practices and use them in the treatment of Aboriginal patients in collaboration with Aboriginal healers and Elders where requested by Aboriginal patients. (65) We call upon the federal government, through the Social Sciences and Humanities Research Council, and in collaboration with Aboriginal peoples,post-secondary institutions and educators and the National Centre for Truth and Reconciliation and its partner institutions, to establish a national research program with multi-year funding to advance understanding of reconciliation.*

Toward a Mutual Creation of Reconciliation

In conclusion, important lessons from improper diagnostic efforts in regards to complex needs of youth can be found in Tait's [17] thesis and other more recent research [30]. FASD among Indigenous people has long been a marker for declining health and intellectual well-being, especially when individuals and families are not treated for complex post-traumatic stress disorders, intergenerational loss, and chronic addictions. Tait continues to warn of a tendency, especially for Indigenous youth, to face the stigma of belonging to a "bio-underclass" or "culture of FASD" by joining rather than fighting family or community dysfunction. The disparity in health, wealth, and lifestyle opportunities between Indigenous peoples and the dominant culture must not continue to be reduced to a perceptual decline rooted in a social-Darwinism paradigm, where failures to adapt and adjust are perceived as inherent personal or genetic weaknesses. The twenty-first-century challenge is to recover ownership of a community wellness model that flows from a holistic context. It is essential to locate cultural survival by examining past successful lifeways, which at one time helped circumvent unhealthy practices in response to colonization. First Nations in the remote north are the last best hope of recovering a living relationship with Mother Earth, and it is therefore critical Canada transitions these populations carefully into today's world while respecting their ability to choose.

There has always been an opportunity to share and respect the strengths of the environment people find themselves living in. As respected Elder Fred Wheatley once stated, "You have to live within the world in which you find yourself," and this means working in a circle with good, strong, and kind minds. Collaboration will be needed to ensure children can go forward without the continuing risk of pain and suffering. This journey will be a humble and compassionate exercise of love, courage, and wisdom, but is the only way to create healthy and fully accessible pathways. Indigenous Peoples are increasingly aware of the genesis of the intergenerational malaise we have carried in our hearts and lives. We know there is a need to expose the absolute truth about the unrelenting and unnecessary hurts that have occurred in our territories and homes. Maladies such as FASD are surely best understood from a broader socioeconomic perspective because the imbalances our children and families have been experiencing are no longer acceptable. Together, as a country, we have an unprecedented opportunity to create reconciliation and ensure the development and sharing of Canada's natural potential is accessible to all. Peace, power, and righteousness (Taiaiake 2008) are gifts the Creator offered to all our relations.[10] The "words before all else" within *Ohe'n:ton Karihwate'hkwen*, the Six Nations Peoples' Thanksgiving Address, [11]can guide our minds to be as one. Indigenous Peoples can thrive once we accept full responsibility to live in gratitude, reciprocity, and with true interdependency.

Principles:*(11)The Hurt of One Is the Hurt of All; The Honour of One Is the Honour of All.*

Call to Action:*(92) We call upon the corporate sector in Canada to adopt the United Nations Declaration on the Rights of Indigenous Peoples as a reconciliation framework and to apply its principles, norms, and standards to corporate policy and core operational activities involving Indigenous peoples and their lands and resources. This would include, but not be limited to, the following:***i.***Commit to meaningful consultation, building respectful relationships, and obtaining the free, prior, and informed consent of Indigenous peoples before proceeding with economic development projects.***ii.***Ensure that Aboriginal peoples have equitable access to jobs, training, and education opportunities in the corporate sector and that Aboriginal communities gain long-term sustainable benefits from economic development projects.***iii.***Provide education for management and staff on the history of Aboriginal peoples, including the history and legacy of residential schools, the United Nations Declaration on the Rights of Indigenous Peoples, Treaties and Aboriginal rights, Indigenous law, and Aboriginal–Crown relations. This will require skills-based training in intercultural competency, conflict resolution, human rights, and anti-racism.*

"Starting from within, working in a circle, in a sacred manner, we heal ourselves, our relationships, and our world."[12]

---

[10] Alfred, Taiaiake (2008) Peace, Power & Righteousness: An Indigenous Manifesto, August 2008

[11] https://danceforallpeople.com/haudenosaunee-thanksgiving-address/

[12] http://www.fwii.net/ Guiding Principles, Retrieved 25 Dec 2015.

References

1. Lane P Jr. Four worlds institute; 2014. http://www.fwii.net/profiles/blogs/sixteen-guiding-principles-for & http://www.fwii.net/
2. Bennett M. Jumping through hoops: a Manitoba study examining the experiences and reflections of mothers involved with child welfare and legal systems respecting child protection matters. Winnipeg, MB: First Nations Child and Family Caring Society of Canada; 2008.
3. Koptie S. Inferiorizing indigenous communities and intentional colonial poverty. First People Child Fam Rev. 2010a;5(2):96–106.
4. Koptie S. Indigenous self-discovery: being called to witness. First Peoples Child Fam Rev. 2010b;4(2):114–25.
5. Absolon K. Indigenous wholistic theory: a knowledge set. First Peoples Child Fam Rev. 2009;5(2):74–87.
6. Ramsden I. Cultural safety and nursing education in Aotearoa and Te Waipounamu. Wellington: Victoria University; 2002. http://culturalsafety.massey.ac.nz/RAMSDEN%20THESIS.pdf
7. Wesley-Esquimaux C, Smolewski M. Historic trauma and aboriginal healing. Ottawa: Aboriginal Healing Foundation; 2004.
8. Johnson H. Firewater: how alcohol is killing my people (and yours), University of Regina Press; 2016.
9. Lewis O. The effects of white settlement upon Blackfoot culture, with special reference to the Fur trade. New York, NY: J. J. Augustin Publisher; 1942.
10. Daschuk J. Clearing the plains: disease, politics of starvation, and the loss of aboriginal life, University of Regina Press; 2014.
11. Smith A. Conquest: sexual violence and American Indian genocide. Brooklyn, NY: South End Press; 2005.
12. Duran E, Duran B. Native American post-colonial psychology. Albany, NY: University Press; 1995.
13. Waldrum J, Herring DA, Young TK. Aboriginal health in Canada: historical, cultural, and epidemiological perspectives. 2nd ed. University of Toronto Press, Scholarly Publishing Division; 2006.
14. Buxton B. Damaged angels: a mother discovers the terrible cost of alcohol in pregnancy. 1st ed. Knopf Canada; 2004.
15. Catterick M, Curran L, Riley E. Understanding foetal alcohol spectrum disorder: a guide to FASD for parents, carers and professionals. Jessica Kingsley Publishers; 2014.
16. Popova S, Lange S, Burd L., Rehm J. The burden and economic impact of foetal alcohol spectrum disorder in Canada, CAMH; 2015.
17. Tait C. Foetal alcohol syndrome among aboriginal people in Canada: review and analysis of the intergenerational links to residential schools. Ottawa, ON: Aboriginal Healing Foundation; 2004.
18. Truth and Reconciliation Commission Report. Published by the Government of Canada; 2015.
19. Helin C. Dances with dependency: indigenous success through self-reliance. Vancouver, BC: Orca Spirit Publishing; 2006.
20. Tait, C.. The tip of the iceberg, The "Making" of foetal alcohol in Canada. Montreal, QC: PhD Thesis, McGill University; 2002.
21. Rapp C. The strengths model: case management with people suffering from severe and persistent mental illness. New York, NY: Oxford University Press; 1998.
22. Chettleburg MC. Young thugs: inside the dangerous world of Canadian street gangs. HarperCollins Publishers Ltd.; 2007.
23. Koptie S. Metaphorical reflections on the colonial circus of the drunken Indian and the kidney machine. First Peoples Child Fam Rev. 2009a;4(1):66–79.

24. Koptie S. Irihapeti Ramsden: the public narrative on cultural safety. First Peoples Child Fam Rev. 2009b;4(1):30–43.
25. Wesley-Esquimaux C, Calliou B. Best practices in aboriginal community development: a literature review and wise practices approach. Alberta: Banff Centre; 2010.
26. Belanger Y, editor. Ways of knowing: an introduction to native studies in Canada. Nelson Education Limited; 2014
27. Dickason OP. A concise history of Canada's first nations. Canada: Oxford University Press; 2006.
28. Vizenor G. Manifest Manners: narratives on postindian survivance; University of Nebraska Press; 1999. 1st Bison Books print edition.
29. Wesley-Esquimaux C. Restoring the balance: first nations women, community and culture. University of Manitoba Press; 2009.
30. Tait CL, Cuthand D. Child welfare—the state as parent. (documentary). Saskatoon, Saskatchewan, Canada: Blue Hill Production; 2011.
31. Blatchford C. It's no accident that what happens at Yellow Quill…happens. Toronto, ON: Globe and Mail: 23/02/08; 2008.
32. Bopp M, Bopp J. Recreating the world: a practical guide to building sustainable communities. 3rd ed. Four Worlds for Development Learning; 2011
33. Conroy J, Fast D. Foetal alcohol syndrome and the criminal justice system. Vancouver, BC: British Columbia Foetal Alcohol Syndrome Recourse Society; 2000.
34. Richard, B. Ashley Smith: a report of the new Brunswick ombudsman and the child and youth advocate on the services provided to a youth involved in the youth criminal justice system. Fredericton, NB: Office of the Ombudsman and Child and Youth Advocate; 2008.
35. Whalen C. Connecting the dots: a report on the condition of youth-at-risk and youth with very complex needs in New Brunswick. Fredericton, NB: Office of the Ombudsman; 2008.

Cynthia Wesley-Esquimaux served as Vice Provost for Aboriginal Initiatives at Lakehead University for 3 years, and effective September 2016 was appointed as the first Indigenous Chair for Truth and Reconciliation in Canada and continues to develop pathways forward to reconciliation in Canada. She is an adjunct assistant professor for the Faculty of Anthropology and maintains a status-only appointment at the University of Toronto's Faculty of Social Work. Her teaching and academic writing are directed toward understanding and resolving the continuing transmission of unresolved intergenerational trauma and grief primarily within the Indigenous community.

Cynthia is a Director of the Teach for Canada nonprofit which addresses the needs of Indigenous schools in Northern Ontario. She was inducted as a "Honourary Witness" by the Truth and Reconciliation Commission of Canada and is a member of the Governing Circle for the National Centre for Truth and Reconciliation at the University of Manitoba.

She is a member and resident of the Chippewa of Georgina Island First Nation in Ontario and has dedicated her life to building bridges of understanding between peoples. She sees endless merit in bringing people from diverse cultures, ages, and backgrounds together to engage in practical dialog and applied research initiatives. Cynthia co-founded the Canadian Roots Exchange (CRE), a youth project out of the University of Toronto, the University of Saskatchewan, and Lakehead University. Information on CRE can be found at: www.canadianroots.ca.

Steven Koptie is an Indigenous man with maternal ties to the Six Nations of the Grand River. He has over 35 years of frontline community service work within child, adolescent, and adult mental health, crisis intervention, addictions counseling, youth living with Fetal Alcohol Spectrum Disorder (FASD), couples and family therapy, family violence prevention, and intervention as well as residential school survivor support. He has worked in urban, rural, and remote First Nation communities as well as in government as a policy advisor.

Steven holds a Masters of Education, Community Development and Counseling Psychology from the University of Toronto (2010) and a Masters of Social Work (MSW) from Wilfred Laurier University (2016). He is registered with the Ontario College of Social Workers. His graduate studies were focused on the intergenerational impacts of colonial trauma, family well-being, and healing as well as culturally safe social work approaches. He is a published author in the areas of Indigenous social work approaches, cultural safety, and reconciliation social work. He presently works as a counselor for the Mamaway Wiidokdaadwin Primary Care Team in Barrie, and Orillia, Ontario.

A Canadian Psychology Task Force Response to the Truth and Reconciliation Commission Report: Summary and Reflections

Christine Maybee, Fern Stockdale Winder, and David Danto

Although the story of the European colonization of North America and the catastrophic impacts upon the Indigenous Peoples living on land that is now Canada is a long one, the stories of the oppressed have only recently come to light. In Canada, in 2008 Prime Minister Stephen Harper apologized to Indigenous Peoples, on behalf of the federal government for the first time. This apology gave rise to the Truth and Reconciliation Commission (TRC). Through a multi-year process of hearings, the TRC guided an investigation into the Residential School System in Canada and recorded accounts of Residential School Survivors, many of whom disclosed horrific accounts of every imaginable type of abuse, within these government-funded, church-run institutions that existed between the late 1800s and 1996, for the purpose of eradicating Indigenous identity and integrating Indigenous Peoples with Euro-Western Settler culture.

The Truth and Reconciliation Commission held its Closing Event in Ottawa, the national capital of Canada, from May 31 to June 3, 2015. That summer, the Canadian Psychological Association annual convention was also in Ottawa only a short distance away, from June 4 to 6. The first part of this chapter will follow three accounts of three people who were impacted by those events and who came together as part of a task force to address Psychology's response to the TRC report of 2015. The second part of this chapter will provide a brief overview of our report with several reflections on the subject matter.

C. Maybee
Payukotayno James and Hudson Bay Family Services, Moosonee, ON, Canada
e-mail: christine.maybee@payukotayno.ca

F. S. Winder
Operational Stress Injury Clinic, Saskatchewan Health Authority, Saskatoon, SK, Canada
e-mail: Fern.StockdaleWinder@saskhealthauthority.ca

D. Danto (✉)
Psychology Department, University of Guelph-Humber, Toronto, ON, Canada
e-mail: david.danto@guelphhumber.ca

D. Danto, M. Zangeneh (eds.), *Indigenous Knowledge and Mental Health*,
https://doi.org/10.1007/978-3-030-71346-1_17

Christine's Introduction

I have been a social worker for many years and for most of my career I have been working in the child welfare field. Throughout the years, I have seen an increase in children coming into care due to substance abuse-related issues, child abuse, and neglect. Due to many reasons, some parents are able to address their issues more quickly than others and some are unwilling to face their multilayered problems stemming from the legacy of Residential School. Unfortunately, a large number of children have chosen to remain in care until they age out or until a family or community member comes forward to take the child/ren into their care.

As a First Nation Social Worker, I take pride in working with my people, as I truly understand why things are the way they are and westernized policies just do not fit when it comes to a First Nation Worldview. It does seem grim, seeing only a small percentage of children returning home even though it is only a small fraction, I still feel joy for those children that return home, that is why I continue to work in this field, it is those moments in the reunification of families. Personally, I did not attend Residential School; however, both of my parents did—my mother attended very briefly and my father attended for a few years.

I attended the initial meeting with the task force. I immediately responded to the invitation because I wanted to make some contribution to positive changes for the people that use the services. I would like to take this opportunity to mention that it made it much easier for me to agree to be part of this group because I have known Dave Danto, a Psychologist for about 10 years. I have assisted in developing the Guelph-Humber, Aboriginal Mental Health Course with Dave. Yes, I can agree this group is amazing, the positive energy allowed me to talk openly and freely about my personal life experiences and current state of being and most of all give some input into the TRC movement. I can truly express my appreciation to others that have shared their pain and personal successes and most of all what this task force will do in methodology in how Indigenous people are treated.

David's Introduction

As a new Psychologist, I worked for Federal Corrections and sadly, for the first time met many Indigenous offenders, quickly recognizing an apparent discrepancy in how frequently I encountered Indigenous people on either side of the prison walls. I also felt that my clinical training was insufficient to address what appeared to be significant sociocultural aspects to client accounts. I enlisted the assistance of the Institutional Elder at my Institution to help with these challenges.

Years later, after a change in careers working in a position overseeing an undergraduate psychology program at a university, I had the opportunity to develop a study-abroad course. I reflected on my experience in corrections and asked for permission to develop a field course within the province to address the topic of

Indigenous knowledge and mental health in northern Ontario. The university was supportive of my request and I began to study this topic. Christine Maybee helped me develop the field course and I came to know her as a pillar of strength in her community. I invited her to join our group. I had found myself on a path of learning, cultural allyship with Indigenous Peoples, and advocacy for reconciliation or working toward righting the wrongs of the past and present. I joined and became active in the Aboriginal Psychology Section of the Canadian Psychological Association.

By the summer of 2015, I was the Chair of the Aboriginal Psychology Section, now the Indigenous Peoples' Psychology Section. Along with our section members, including Associate Chair at the time, Dr. Suzanne Stewart and allies from other sections, we took that opportunity to raise the subject to the CPA Board of Directors and the Accreditation Committee to address the quality, accessibility, and appropriateness of psychological services available to Indigenous Peoples in Canada.

Fern's Introduction

I joined the CPA Board in July 2016, and one of my hopes was to work with other Board members to find ways to begin to address the recommendations from the Truth and Reconciliation Commission's report. I had the privilege of attending the TRC hearings in Saskatoon in 2012. As a volunteer, I was given the responsibility of entering a subset of the names of people who had attended residential school. There was a solemnity in entering names and schools of person after person whose lives and their children's lives had been substantially altered by their attendance at the schools. As a clinician, I also had the honor of journeying beside some people who chose to tell their stories at the hearings or in other settings—for some a journey of healing, and for others an ordeal that they chose to move through in order to bring Truth forward. I felt it was tremendously important for their generosity of story, which then informed the recommendations, to be heeded by listening to the Truth and beginning the action of Reconciliation. I was fortunate to be part of a Board that was also wishing to find ways to acknowledge and act on the TRC report, and in March of 2017, I contacted Dr. David Danto.

David's Reflection

In March of 2017, I was invited by Dr. Fern Stockdale Winder, on behalf of the CPA Board of Directors, to Chair a task force to address Psychology's response to the Truth and Reconciliation Commission report. In consultation with our section members as well as Indigenous Knowledge Keepers, we assembled the task force. Membership consisted of 17 participants, 10 who self-identified as Indigenous and 7 who were registered psychologists. Four members of the task force were Trustees for the Psychology Foundation of Canada in addition to their involvement with the CPA.

In addition to CPA and PFC support, I reached out to the University of Guelph-Humber, where I work, to assist with funding. The university covered the costs of bringing the 17 members together in Toronto for 3 days at the Native Canadian Centre. Along with the assistance of six UofGH undergraduate Psychology student volunteers who took copious notes and minutes, that three-day meeting in August 2017, after about eight iterations, ultimately developed into our 35-page report, published jointly by CPA and PFC in May, 2018.

Fern's Reflection

These were an emotional 3 days. Laughter was important. One Elder noted to me, "We're not on city time (although we were in the heart of Toronto), you can slow down," as we walked along the sidewalk, which proved to be an important truth to remember through all our conversations. Tears, vulnerability, and an openness to different ways of knowing fostered a sense of sharing and truth-telling. The Elders and Indigenous members of the Task Force were persistent, patient, and kind. Sometimes as someone rooted in non-Indigenous ways of knowing I was slow, and I acknowledge many continued blind spots because of my cultural background. I am so thankful for their patience in sharing their knowledge and experience.

Christine's Reflection

I have known Dave for about 10 years. He and Guelph-Humber Psychology students have come to our territory to learn about our local health services and modalities used in helping our people heal. Before, inviting Dave and students to our community, it took some time to build that trust relationship and connection which is very important when beginning a relationship and most of all Dave seemed to have a willingness to learn our Cree way of life. Therefore, cultural allyship is so important to establish with our outside professional partners. Without trust and connection, one cannot even begin to work with the people that need help.

Christine, Fern, and David: We all encourage you to read the full report but will provide a brief overview of the document and present a bit about our next steps in the paragraphs that follow, largely drawn from the original report.

Summary of Report

The scope of the report includes psychology's role in service delivery, research, and mental health program development and evaluation. The task force developed its report with the intention that it would directly and quickly be of assistance to Indigenous communities, by providing direction and guidelines for the profession of psychology and by leading to further self-reflection, recommendations, and cultural literacy development by those who practice psychology.

The task force created a statement of accountability and responsibility to Indigenous Peoples on behalf of the profession of psychology in Canada and developed guiding principles for psychological practice with Indigenous Peoples. The objectives included creating recommendations and guiding principles that acknowledge and respect Indigenous concepts of the person, health, family, and ways of knowing. The task force also addressed: assessment, treatment, research, education, clinical training at the graduate level, continuing education for practicing psychologists, program development and evaluation, and advocacy.

Professional Ethics as a Starting Point

The Truth and Reconciliation Commission of Canada report published in 2015 [1] has provided evidence and details of the cultural and physical genocide of Indigenous Peoples in Canada, particularly through the residential school system which began in the late 1800s. Throughout the nineteenth and twentieth centuries, the Government of Canada developed and enforced policy and legislation that contributed to the marginalization and oppression of Indigenous Peoples in Canada, through enforcement of the Indian Act, forced relocations of communities, and the ongoing control and subjugation of Indigenous Peoples and families. The profession of psychology in Canada developed in the same political climate and colonial context that gave rise to the residential school system and participated in the process of cultural genocide. A useful lens for seeing the impact of that context is to juxtapose the ideals of the profession of psychology with the historical and present reality of Indigenous peoples in Canada. The profession of psychology in Canada highly values its code of ethics. It is with a sense of pride that we use its four principles to assist in ethical decision-making, to assist us in the complex responsibilities involved in our activities. The *Canadian Code of Ethics for Psychologists* has four main principles:

1. Respect for rights of the dignity of persons and people
2. Responsible caring
3. Integrity in relationships
4. Responsibility to society

As we examined these four principles within the context of the TRC report and immersed ourselves in discussion with Task Force members, it became apparent that in psychology's interaction with Indigenous Peoples in Canada we have contravened our own code of ethics. It was an impactful and powerful dissonance to look at the ethical code against the historical and present reality of Indigenous peoples in Canada. As a group, we identified the following failures:

Respect for Rights and Dignity of Persons and People

Historically, the profession has failed to respect the rights and dignity of Indigenous Peoples by failing to acknowledge the social injustice of over a century of federal policy aimed at the eradication of Indigenous culture and peoples through residential schooling and forced adoption initiatives, among others, and the impact that those policies have had both directly and inter-generationally on the mental health of Indigenous Peoples.

Responsible Caring

In relying on methods and epistemologies that are foreign and potentially harmful to Indigenous Peoples in Canada, much of the care that has been provided has not been grounded in appropriate cultural understandings that include Indigenous concepts of self, Indigenous concepts of health and illness, Indigenous views of family, and Indigenous cultural values. As a result, the treatment that has been provided has not been responsible, and in many instances, has been traumatizing and re-traumatizing to already marginalized Indigenous Peoples. In addition, as a health-related discipline, psychology has the moral obligation to welcome research that identifies culture and tradition as aspects of empowerment and treatment. Psychology, as a collective profession, has failed to meet these basic standards of care.

Integrity in Relationships

This ethical principle mandates that, in providing treatment in their particular areas of competence, psychologists in Canada are called upon to evaluate how their "experiences, attitudes, culture, beliefs, values, individual differences, specific training, external pressures, personal needs, and historical economic and political context might influence their activities." As a discipline, psychology has not done this in relation to Indigenous Peoples in Canada. Psychologists have not, as a profession, engaged in the essential cultural safety and cultural competence training required to reflect on cultural values, implicit biases, and ethnocentrism that dominate the field, in order to engage in these relationships with true integrity.

Responsibility to Society

Psychology as a discipline has not demonstrated a respect for the social structures of Indigenous communities in Canada that have evolved since time immemorial. Approaches to assessment and treatment have not been normed or validated in partnership with Indigenous populations. Assessments that do not acknowledge or draw from Indigenous epistemologies have caused unnecessary disruption to already marginalized family and community structures. Psychological tools that are inappropriate have been used to support discriminatory policies that pathologize Indigenous Peoples, as well as practices that are neither just nor beneficial to Indigenous communities in Canada. These behaviors fail Indigenous communities and thus are irresponsible to Canadian society as a whole.

Statement of Acknowledgment from the Task Force

The acknowledgment of the contravention of psychology's own ethical principles led us to a sense of sadness and regret, and to the need to acknowledge and offer apology:

> As we acknowledge a failure to meet our own ethical standards, the profession of psychology in Canada must also acknowledge our history of having caused harm toward Indigenous Peoples. We acknowledge that these failings have roots as far back as the development of this profession in Canada. We apologize for not opposing discriminatory governmental policy. We apologize for colluding with policies and laws that have promoted the marginalization and oppression of Indigenous Peoples. We apologize for grounding our approaches to assessment and treatment in epistemologies and research that have little relevance to Indigenous Peoples. We apologize for the lack of acknowledgement of cultural and historical contexts of Indigenous Peoples in Canada in our professional work, and our failure to name the unjust impacts of our governmental policies on Indigenous Peoples. Although as a profession we have a strong commitment to healing in ways that are empirically supported, we have been biased, irresponsible and disrespectful to Indigenous Peoples in Canada in the manners described here. We apologize for failing to be supportive allies and advocates to Indigenous Peoples ([2] p. 9).

A Path Toward Accountable Practices

The Elders in our Task Force were incredibly generous in continuing to believe that psychology could provide additional assistance to enhance the greater well-being of Indigenous Peoples in Canada despite the past and present harms inflicted by the discipline. They were powerful healers themselves but stated that psychology and what it offered in knowledge of mental health had the potential to assist Indigenous communities and individuals in healing. They encouraged us to look for paths of action, and practical ways that we could change to reflect a truly ethical approach to working with Indigenous Peoples. As a Task Force, we developed six important guiding principles for psychology as a profession and for individuals within it.

Guiding Principles Applying to the Study and Practice of Psychology in General

The task force proposed six guiding principles relevant to those involved in the discipline of psychology in general. These guiding principles are intended to provide practical direction to members of the field of psychology in their day-to-day work whether that work is in education, research, or applied psychology.

Cultural Allyship

Whether the topic is treatment, assessment, research, education, or program development and evaluation, psychologists in Canada are called to stand with Indigenous Peoples, rather than simply knowing about them. The task force related a number of topics to cultural allyship including cultural safety and literacy, understanding Indigenous epistemologies, the role of ceremonies, traditions, Indigenous spirituality, the impacts of colonization, the residential school system, the 60's scoop, the present-day dominant culture, as well as training in deconstructing the cultural assumptions of mainstream psychology.

The Task Force concluded that whether one is an academic, a researcher, or an applied psychologist, the discipline of psychology should embrace familiarity with Indigenous culture through Indigenous cultural safety training, for example. Psychologists should be able to communicate with clients in culturally appropriate terms. Clinicians unaware of the historical and intergenerational trauma and social and historical context in which pathology arises, or who lack an understanding of Indigenous concepts of self or health are at risk of traumatizing Indigenous clients. Similarly, psychological assessments in the absence of a culturally competent assessor; education and training provided by faculty who lack cultural literacy; research or program development initiated and carried out by those lacking appropriate cultural understanding; and those who believe that their approach to treatment, assessment, or research is culture or value free are all problematic.

In addition to general Indigenous cultural allyship, which gives a broader perspective regarding Indigenous knowledge and history, it is important to have localized knowledge regarding each community's unique views of distress or mental health. General cultural literacy is necessary but not sufficient.

Humility

Psychologists have been trained in particular ways of knowing. Historically, ways of knowing that are foreign to our training have been seen as less valid. Whether providing treatment or engaging in research or assessment, those in the discipline should be guided by humility and address Elders, traditional knowledge and approaches with respect and a spirit of genuine learning and collaboration.

Humility is not necessarily something we teach psychology students or other health professionals. It is becoming increasingly recognized that it is an essential component of care. Dr. Evan Adams, Chief Medical Officer, First Nations Health Authority stated, "To provide culturally 'safe' care, or care where those we serve feel safe and respected, we need to be humble enough to admit that we don't know everything about everyone's life experiences, culture and feelings, and that health care providers don't know it all" ([3], p.1).

Working with cultural humility requires knowledge of local culture, collaboration, and critical self-reflection, and such goes hand in hand with the other guiding principles noted below.

Collaboration

Services should be the product of community collaboration and ongoing discourse, not post hoc consultation. Planning with community leaders, Elders, and healers about what is needed and for whose sake it is needed should occur prior to engagement with community members. Psychologists should visit with participants and discuss collaboration at the outset of assessment, treatment, data collection, etc. Furthermore, those engaging with a community should develop ways for the community to provide feedback to psychologists regarding the degree to which they have been helpful, whether the treatment was culturally appropriate, and how services could be improved. It is important for communities to evaluate the services provided by psychologists. Psychologists should work toward bridging Western and Indigenous cultures, making efforts to understand the person's cultural worldview in trying to arrive at shared agreements and understandings.

Critical Reflection

It is incumbent on the psychologist, in whatever capacity service is being provided, to not only be culturally literate with regard to the population but also to be able to 'self-locate', in terms of what are their credentials, who are their ancestors, what is their family's role in colonization, etc. Additionally, psychologists working with Indigenous Peoples must have a commitment to unlearn some of their training and be comfortable not knowing, keeping an open mind toward Indigenous approaches, and identifying those times when the rigidity a particular trained perspective limits rather than illuminates.

Critical reflection occurs for us as psychologists on many levels, and it may be helpful when considering how to approach critical reflection to think of three levels (an artificial but possibly useful distinction): individual, professional, and societal. As noted in the report, we all have individual experiences including family, culture, and education that influence how we approach others. The profession of psychology has inherent frameworks and biases that can be difficult to discern when one is steeped in that culture, and it can be equally or more difficult to reflect on societal biases—especially if we do not purposefully have diverse feeds on our social media! Critical reflection takes time. In the busy lives of clinicians, academics, researchers, administrators, we may get caught up and forget to reflect. In Saskatchewan, we are fortunate to have psychology-specific Talking Circles, which can slow us down, and give space for reflection, as well as having people in the Circle speak their truths which can help us to see the hidden to self/visible to others corner of the Johari Window. Mindfulness, distance from media, purposefully seeking out environments which are uncomfortable and challenge assumptions, can all be ways to critically reflect. A recent news story highlighted the values of self-reflection for psychology students who attended Talking Circles and worked with Indigenous Knowledge Keeper Brenda Dubois. She is quoted in an article by Melnychuk [4], "Dubois explained that she tried to help the students look at things through a different world view. That Indigenous perspective, she said, should be fluidly incorporated into the work a psychologist does, rather than be seen as a side piece. [Dubois stated] 'It's like what they say, culture saves lives'."

Respect

This term is used to denote respect not only for the specific person or people with whom the psychologist interacts but also for Indigenous culture that has been resilient and has survived, as well as that which has been taken and lost, including knowledge, wisdom, and societal structures. Whether engaging in research or assessment, psychologists are at much greater risk for misunderstanding, misconstruing, mistreating, or misdiagnosing Indigenous clients. Psychologists must understand this risk.

The ways Indigenous people validate their knowledge are rigorous and grounded in their community and epistemology—some have used the term 'Indigenous science' to capture the rigorous aspect of this knowledge. Psychologists have an important role in facilitating the healing reconnection of clients with the culture and traditions that were taken from them by the dominant Western Euro-settler culture. Research, treatment, assessment, and programs are needed in Indigenous languages, in part because language connects Indigenous Peoples to their land, traditions, worldviews, and future well-being.

Social Justice

Psychologists should strive for a greater understanding of the social justice context when providing services in general. The question of who will benefit from a particular program, research project, assessment, or treatment modality should be examined and explored carefully with community members and participants with particular emphasis on vulnerability, power dynamics, and the historical impact of the profession of psychology on the population. Communities should have ownership, control, access, and possession (OCAP) of data. The CPA can take a greater role in social justice for Indigenous Peoples in Canada.

Dr. Suzanne Stewart, at the CPA Convention in 2017 led a participatory session that included discussion about the agreements and treaties with Indigenous peoples of Canada. Dr. Stewart asked us all to consider, what we had that comes from the agreements made in the Treaties with Indigenous Peoples of Canada. The non-Indigenous people in the room came up with some answers that seemed inadequate, although each accurate in their own context. Dr. Stewart then answered, "Everything." It was an incredibly powerful moment of learning. We do owe everything to the Indigenous Peoples of Canada, and the agreements made in our treaties. It is important then, that we work as individuals or as part of the profession of psychology, as cultural allies to support our larger society in respecting the agreements made in the Treaties or agreements made across Canada.

Guiding Principles that Relate to Specific Areas Within the Discipline

The full report then details guiding principles that relate to specific areas within Psychology. These areas include assessment, treatment, research, education, training, program development, program evaluation, advocacy, and social justice. Although not viable to summarize in this overview, once again, we direct you to the actual report for the specific guiding principles.

Directions Forward

The report makes a number of recommendations directly to psychology organizations in Canada. One such recommendation was for the creation of a knowledge sharing group/standing committee comprised of Indigenous and non-Indigenous psychologists and community members to continuously respond to questions, challenges, and opportunities regarding the interaction between the discipline of psychology and Indigenous Peoples. Its goals are to facilitate and build relationships to work for and with Indigenous people to build better understandings and supports that meet their health and well-being needs and to continue to explore and understand truth from an Indigenous perspective on the road to reconciliation. An important function of the group would be to take the burden of educating the general population of the CPA off of Indigenous members of the CPA and the Indigenous Peoples section.

The CPA Board of Directors accepted the Task Force recommendation to create this Knowledge Sharing Group (KSG). The Terms of Reference for the KSG were ratified in the summer of 2018. The release of the report and the creation of the KSG seemed to come at a time when there was openness for hearing the truth and moving toward reconciliation. We have been encouraged by the actions taken recently within the landscape of Canadian Psychology, and the continued calls for change, which will provide direction for the future. Recent actions and calls for change include:

1. Psychology educational institutions are one of the organizations that are called to make changes. Drs. Ansloos and Stewart and several other Indigenous scholars [5] published a paper which reflects the voices of Indigenous scholars and their perspectives on what needs to change or stay the same:

   > To date, there has been almost no research conducted at the intersection of Indigenous communities and professional training in psychology in Canada ....Through first-person editorial reflections, the authors identify key challenges and opportunities in professional training in psychology relevant to Indigenous peoples; and the changes that are needed to advance Indigenous peoples in the field (p. 265).

   This paper offers an incredibly important starting point for programs seeking to make changes in their educational institutions.
2. Regulatory Bodies and Associations:

   All across Canada, regulatory bodies and psychology associations are reviewing their requirements for practice, and beginning to incorporate the recommendations from the CPA Task Force Report and from the TRC Report. Two examples are below.

   In Saskatchewan, the emphasis on cultural humility has now been placed into the professional practice guidelines for the Saskatchewan College of Psychologists:

   > The Guidelines must be interpreted with cultural humility, recognizing that they may not be universal across cultures. Psychologists are encouraged to approach any apparent conflicts of the Guidelines and best cultural practices with careful consideration of the relevant ethical and cultural factors that may influence a course of action, and to consult with colleagues, the College, and respected cultural group leaders or healers in establishing appropriate courses of action ([6], p. 6).

   In Alberta, "The College of Alberta Psychologists (CAP) and the Psychologists' Association of Alberta (PAA) have formed a joint working group, sanctioned by both boards, to impact change in our province specific to realizing truth and reconciliation considerations relevant to our profession, to Indigenous psychologists who live and work in our communities, and to our clients" ([7], p. 8). At the time of the article, they were moving quickly toward actions, such as CAP drafting practice standards and guidelines for work with Indigenous people, and requiring registering psychology providers in Alberta to have a foundational knowledge of the TRC report. There are more examples in the article, and it is an inspiring and practical article in how we can move to action.
3. Changes in psychological assessments.

   Barker [8] writes of the importance of doing psychoeducational assessments in a Good Way. He notes this includes being "strength-based, trauma-informed, community-oriented, and respectful of Indigenous ways of knowing," ([8], p. 21). He then continues with several practical suggestions for psychological assessments to bring them closer to these ideals. Gale [9] likewise brings a series of practical suggestions from her work in the Yukon Territory, such as prioritizing formal cultural safety training, budgeting significantly for significantly more assessment time, working with and remunerating Elders in the process, planning for the involvement of the community, being mindful of community norms for communication and listening with respect to that different communication style (e.g., storytelling and silence).

4. Bringing together ideas for change. The astute reader will have noticed that this chapter quotes several articles from the 2019 Psynopsis edition, Indigenous Peoples mental health and wellbeing: Updates in Canadian psychology practice, with guest editors Danto and Ansloos [10]. This issue brought together many examples of work that is happening across Canada, and it both summarizes action taken and leads us toward more action. Through the continued work of the KSG, ongoing idea sharing at the local, provincial, and national level, we give ourselves both ideas and energy for change as well as continuous connection with Indigenous knowledge keepers. Creating this collaboration and action impetus needs not to be a one-time initiative, but rather a continued encouragement in order to see change in practice, teaching, and social justice that is sustained and meaningful. Through ongoing dialog within an atmosphere of allyship, humility, collaboration critical reflection, respect, and social justice, it is our hope that psychology in Canada can address its failings and support Indigenous Peoples in the many appropriate ways that are long overdue.

Christine's Closing Thoughts

The message is that treatment cannot come from a place that is unrecognizable to Indigenous people, it must come from a place where we can recognize the same worldview, to share an understanding. Whoever is speaking must convey their thoughts in a way that is understood by all and about a topic that the group wants to discuss. It will have to come from a place that uses the language that everyone understands and can agree to, not from a place of austerity but from a place of simplicity that is straight to the point. This is when everyone speaks and everyone is heard. A view that is called being humble.

When I first was introduced to this task force the goals that were presented seemed like large subject matter that would or could be a nearly insurmountable topic. The group could be heading toward a rabbit hole that would be a never-ending contradiction in work for praise or on the other hand it could be work toward achievements. The future will tell if the latter will be achieved. I am hoping to see that the results we set for ourselves are in fact achieved, and not in some paper that sits within a bureaucracy of political scrutiny where ambiguous thoughts lead to the crossing off of goals for some political objective. It is difficult to see our course and direction as we strive for change in the betterment of Indigenous well-being and a focus toward reconciliation. Only time will tell.

References

1. Truth and Reconciliation Commission of Canada. Truth and Reconciliation Commission of Canada: calls to action; 2015. http://trc.ca/assets/pdf/Calls_to_Action_English2.pdf
2. Canadian Psychological Association. Psychology's response to the truth and reconciliation commission of Canada's report; 2018. https://cpa.ca/docs/File/Task_Forces/TRC%20 Task%20Force%20Report_FINAL.pdf
3. Adams, E (Tiesla II). Quoted in FNHA's policy statement on cultural safety and humility "It Starts with Me"; 2000. https://www.fnha.ca/documents/fnha-policy-statement-cultural-safety-and-humility.pdf. Accessed 20 February 2020
4. Melnychuk M. Healing the relationship between psychology and indigenous peoples; 2018. https://leaderpost.com/news/local-news/healing-the-relationship-between-psychology-and-Indigenous-peoples. Accessed 11 April 2020.
5. Ansloos J, Stewart S, Fellner K, Goodwill A, Graham H, McCormick R, Harder H, Mushquash C. Indigenous peoples and professional training in psychology in Canada. Can Psychol. 2019;60(4):265–80. https://doi.org/10.1037/cap0000189.
6. Professional Practice Guidelines for Psychology in Saskatchewan; 2019. http://www.skcp.ca/wp-content/uploads/PROFESSIONAL-PRACTICE-GUIDELINES-20193.pdf.
7. Malone JL, Fellner K, Spelliscy R. Workin together: truth and reconciliation starts with us. Psynopsis. 2019;41(3):8–9.
8. Barker C. Psychoeducational assessments with indigenous students in postsecondary settings: moving forward in a good way. Psynopsis. 2019;41(3):21–2.
9. Gale R. Approaching psychological assessment with northern indigenous peoples: suggestions from a psychologist in the Yukon territory. Psynopsis. 2019;41(3):20, 22
10. Danto, D., Ansloos, J., editors. Indigenous peoples mental health and wellbeing: updates in Canadian psychology practice, Psynopsis. Vol 41(3); 2019.

Christine Maybee is the Director of Services, Child Welfare Department, Payukotayno: James and Hudson Bay Family Services in Moosonee, Ontario. Christine is Cree and is a member of Fort Albany First Nation. She holds an Honors Bachelor of Social Work from Carleton University.

For the past 15 years, Christine Maybee has worked in the Child Welfare sector in many capacities, such as Intake and Assessment, Youth Probation, Child Protection, and Supervised Child Protection Unit. Christine also worked for Weeneebayko Area Health Authority (WAHA) for 7 years as the Director of Mental Health and Addiction Services in Moosonee.

Christine is involved in various committees, both internally and externally. Some of these include the Association of Native Child and Family Services, Ontario Association of Children's Aid Societies, Deputy Chiefs and Band Representative Committee, Omushkegiskwew House Family (VAW) Collaboration Agreement Committee.

Christine enjoys working with her people in the James and Hudson Bay Region. The most rewarding experience in her role is seeing children return home to their caregiver/s whether that be mother, father, grandparent, and other members of the family or community member within the region.

Christine hopes to see that less or no children come into care and see more families and communities take responsibility for the welfare of their children!

Fern Stockdale Winder is a Registered Doctoral Psychologist in Saskatoon, Saskatchewan. She has practiced psychology for over 20 years with significant experience in health psychology, geriatrics, and more recently Operational Stress Injuries. She has a cross-appointment as a Professional Affiliate in the Psychology Department at the University of Saskatchewan. Dr. Stockdale Winder was a member of the inaugural Board of Directors of the Mental Health Commission of Canada and served for 6 years, the Commissioner for the Mental Health and Addictions Action Plan in Saskatchewan from 2013 to 2014, and a Director on the Board of the Canadian Psychological

Association from 2016 to 2018. It was during that time that she had the pleasure of working with the Task Force referred to in this chapter. Throughout her career, she has worked to acknowledge her own cultural context, to respect the journeys of others, and to find ways to be an ally for change.

David Danto is a clinical psychologist, registered in the Province of Ontario. He is the Head of Psychology at the University of Guelph-Humber. Dr. Danto serves on the Board of Directors of the Canadian Psychological Association (CPA), is Board Liaison to the CPA Committee on Ethics, and is a Trustee for the Psychology Foundation of Canada (PFC). He recently chaired the CPA and PFC Task Force on Responding to the Truth and Reconciliation Commission Report, and he currently Chairs the CPA Standing Committee on Reconciliation. Dr. Danto has worked in psychiatric hospitals, university counseling centers, private practice, and correctional facilities in Canada and the United States. In collaboration with Christine Maybee and community members in Mushkegowuk Territory along the James and Hudson Bay coast, Dr. Danto has delivered a course on Indigenous knowledge and mental health for the last 9 years. Dr. Danto researches the role of the land in healing the impacts of colonialism and trauma within Indigenous communities.

Index

D. Danto, M. Zangeneh (eds.), *Indigenous Knowledge and Mental Health*,
https://doi.org/10.1007/978-3-030-71346-1

GPSR Compliance

The European Union's (EU) General Product Safety Regulation (GPSR) is a set of rules that requires consumer products to be safe and our obligations to ensure this.

If you have any concerns about our products, you can contact us on ProductSafety@springernature.com

In case Publisher is established outside the EU, the EU authorized representative is:

Springer Nature Customer Service Center GmbH
Europaplatz 3
69115 Heidelberg, Germany

Batch number: 10732090

Printed by Printforce, the Netherlands